Hernia
Updates and Approaches

Edited by Selim Sözen

Published in London, United Kingdom

Hernia Updates and Approaches
http://dx.doi.org/10.5772/intechopen.1000397
Edited by Selim Sözen

Contributors
Kastriot Haxhirexha, Agron Dogjani, Aulona Haxhirexha, Dritan Alushani, Labeat Haxhirexha, Aferdita Ademi, Blerim Fejzuli, Teuta Emini, Fotios Seretis, Paraskevi Dedopoulou, Nikiforos Rodis, Konstantina Soukouli, Nikolaos Bogiatzopoulos, Charalampos Seretis, Georgios Zacharis, Suat Benek, İlhan Bali, Seyfi Emir, Selim Sözen, Mohamed Alfatih Hamza, Mekki Hassan, Sean Johnston, Bachir Elias, Carine El Hajj, Caline Zeaiter, Athanasios Pantelis, Mohit Bhandari, Igors Ivanovs, Fabrizio Ferranti, Kumar Hari Rajah, M. Somanathan, George Sakellaris, Konstantinos Zachos, Maria Athanasopoulou, Antonios Panagidis, Vasileios Alexopoulos, Ioannis Spyridakis, Anastasia Vareli, Xenophon Sinopidis, Mohamed Arif Hameed Sultan, Dayang Corieza Febriany, Suphakarn Techapongsatorn, Eren Tuncer, Fatih Cınar, Percin Karakol, Gabriel Paiva de Oliveira, Carmen Maillo, Krzysztof Balawender, Anna Pliszka, Omar Alhafidh, Matteo Bonetti, Gian Maria Ottaviani, Luigi Simonetti, Giannantonio Pellicanò, Francesco Bonetti, Mario Muto

First published in London, United Kingdom, 2023 by IntechOpen
IntechOpen is the global imprint of INTECHOPEN LIMITED, registered in England and Wales, registration number: 11086078, 5 Princes Gate Court, London, SW7 2QJ, United Kingdom

British Library Cataloguing-in-Publication Data
A catalogue record for this book is available from the British Library

Additional hard and PDF copies can be obtained from orders@intechopen.com

Hernia Updates and Approaches
Edited by Selim Sözen
p. cm.
Print ISBN 978-1-83769-664-2
Online ISBN 978-1-83769-663-5
eBook (PDF) ISBN 978-1-83769-665-9

Meet the editor

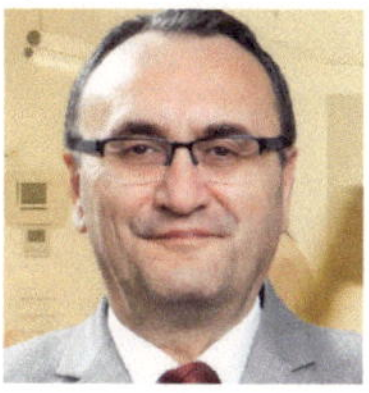

Dr. Selim Sözen is an expert in general surgery who received his medical degree from Ondokuz Mayıs University, Turkey, in 1998. From 1999 to 2004, he was an assistant doctor at Ankara Atatürk Education and Research Hospital, Turkey. From 2004 to 2013, he worked as a specialist at different government hospitals in Turkey. He joined the Medicine Faculty, Department of General Surgery, Namık Kemal University, Turkey, as an associate professor in 2013. He completed liver transplantation surgery at İnönü University, Turkey, in 2014–2015. Since 2016, Dr. Sözen has run his own surgery clinic in İstanbul, Turkey. He is a member of the Turkish Surgical Association and a review board member for several journals. He has published several articles in scientific journals and presented sixty-four poster papers at scientific congresses. His research interests include general, gastrointestinal, emergency, and trauma surgery, bacterial translocation, liver disease, and hernia surgery.

Contents

Preface

This book is a collection of review papers on hernia treatments. In addition to sharing their knowledge, the chapter authors provide their personal clinical experiences, making this book a useful resource for scientists and physicians practicing in the field. The book presents essential knowledge and key facts about hernia surgery.

Chapter 1, "A Brief Overview of Incisional Hernias through the Ages: Etiology, Treatment, and Complications" by Aulona Haxhirexha et al., discusses incisional hernias.

Chapter 2, "Approaching the Complex Abdominal Wall Hernia: General Principles of Component Separation Techniques" by Charalampos Seretis et al., discusses general principles of component separation techniques. Anterior component separation and posterior component separation are expansions of the retrorectus Rives-Stoppa repair.

Chapter 3, "Clinical Features, Diagnosis, Prevention and Management of Incisional Hernias" by Suat Benek, examines the techniques of separating into anterior or posterior components for large and complex incisional hernias.

Chapter 4, "Controversies in Laparoscopic Ventral Hernia Repair" by Mohamed Alfatih Hamza et al., provides an overview of ventral hernias, their causes, risk factors, symptomatology, diagnosis, and different approaches to their management, focusing mainly on laparoscopic surgery.

Chapter 5, "Management of Ventral Hernia in Obese Patients: Before or After Bariatric Surgery?" by Bachir Elias et al., focuses on ventral hernia in obese patients during the management of their obesity. The laparoscopic approach is recommended to allow an exploration of the trocar sites and a second look after obesity surgery.

Chapter 6, "Hernia as a Complication of Metabolic Bariatric Surgery" by Athanasios Pantelis and Mohit Bhandari, discusses the approach to hiatal hernias post metabolic bariatric surgery (MBS), internal hernias, and abdominal wall hernia.

Chapter 7, "Hiatal Hernia Surgery" by Igors Ivanovs, discusses the classification, clinical features, investigations, and management of hiatal hernias.

Chapter 8, "Incarcerated Inguinal Hernia in the Elderly: Surgical Implication" by Fabrizio Ferranti, focuses on incarcerated inguinal hernia in the elderly. Elective surgical hernia repair is considered the treatment of choice in elderly patients. The use of mesh in incarcerated inguinal hernia is disputed because of the increased risk of post-operative wound infection.

Chapter 9, "Open Hernia Repair" by Kumar Hari Rajah and M. Somanathan, discusses various open hernia techniques with an emphasis on tension-free repairs, which may involve the use of mesh (Lichtenstein) or may not (Desarda). The chapter also reviews older tension repairs like the Shouldice and Bassini repairs.

Chapter 10, "Individualized Treatment of Inguinal Hernia in Children" by George Sakellaris et al., examines the evolution of hernia surgery in children from the classical operative methods to the modern laparoscopic techniques.

Chapter 11, "Management of Strangulated Inguinal Hernia" by Mohamed Arif Hameed Sultan and Dayang Corieza Febriany, provides information about strangulated inguinal hernia. Management strategy differs and depends on the presentation of the hernia, duration, patient, and surgical factors. Conservative management is not recommended for strangulated inguinal hernia, as it always requires surgical intervention. Prompt diagnosis and management are required to reduce the morbidity and mortality associated with strangulated inguinal hernia.

Chapter 12, "Hernia Mesh Fixation" by Suphakarn Techapongsatorn, discusses mesh fixation techniques. There are a variety of mesh fixation methods, materials, and devices currently available. However, there is no consensus or evidence regarding the most effective mesh fixation. Mesh fixation techniques have been demonstrated to be equally safe in terms of recurrence; however, tissue adhesives are associated with a lower incidence of chronic pain. Chapter 13, "Advances in Hernia Management in Plastic Surgery" by Eren Tuncer et al., provides an overview of the latest updates in hernia management within the context of plastic surgery.

In Chapter 14, "Prehabilitation: Enhancing Recovery and Outcomes in Hernia Surgery," Gabriel Paiva de Oliveira and Carmen Maillo believe the implementation of a structured multimodal preoperative intervention is essential to improve hernia care outcomes in patients with identifiable risk factors and potentially complex hernias.

Chapter 15, "Male Fertility Following Inguinal Hernia Repair" by Krzysztof Balawender and Anna Pliszka, discusses male fertility. There are theories of a negative impact on male fertility following inguinal hernia repair surgery. A preoperative and postoperative semen analysis will help exclude or confirm its impact on patient fertility in the future.

Chapter 16, "Parastomal Hernia – Latest Knowledge and Approach" by Omar Alhafidh, discusses the latest on the diagnosis, complications, and repair techniques in parastomal hernia.

Chapter 17, "Treatment of Low-Back Pain with Oxygen-Ozone Therapy" by Matteo Bonetti et al., provides information about oxygen-ozone therapy for the treatment of low back pain. The authors have been carrying out these treatments for more than 25 years, and in this chapter, they report their experience with oxygen-ozone therapy for discogenic and non-discogenic low back pain caused by pathology of the posterior compartment (facet synovitis, Baastrup syndrome, spondylolysis and spondylolisthesis, facet degeneration).

I thank the authors for their professional dedication and outstanding work in summarizing their clinical and research practices.

Selim Sözen
Associate Professor of General Surgery,
Sözen Surgery Clinic,
Tekirdağ, Turkey

Chapter 1

A Brief Overview of Incisional Hernias through the Ages – Etiology, Treatment, and Complications

Kastriot Haxhirexha, Agron Dogjani, Aulona Haxhirexha, Dritan Alushani, Labeat Haxhirexha, Aferdita Ademi, Blerim Fejzuli and Teuta Emini

Abstract

Among the most frequent pathologies of the abdominal wall are hernias, which are defined as a protrusion of the abdominal organs through any of the weak points of the abdominal wall. They can be spontaneous appearing in weak points of the abdominal wall or along the site of surgical incisions. Even though hernias have been acknowledged since ancient times, the topic of incisional hernias was rarely discussed until the advent of modern surgery. After the introduction of anesthesia and antisepsis, abdominal interventions became common, and with this, the incidence of incisional hernias significantly increased. Until after the second world war, the correction of incisional hernias was done using simple sutures, continuous fascial sutures, etc. The large variety of prosthetic materials that are in use today, both dual and biological, helps in the successful correction of incisional hernias. A new era in the treatment of hernias began with the introduction of laparoscopic techniques in 1993 by Le Blanc. However, the correction of incisional hernias continues to remain a real challenge that requires a personalized approach for each patient with the aim of achieving good results and avoiding postoperative complications, of which hernia recurrence remains one of the most serious.

Keywords: hernia, incisional, correction, recurrence, meshes

1. Introduction

Hernias are a common pathology of the abdominal wall, affecting a large number of people worldwide. They are defined as the protrusion of abdominal organs through any weak point in the abdominal wall. Although there are different types of hernias, including spontaneous hernias that develop in weak points of the abdominal wall, there is another group of hernias that can occur along the site of a previous surgical incision in the abdominal cavity. These are called incisional hernias and can occur after any surgical intervention that involves a cut in the abdominal wall, such as a laparotomy or a cesarean section.

Incisional hernias can be a challenging problem to manage, and their treatment often requires a multidisciplinary approach. In recent years, several advances have been made in the diagnosis and treatment of incisional hernias, leading to better outcomes for patients.

2. History

Hernias have been a concern since ancient times, but the concept of hernias was initially focused only on inguinal and umbilical hernias until the second half of the nineteenth century, when the era of modern surgery began [1].

The Edwin Smith papyrus, one of the oldest medical documents and a surgical treatise, does not mention any of the hernias of the abdominal wall [2]. Similarly, the papyrus of Ebers, which dates back to approximately 1500 years before Christ, describes swellings and tumors of the abdominal wall, including the first recorded instance of epigastric hernias [3].

Abdominal hernias were briefly mentioned in the Corpus Hippocraticum, the most famous medical work of ancient Greece, while incisional hernias were not mentioned at all [3]. However, the writings of Celsus in ancient Rome (first century AD) highlighted the importance of correcting abdominal hernias and described the method of closing the abdominal wall with layers to prevent incisional hernias [4]. Galen of Pergamon, another prominent Roman physician nearly a century later, described the mass closure technique for the closure of the abdominal wall and suggested the paramedian incision as the optimal technique for preventing incisional hernias [5].

During the Renaissance period, there were remarkable advances not only in art, literature, and science but also in the field of human anatomy, which led to the age of the anatomist surgeon. In 1721, La Chausse described in his dissertation "de Hernia Ventralis" a case of abdominal trauma that resulted in an incisional hernia, along with the different types of abdominal hernias. These findings represented a significant contribution to the understanding of abdominal wall hernias [6].

The development of surgery also saw remarkable advancements in France, where in 1768, during the reign of King Louis XV, surgeons were separated from barbers, and all surgeons had to attend the College of Surgeons [7]. The first documented correction of incisional hernias was performed by the French surgeon Pierre Nichollas Gerdy in 1836. Gerdy's work in correcting incisional hernias represented a significant breakthrough in the field of surgery [8].

In 1896, the French surgeon Quenu made a significant contribution to the field of hernia repair by differentiating postoperative eventration from other types of eventration in his work "Traitement opertoire de l'éventration." This is regarded as the first detailed description of incisional hernias [9].

After the advent of anesthesia and antisepsis, the incidence of incisional hernias increased substantially with the growing number of abdominal interventions [10–12]. Consequently, various techniques for correcting these hernias were developed, including simple sutures by Quenu, transverse overlapping technique by Mayo, and continuous fascial sutures from the external oblique by Witzel, Goepel, and Bartlet, among others [13–16]. In 1954, the Keel technique was introduced by the renowned surgeon Maingot as a new technique for correcting large incisional hernias [17].

At the start of the twentieth century, homologous and autologous materials were introduced for the successful closure of large defects in the abdominal wall. During this time, well-known surgeons such as Kirschner, Loewe, Nuttall, and Judd described hernia repair using various structures of the abdominal wall, including fascia, peritoneum, muscles, and even skin. The results they reported in their papers were satisfactory [11, 18–21].

The first hernia repair with metallic prosthetic materials was reported by Goepel and Witzel in 1900. The material used for these purposes was silver mesh. Other surgeons of this period such as Douglas, Koontz, and Throckmorton also referred to hernia repair through metal meshes, either silver or steel [22–26].

After the second world war, different plastic materials were synthesized, some of which began to be used for the correction of abdominal hernias. The first synthetic materials that were used for these purposes were nylon and perlon, which due to their poor characteristics were quickly withdrawn from use. Soon after that, other synthetic meshes with very good characteristics were synthesized and began to be widely used for the correction of hernias. Some of these materials that remain preferred for hernia repair are polypropylene, mersilene, polytetrafluoroethylene (ePTFE), etc. [27–29].

In 1993, for the first time, the correction of ventral hernias with laparoscopic techniques was reported by Le Blanc. The correction is done using synthetic meshes from prolene. Laparoscopic techniques are gaining more and more space in the correction of abdominal hernias, including incisional ones [30].

Great advances in the correction of hernias have been noted after the synthesis of dual and biological meshes, which enable their intraperitoneal placement without risking the appearance of adhesions or enterocutaneous fistulas [7, 31–33].

3. Anatomy of the anterior abdominal wall

The abdomen is the part of the body between the thorax and the pelvis. For hernias and their correction, the anterior abdominal wall is more important, because most of them are located in this part. The anterior abdominal wall is made up of different structures such as the skin, the oblique, transverse, and rectus muscles as well as their fascias and the parietal peritoneum.

The blood supply of the superficial layers of the abdominal wall is done through the arteries that originate from the femoral artery. The other three arteries that supply blood to the abdominal wall are two branches from the external iliac artery and one branch from the internal thoracic artery.

The sensory and motor innervation of the abdominal wall is done through several nerves such as the anterior and lateral cutaneous branches of the ventral rami of the 7th to 12th intercostal nerves and the ventral rami of the first and second lumbar nerves. The musculature of the abdominal wall consists of four paired muscles and their respective aponeuroses.

The external oblique muscle makes up the superficial layer of the abdominal wall. This muscle takes its origin from the lower eight ribs posteriorly to interdigitate with both the serratus and latissimus muscles. The fascia of this muscle takes part in the creation of the anterior portion of the rectus abdominis sheath, while together with the medial termination of all the aponeuroses of the three muscles, form the linea alba. External and internal oblique muscles support the abdominal organs as well as take part in the flexion and rotation of the body.

The internal oblique muscle takes its origin from the thoracolumbar fascia, iliac crest, and the lateral two-thirds of the inguinal ligament and inserts on the 10th and 12th ribs inferiorly. Studies show that incisional hernias in most cases are the result of disinsertion of these lateral muscles in the midline, thus resulting in retraction and subsequent atrophy.

The transversus abdominis muscle takes its origin from the 7th to 12th costal cartilages, iliac crest, and the lateral third of the inguinal ligament.

The rectus abdominis muscle originates from two different points. Its lateral head originates from the crest of the pubis, between the pubic symphysis and the pubic tubercle, while its median head originates from the pubic symphysis, being crossed with the fibers of the muscle on the contralateral side. The rectus sheath is formed from the aponeuroses and fasciae of the external oblique, internal oblique, and transversus abdominis. The anterior sheath of the rectus muscle superior to the umbilicus is composed only of aponeuroses from the internal and external oblique muscles, while the aponeurosis of the transverse muscle does not take part in this. The anterior sheath consists of all three aponeurotic layers only below the umbilicus. Even the posterior sheath of the rectus muscle is described in relation to the umbilicus. Above the umbilicus, it is built from the aponeuroses of the internal oblique and the transversus abdominis muscles, while below the umbilicus the internal abdominal aponeurosis does not participate in the construction of the posterior rectus sheath.

4. Incisions in the abdominal wall

The midline incision is the most commonly used incision in abdominal surgery due to its ease of performance and minimal blood loss, as the linea alba is poorly vascularized. This incision provides excellent exposure to the abdominal organs and can be easily extended superiorly or inferiorly as needed. However, the paramedian incision may be used in special cases, either as a conventional paramedian incision near the linea alba or a lateral paramedian incision made on the anterior side of the rectus muscle sheath's lateral edge. The rectus muscle fibers are displaced to avoid damage to the epigastric vessels, and a longitudinal incision is made above the arcuate line to open the abdominal cavity. The paramedian incision has limitations and difficulties and takes longer to perform than the midline incision.

The transverse supraumbilical incision is often used in conventional interventions in the right upper quadrant, but it is associated with greater blood loss and takes longer to complete due to the need to cut the external and internal oblique muscles, the transverse muscle, and part of the rectus muscle. Pfannenstiel incision is a transverse incision in the lower abdomen widely used in gynecology and some urological procedures, where the muscles can be cut either transversely parallel to the skin or along the linea alba.

Kocher's incision is an oblique subcostal incision widely used in surgical interventions of the biliary tract or bariatric surgery. It can be extended from both sides if necessary, and during this incision, the oblique, transverse, and rectus muscle fibers are cut, and many nerve fibers and segmental blood vessels are dissected.

McBurney's incision is another mid-caudal incision used in the lower right quadrant during appendectomies. The muscle fibers of the three abdominal wall muscles are separated to avoid damage to them, as well as to the nerve fibers and blood vessels.

5. Etiology of incisional hernias

Incisional hernias are a common complication of surgical procedures and can result from inadequate closure of operative wounds or traumatic injury. Despite advancements in wound closure materials and surgical techniques, incisional hernias continue to pose a challenge in open abdominal surgery and are also observed in laparoscopic surgery albeit at a lower frequency.

Etiological factors for incisional hernias can be grouped into patient-related factors, factors related to the disease treated with surgical intervention, and those related to the surgical technique used for incision closure.

Certain health disorders, particularly chronic ones, have a direct impact on the closure of operative wounds, thereby affecting the strength of the newly formed scar tissue, which is crucial for resisting high abdominal pressure. Chronic diseases such as diabetes mellitus, autoimmune disorders, and malignant diseases, as well as long-term use of corticosteroids, immunosuppressors, or cytostatics, can impair wound healing [34, 35]. Additionally, morbid obesity is a major risk factor for the development of incisional hernias [34, 36]. Advanced age, which weakens the abdominal wall muscles and can result in changes in connective tissue, is another significant risk factor for incisional hernia development.

Malnutrition, smoking, radiotherapy, and frequent surgical interventions in the abdomen are major factors that can hinder good wound healing and promote the development of incisional hernias [34, 37, 38]. Infection of the operative wound is one of the most critical factors that can cause dehiscence of the wound and increase the likelihood of incisional hernias [39]. Several preventive measures can help reduce the risk of infection, such as atraumatic surgical techniques, careful handling of the gastrointestinal organs, good hemostasis, and removal of all necrotic tissue.

The second group of factors that can increase the risk of developing incisional hernias is that related to the disease treated through surgical intervention. This group of factors includes the site and size of the incision, the nature of the disease (malignant or benign), the duration of the intervention, the opening of any part of the digestive system, the amount of blood loss, and the presence of any complications during the surgery. Acute abdominal diseases and emergencies have a higher risk of causing incisional hernias.

Multiple studies have shown that certain surgical interventions, such as those for aortic aneurysms, liver pathologies, and colorectal cancer, are associated with a higher incidence of incisional hernias [40, 41]. The type of incision used during the surgical procedure is also a significant factor in the development of incisional hernias. Studies have demonstrated that incisions such as the lateral paramedian and transverse incisions pose a lower risk for the development of incisional hernias, owing to the fact that well-vascularized structures heal faster. Therefore, during the opening of the abdominal cavity, maximum care must be taken not to injure the large arteries supplying abdominal muscles [36, 42].

The direction of the pulling force of the abdominal muscles is another factor that affects the appearance of incisional wounds, mainly transverse. This leads to the edges of vertical incisions moving away from each other during exercises and pulling forces, while transverse incisions come closer to each other. If the lips of the muscle fascia are not properly sewn together using strong sutures with the appropriate length in relation to the incision (at least four times longer than the wound), there is a high risk of incisional hernias [43, 44].

Surgical wounds require time to restore their tensile strength. It is estimated that at least 4 weeks are needed for the wound to return around 50% of its strength, while after 12 months, the wound returns 80% of its tensile strength [43]. Therefore, suture materials must be strong and durable for at least 6 weeks until the damaged tissues regain sufficient tensile strength [44, 45].

6. Clinical presentation

The causes of incisional hernias vary and depend on factors such as the size, positioning, and contents of the hernial sac. Patients with incisional hernias are more prone to complications than those with primary hernias. Incisional hernias occur at the incision site and are clinically manifested by swelling due to the protrusion of abdominal organs through the abdominal wall defect. In the case of small hernias, patients may experience discomfort or moderate pain, although even small hernias can become incarcerated. In the case of large hernias, there is a risk of intestinal incarceration or, in severe cases, strangulation, which requires immediate surgical intervention.

Incarceration as a complication occurs in about 1.24 to 2.59% of patients with incisional hernia, while strangulation is the most serious complication and is recorded in about 2% of all patients with incarcerated incisional hernia [46].

Generally, early postoperative hernias are a consequence of wound infection or problems with suturing, while the causes of late postoperative hernias are not entirely known, although some are related to connective and fibrotic tissue disorders [42].

7. Diagnosis

Diagnosing incisional hernias is typically straightforward, as there is often a visible swelling above or near the site of the operative wound that can be reduced with manual pressure. The edges of the hernia can often be felt, allowing for determination of the size of the abdominal wall defect. Coughing or straining can also help to provoke the displacement of abdominal organs into the hernial sac and facilitate diagnosis.

In some cases, however, such as extreme obesity or complex cases, a CT scan of the abdomen may be necessary to confirm the diagnosis. This examination can also aid in planning the surgical intervention, identifying potential challenges for the surgeon during the repair of the defect and determining the appropriate incision size for correction.

Ultrasonography examinations can also provide important information about the size of the hernia, the contents of the hernial sac, and the condition of the abdominal wall muscles.

8. Treatment

Except in special cases when incisional hernias must be treated conservatively, such as in elderly patients or those with chronic diseases that may worsen their condition in the postoperative period or even threaten their life, surgical intervention is required to correct incisional hernias. This is especially true for large hernias, as correcting them eliminates the patient's discomfort and avoids the risks of incarceration or strangulation, thus significantly improving their quality of life.

At the beginning of modern surgery, for a long time, the correction of incisional hernias was conventional, which involved closing the abdominal defect by approaching and suturing the edges of the wound. Later, with a better understanding of the nature and mechanisms of the development of incisional hernias, other correction techniques began to be used, such as the Mayo technique, which involves overlapping a part of the hernial sac on the incisional wound [47, 48]. Another successful technique for correcting incisional hernias is the separative technique, also known as the Ramirez technique [49].

However, great progress has been made in the correction of incisional hernias after the introduction of prosthetic materials, specifically the use of meshes for correcting abdominal wall defects.

These materials not only make it possible to close abdominal wall defects without tension but they also strengthen the abdominal wall. Among the first meshes used to correct incisional hernias were those made of prolene, which Usher introduced in 1963. The correction of hernias with simple meshes, while showing good results in terms of reducing recurrence rates, was often accompanied by complications resulting from contact with visceral organs and the development of intestinal adhesions and enterocutaneous fistulas. However, the introduction of dual meshes, which have one side covered with an absorbable layer that prevents the mesh from adhering to abdominal organs and another side made of a nonabsorbable layer that maintains proper abdominal wall strength after closing the defect, significantly reduced the incidence of these severe complications, such as adherent ileus and enterocutaneous fistulae.

The most commonly used meshes for incisional hernia correction are those made of prolene. There are two types of prolene meshes in use: lightweight with a weight < 50 g/m^2, which are superior to heavy-weight ones (with a weight > 50 g/m^2), in terms of reducing postoperative pain and enabling a faster return to daily activity. In recent years, coated or barrier meshes have become increasingly popular for incisional hernia correction. In these meshes, the surface that contacts the abdominal organs should prevent their adhesion to the mesh, while the other surface should integrate as best as possible with the abdominal wall. The first meshes with these characteristics to be put into use were those made of ePTFE [48].

Currently, there are many types of meshes available that have better antiadherence properties than ePTFE. Biological meshes have also been developed, which are made of collagen obtained from living tissues such as skin, submucosa of small intestines, and pericardium. These meshes can be left in their natural state or chemically reinforced. Unreinforced meshes were destroyed within 3 months and strengthened ones remained unchanged for over a year. They are useful in infected wounds and prevent intestinal adhesions to the mesh [50].

When it comes to using prosthetic materials to correct incisional hernias, there is no one-size-fits-all approach. It depends on various factors, such as the size and location of the hernia, the patient's constitution and clinical condition, the surgeon's experience, and the available types of meshes.

Laparoscopic correction of hernias, which involves inserting a dual mesh over the hernial defect and fixing it to the abdominal wall, has become increasingly popular since Le Blanc reported the first case in 1993. Studies indicate that the incidence of postoperative complications, such as pain, wound infection, and seromas, is significantly lower when using laparoscopic techniques for incisional hernia repair [40, 41, 49, 51].

9. Post operative complications

Postoperative complications following the correction of incisional hernias may include various issues, such as postoperative pain, wound bleeding, wound infection, seroma formation, dehiscence, and hernia recurrence.

Regarding the incidence and intensity of pain in the postoperative period, several randomized studies have shown that patients with incisional hernias along the linea alba experience a lower intensity of pain compared to those with transverse incisional hernias [52]. Furthermore, numerous studies have shown a higher incidence of postoperative pain after hernia correction with prosthetic materials [53]. However, the precise factors that cause pain after incisional hernia correction are still not known [53].

Postoperative pain, especially if it is of greater intensity and lasts longer, can increase the level of morbidity and patients' need for analgesics, including potent ones such as opioids [54].

Moreover, there is a difference in the intensity of pain between open hernia correction techniques and laparoscopic procedures. Several studies show that the intensity of postoperative pain is higher in patients who underwent hernia correction with laparoscopic procedures compared to those who underwent hernioplasty with an open method [55]. The reason for the greater intensity of the pain in laparoscopic procedures is thought to be due to the way the mesh is fixed. The fixation of the mesh with transfascial sutures, which penetrate the abdominal muscles, can capture nerve fibers and blood vessels, inducing muscle ischemia and intense pain [56].

However, there are also studies that do not show any difference in pain intensity between open and laparoscopic techniques in the correction of incisional hernias [57].

One of the most serious problems in the early postoperative period after correction of incisional hernias, especially in cases where prosthetic materials are used, is the infection of the operative wound. This complication is not only difficult to eradicate because the mesh represents a foreign body, but it also makes it difficult for the wound to heal quickly, thereby significantly increasing the risk of hernia recurrence.

While pain is more frequent in patients with incisional hernias along the linea alba, numerous retrospective studies show that the risk of surgical wound infection after incisional hernia repair does not depend on its location.

The most serious complication after incisional hernia repair is hernia recurrence, and one of the main reasons for its appearance is considered to be infection of the operative wound. According to numerous studies, this complication shows a slightly higher incidence in midline hernias compared to hernias in other locations, while transverse hernias show a lower incidence compared to paramedian or medial ones.

The highest incidence of incisional hernias along the linea alba has several reasons, the most important of which seem to be the poor blood supply of this part of the abdominal wall, as well as the fact that the contraction of abdominal wall muscles during coughing, vomiting, or erecting retracts wound edges laterally and thereby facilitating wound dehiscence.

The type of incision with the lowest incidence for the development of hernias is transverse one, but this applies only if the defect is located in one quadrant of the abdominal wall. However, if these apertures extend beyond the midline, then this incidence does not differ from those along the linea alba.

While transverse incisions have the advantage of producing less scarring, they offer limited exposure to the abdominal cavity, which restricts their use in many surgeries. In addition, these incisions can damage the nerve fibers that innervate the abdominal muscles, leading to muscle weakness and numbness.

On the other hand, premedian incisions provide excellent exposure of the abdominal cavity similar to median incisions and can be expanded in both directions if necessary. During this type of incision, the rectus muscles can be displaced laterally, preserving not only the muscles but also the neurovascular structures of the abdomen. The low incidence of hernias in paramedian incisions is attributed to well-vascularized wound beds, as well as to other features such as wound reinforcement by the rectus muscle and the so-called shutter mechanism.

10. Factors affecting wound healing in incisional hernias

In the appearance of incisional hernias, many factors have an impact, some of which cannot be influenced by the surgeon, such as the age of the patients, obesity, the degree of urgency, the degree of contamination of the operative field, and the type of surgical intervention [58]. However, there are some factors on which the surgeon has a great impact, such as the type of incision, suture material, careful tissue handling, the type of meshes that will be used if it is necessary, and the surgical technique with which the intervention will be performed, i.e., conventional or laparoscopic.

Numerous studies have demonstrated that transverse and paramedian incisions, along with the Pfannenstiel incision, exhibit superiority in decreasing the likelihood of incisional hernias [59–61].

Furthermore, the speed and quality of wound healing play a critical role in mitigating the risk of incisional hernias. The more vascularized the tissues are, the faster the wound healing will be [62].

Conversely, the presence of bacteria and their toxins within the wound may trigger a pro-inflammatory cytokine response, hindering timely and effective healing [63].

Advancing age may also impede wound healing, given the observed delay in epithelialization, collagen synthesis, and angiogenesis in elderly individuals [64, 65].

Additionally, stress has recently emerged as a noteworthy factor in wound healing [66].

The latest estimates suggest that due to the hormonal action of estrogens, wound healing in women is slightly faster compared to men. This is because estrogens regulate a variety of genes associated with regeneration [67].

Diabetes has a great impact on wound healing through several complex mechanisms such as hypoxia and venous stasis [68, 69]. Other factors that prevent wound healing in diabetics are defects in leukocyte chemotaxis, phagocytosis, and bactericidal destructive capacity [70]. Diabetic neuropathy, a severe problem in diabetic people, also affects the timely healing of wounds [71].

Obese individuals, due to accompanying conditions such as diabetes, hypertension, dyslipidemia, and respiratory problems, have a higher risk of wound infection, hematomas, seromas development, and pressure and venous ulcer formation, thereby negatively affecting wound healing [72, 73].

The prolonged use of certain medications, particularly glucocorticoids, can affect fibroblast proliferation and collagen synthesis, resulting in difficult wound healing [74].

Additionally, cytostatic drugs inhibit DNA, RNA, or protein synthesis, which leads to decreased fibroplasia and neovascularization of wounds [75].

Finally, malnutrition and inadequate daily protein intake can also impede wound healing since proteins play a crucial role in capillary formation, fibroblast proliferation, collagen synthesis, and wound remodeling [76].

11. Discussion

Currently, incisional hernias not only represent a health problem but also an economic one. Their treatment remains a real challenge for surgeons, requiring good knowledge of the surgical techniques used for their correction, as well as sufficient experience and skills. According to many studies, the incidence of incisional hernias after abdominal surgical interventions ranges from 2 to 20%. This great difference in incidences is not only due to the experience that surgeons have in the treatment of these complications but also to many other factors, such as the different techniques used to correct them, the materials used to close the defect, the patient's condition, and the incidence of nosocomial infections.

The etiological factors that affect the appearance of incisional hernias are different. Among those that have to do with surgical intervention, the most important is the type of incision, the infection of the operative wound, the technique used to repair the defect, and the type of sutures used for hernia correction, as well as the use or non-use of prosthetic materials for closing the operative wound.

Regarding incision and localization, the experience referred to by many researchers shows an advantage of transversal incisions compared to median ones in terms of the risk of developing incisional hernias. However, this remains correct only as long as they are located only in one quadrant of the abdominal wall and do not cross the linea alba. The incidence of hernias after transverse incisions is about 5% if they are unilateral and up to 10% if they cross the linea alba. Other incisions that show a low degree of risk for the appearance of incisional hernias are the paramedian one and that of Pfannenstiel.

Pfannenstiel transversal incisions, which are mainly used by gynecologists and obstetricians, also show a low incidence of hernia development. However, the negative side of all these incisions is that they do not allow for a good exposure of the abdominal cavity. The medial incision enables better exposure of the abdominal cavity in general and is particularly preferred in emergency abdominal interventions where quick exploration of the abdominal cavity is necessary for the treatment of the patient and a fast and safe diagnosis of abdominal organ damage should be made.

In addition to localization, the size of the operative wound also has a significant impact on the occurrence of incisional hernias. Large wounds are more prone to the development of this complication, as shown in almost every study on incisional hernias.

The incidence of incisional hernias is affected by suture materials and the technique used to close the operative wound, which is confirmed by many meta-analytical studies and researchers. Nonabsorbable materials such as prolene and continuous suturing have advantages in minimizing the incidence of incisional hernias compared to other materials and techniques used for closing wounds after laparotomy. Of the absorbable sutures, only polydioxanone (PDS) gives similar results to prolene regarding the risk of incisional hernias, although there are no convincing studies for this yet. The ratio between the length of the wound and the length of the suture used to close it also seems to be important in the risk of developing incisional hernias, which is related to the distance between the two stitches and should preferably be approximately 5 mm.

In recent decades, laparoscopic surgery is increasingly used for the treatment of incisional hernias, especially after the manufacturing of the so-called dual meshes, which have one side made of materials that do not adhere to the organs of the abdominal cavity. The incidence of recurrence of hernias treated with laparoscopic techniques is low, estimated to be somewhere between 0.2–2%, which is also due to the small wounds created during these interventions.

The incidence of recurrence after the correction of incisional hernias with prosthetic materials is also significantly lower compared to the classical closure by suturing the wound using any of the referred conventional techniques.

Regarding the positioning of the mesh during the correction of incisional hernias, specifically the onlay, inlay, and intraperitoneal technique, most studies show an advantage of the intraperitoneal technique over the other two, not only in terms of the rate of recurrence but also in terms of other complications such as the incidence of seromas, surgical wound infections, and postoperative pain.

Studies show that there is no difference in the recurrence rate of incisional hernias between laparoscopic and conventional techniques, as long as prosthetic materials are used for their correction. On the other hand, the laparoscopic technique has clear advantages in minimizing some postoperative complications, such as wound infections, seromas, recurrence, morbidity, hospitalization, and postoperative pain, according to various studies.

However, there are some disadvantages to laparoscopic techniques for treating incisional hernias, including the longer operative time required for correction and a slightly greater risk of intestinal damage that can be complicated by peritonitis, which can be life-threatening. Despite these potential risks, laparoscopic techniques remain effective and safe for treating not only incisional hernias but also other types of hernias.

The type of sutures used to close the defect or fix the mesh in the abdominal wall also has a significant impact on the incidence of postoperative complications after mesh hernia correction. The critical period for fixing the mesh to the abdominal wall is around 1 year, which is why the sutures used to fix the mesh should not be absorbed before this time. As a result, most authors prefer to use nonabsorbable sutures or a combination of absorbable and nonabsorbable sutures to ensure sufficient tensile strength during this critical period until the mesh is well integrated into the host's tissues.

In recent years, biological meshes have also been used in the treatment of incisional hernias. Studies on the results of the correction of incisional hernias with these meshes are different and sometimes controversial. Some authors argue that biological meshes are superior to synthetic meshes in terms of recurrence rate and other complications, while others suggest a higher incidence of complications in cases corrected with biological meshes.

12. Conclusion

In conclusion, the treatment of incisional hernias requires careful consideration of various factors, such as the choice of suture material and technique for closing the operative wound, as well as the type and positioning of the mesh used for correction. Laparoscopic techniques have advantages in terms of minimizing certain postoperative complications but also carry some risks, such as longer intraoperative time and the potential for intestinal damage. Prosthetic materials for mesh hernia correction generally have a lower recurrence rate compared to traditional suturing techniques, and the type of suture used to fix the mesh also plays an important role in the prevention of postoperative complications. Furthermore, the use of biological meshes in incisional hernia correction remains controversial, with some studies reporting superior results compared to synthetic meshes, while others indicate a higher incidence of complications. Ultimately, the selection of the most appropriate technique and materials for the treatment of incisional hernias should be tailored to the individual patient's needs and preferences and based on a thorough evaluation of available evidence and clinical experience.

Acknowledgements

The authors thank their surgeon colleagues from Albania and Macedonia for the valuable advice and suggestions for the successful completion of this work.

Author details

Kastriot Haxhirexha[1], Agron Dogjani[2], Aulona Haxhirexha[2*], Dritan Alushani[2], Labeat Haxhirexha[2], Aferdita Ademi[1], Blerim Fejzuli[1] and Teuta Emini[1]

1 Faculty of Medical Sciences, University of Tetova (Republic of North Macedonia) Clinical Hospital, Tetova

2 University Hospital Center "Mother Teresa", Tirana, Albania

*Address all correspondence to: aulona.haxhirexha@gmail.com

References

[1] Mulvany NJ. History of abdominal wall hernia repair. Surgical Clinics. 2018;**98**(2):153-163

[2] Bendavid R. Abdominal Wall Hernias: Principles and Management. New York: Springer; 2001

[3] Bryan CP. Ancient Egyptian Medicine: The Papyrus Ebers. Ares, Chicago; 1930 (1974 [printing])

[4] Breasted JH. The Edwin Smith Surgical Papyrus. Chicago: University of Chicago Press; 1980

[5] Nahai F. The Craft of Surgery. 4th ed. Philadelphia, PA: Lippincott Williams & Wilkins; 2013

[6] Zimmerman LM. A brief history of hernias and their repairs. Hernia. 2015;**19**(2):153-159

[7] Badylak SF. The extracellular matrix as a scaffold for tissue reconstruction. Seminars in Cell & Developmental Biology. 2002;**13**(2):377-383

[8] Leven K-H. The Invention of Hippocrates: Oath, Letters and Hippocratic Corpus. Aldershot: Ashgate; 1998

[9] Reiffel AJ. The pioneers of hernia repair: Bassini and Halsted. Journal of the American College of Surgeons. 2009;**209**(6):831-833

[10] Papavramidou N, Christopoulou-Aletra H. The ancient technique of "gastrorrhaphy". Journal of Gastrointestinal Surgery. 2009;**13**(7):1345-1341

[11] Dunn KA. A glimpse into the past: Two millennia of inguinal hernia repair. Hernia. 2017;**21**(1):1-10

[12] Toledo-Pereyra LH. Galen's contribution to surgery. Journal of the History of Medicine and Allied Sciences. 1973;**28**(4):357-375

[13] Rutkow IM. A selective history of groin hernia repair from ancient Egypt to the end of the 18th century. Hernia. 2013;**17**(3):305-312

[14] La Chausse BI. Dissertatio chirurgica de hérnia ventrali [Dissertation of surgical ventral hernia]. Naples: Gessare; 1756. Italian

[15] Tintinalli JE. Tintinalli's Emergency Medicine: A Comprehensive Study Guide. 9th ed. New York, NY: McGraw-Hill Education; 2020

[16] Gerdy P. Nouvelles operations pour guerir radicalement les hernies du ventre. Gaz Hop. 1836;**1**:10-14

[17] Rutkow IM. A selective history of groin hernia repair from ancient Egypt to the end of the 18th century. Surgical Clinics. 2003;**83**(6):1165-1172

[18] Quenu E. Traitement opertoire de l'é ventration. Mémoires. Académie de Chirurgie. 1896;**22**:2

[19] Witzel O. Uber den Verschluss van Bauchwunden und Bruchpforten durch versenkte Silberdrahtnetze. Centralblatt für Chirurgie. 1900;**27**(3):36

[20] Goepel R. Uber die Verschliessung von Bruchpforten durch Einheilung geflochtener fertiger Silberdrahtnetze. Zentralblatt für Chirurgie. 1900;**17**:3

[21] Shulman AG, Amid PK, Lichtenstein IL. Maingot's Abdominal Operations. Vol. 1. London: Prentice-Hall International; 1994

[22] Maingot R. Abdominal Operations. 3rd ed. London: Lewis; 1955

[23] Judd E. The prevention and treatment of ventral hernia. Surgery, Gynecology & Obstetrics. 1912;**14**:7

[24] Zimmerman LM, Anand KJ. History of hernia mesh. Surgical Technology International. 2007;**16**:131-137

[25] Loewe O. Uber Hautimplantation an Stelle der freien Fascienplastik. Muncher Med Wochenschr. 1913;**60**:1320-1321

[26] Throckmorton TD. Tantalum gauze in the repair of hernias complicated by tissue deficiency; a preliminary report. Surgery. 1948;**23**(1):32-46

[27] Smith DR. Hernia surgery on coins from antiquity to the renaissance. Hernia. 2014;**18**(4):617-622

[28] Koontz AR, Kimberly RC. Tantalum and marlex mesh (with a note on marlex thread): An experimental and clinical comparison—Preliminary report. Annals of Surgery. 1960;**151**:796-804

[29] McBride ED. Synthetic mesh in hernia repair. Annals of Surgery. 1953;**137**(4):482-487

[30] Usher FC, Wallace SA. Tissue reaction to plastics; a comparison of nylon, orlon, dacron, teflon, and marlex. A.M.A. Archives of Surgery. 1958;**76**(6):997-999

[31] Grannell JP, Leonard JN. Hernia repair with Mersilene mesh. Surgery, Gynecology & Obstetrics. 1956;**103**(1):97-100

[32] LeBlanc KA, Booth WV. Laparoscopic Repair of Incisional Abdominal Hernias Using Expanded Polytetrafluoroethylene: Preliminary Findings. Surg Laparoscopy; 1993

[33] Davies SW, Turza KC, Sawyer RG, et al. A comparative analysis between laparoscopic and open ventral hernia repair at a tertiary care center. The American Surgeon. 2012;**78**:888-892

[34] Sorensen LT, Hemmingsen UB, Kirkeby LT, et al. Smoking is a risk factor for incisional hernia. Archives of Surgery. 2005;**140**(2):119-123

[35] Sugerman HJ, Kellum JM Jr, Reines HD, et al. Greater risk of incisional hernia with morbidly obese than steroid-dependent patients and low recurrence with prefascial polypropylene mesh. American Journal of Surgery. 1996;**171**(1):80-84

[36] Hoer J, Lawong G, Klinge U, et al. Factors influencing the development of incisional hernia. A retrospective study of 2,983 laparotomy patients over a period of 10 years. Der Chirurg. 2002;**73**:474-480

[37] Israelsson LA. Wound failure and incisional hernia: Mechanism and prevention. In: Fitzgibbons RJ Jr, Greenburg AG, editors. Nyhus and Condon's Hernia. Philadelphia: Lippincott Williams & Wilkins; 2002. pp. 3-8

[38] Klinge U, Prescher A, Klosterhalfen B, et al. Development and pathophysiology of abdominal wall defects. Chirurg. 1997;**68**(4):293-303

[39] Walming S, Angenete E, Block M, Bock D, Gessler B, Haglind E. Retrospective review of risk factors for surgical wound dehiscence and incisional hernia. BMC Surgery. 2017;**17**:19

[40] Ahonen-Siirtola M, Rautio T, Ward J, Kössi J, Ohtonen P, Mäkelä J. Complications in laparoscopic versus open incisional ventral hernia repair.

A retrospective comparative study. World Journal of Surgery. 2015;**39**:2872-2877

[41] Heniford BT, Park A, Ramshaw BJ, Voeller G. Laparoscopic ventral and incisional hernia repair in 407 patients. Journal of the American College of Surgeons. 2000;**190**:645-650

[42] Höer J, Junge K, Schachtrupp A, Klinge U, Schumpelick V. Influence of laparotomy closure technique on collagen synthesis in the incisional region. Hernia. 2002;**6**(3):93-98 Epub 2002 Jul 20

[43] Editorial: Ten commandments of safe and optimum Abdominal Wall closure. Indian Journal of Surgery. 2018;**80**(2):105-108

[44] Patel SV, Paskar DD, Nelson RL, Vedula SS, Steele SR. Closure methods for laparotomy incisions for preventing incisional hernias and other wound complications. Cochrane Database of Systematic Reviews. 2017;**11**(11):CD005661. DOI: 10.1002/14651858.CD005661.pub2

[45] Henriksen NA, Deerenberg EB, Venclauskas L, Fortelny RH, Miserez M, Muysoms FE. Meta-analysis on materials and techniques for laparotomy closure: The MATCH review. World Journal of Surgery. 2018;**42**(6):1666-1678. DOI: 10.1007/s00268-017-4393-9

[46] Dadashzadeh ER, Huckaby LV, Handzel R, Hossain MS, Sanin GD, Anto VP, et al. The risk of incarceration during nonoperative Management of Incisional Hernias. Annals of Surgery. 2022;**275**(2):e488-e495

[47] Welty G, Klinge U, Klosterhalfen B, et al. Functional impairment and complaints following incisional hernia repair with different polypropylene meshes. Hernia. 2001;**5**(3):142-147

[48] Bauer JJ, Salky BA, Gelernt IM, et al. Repair of large abdominal wall defects with expanded polytetrafluoroethylene (PTFE). Annals of Surgery. 1987;**206**(6):765-769

[49] Eker HH, Hansson BME, Buunen M, Janssen IM, Pierik RE, Hop WC, et al. Laparoscopic vs. open incisional hernia repair: A randomized clinical trial. JAMA Surgery. 2013;**148**:259-263

[50] Franklin ME Jr, Gonzalez JJ Jr, Michaelson RP, et al. Preliminary experience with new bioactive prosthetic material for repair of hernias in infected fields. Hernia. 2002;**6**(4):171-174

[51] Lavanchy JL, Buff SE, Kohler A, Candinas D, Beldi G. Long-term results of laparoscopic versus open intraperitoneal onlay mesh incisional hernia repair: A propensity score-matched analysis. Surgical Endoscopy. 2019;**33**:225-233

[52] Erritzøe-Jervild L, Christoffersen MW, Helgstrand F, et al. Long-term complaints after elective repair for small umbilical or epigastric hernias. Hernia. 2013;**17**:211-215

[53] Gronnier C, Wattier JM, Favre H, et al. Risk factors for chronic pain after open ventral hernia repair by underlay mesh placement. World Journal of Surgery. 2012;**36**:1548-1554

[54] DeLong CG, Doble JA, Schilling AL, Pauli EM, Soybel DI. Delineating the burden of chronic post-operative pain in patients undergoing open repair of complex ventral hernias. American Journal of Surgery. 2018;**215**(4):610-617. DOI: 10.1016/j.amjsurg.2018.01.030

[55] Muysoms F, Vander Mijnsbrugge G, Pletinckx P, et al. Randomized clinical trial of mesh fixation with "double crown" versus "sutures and tackers"

in laparoscopic ventral hernia repair. Hernia. 2013;**17**(5):603-612

[56] Gillian GK, Geis WP, Grover G. Laparoscopic incisional and ventral hernia repair (LIVH): An evolving outpatient technique. JSLS : Journal of the Society of Laparoendoscopic Surgeons. 2002;**6**:315-322

[57] McGreevy JM, Goodney PP, Birkmeyer CM, Finlayson SRG, Laycock WS, Birkmeyer JD. A prospective study comparing the complication rates between laparoscopic and open ventral hernia repairs. Surgical Endoscopy. 2003;**17**:1778-1780

[58] Rutkow IM. Demographic and socioeconomic aspects of hernia repair in the United States in 2003. The Surgical Clinics of North America. 2003;**83**(5):1045-1051 v–vi

[59] Grantcharov TP, Rosenberg J. Vertical compared with transverse incisions in abdominal surgery. The European Journal of Surgery. 2001;**167**:260-267

[60] Burger JWA, van't Reit M, Jeekel J. Abdominal incisions: Techniques and postoperative complications. Scandinavian Journal of Surgery. 2002;**91**:315-321

[61] Orcutt ST, Balentine CJ, Marshall CL, Robinson CN, Anaya DA, Artinyan A, et al. Use of a Pfannenstiel incision in minimally invasive colorectal cancer surgery is associated with a lower risk of wound complications. Techniques in Coloproctology. 2012;**16**:127-132

[62] Edwards R, Harding KG. Bacteria and wound healing. Current Opinion in Infectious Diseases. 2004;**17**:91-96

[63] Davis SC, Ricotti C, Cazzaniga A, Welsh E, Eaglstein WH, Mertz PM. Microscopic and physiologic evidence for biofilm-associated wound colonization in vivo. Wound Repair and Regeneration. 2008;**16**:23-29

[64] Swift ME, Burns AL, Gray KL, DiPietro LA. Age-related alterations in the inflammatory response to dermal injury. The Journal of Investigative Dermatology. 2001;**117**:1027-1035

[65] Swift ME, Kleinman HK, DiPietro LA. Impaired wound repair and delayed angiogenesis in aged mice. Laboratory Investigation. 1999;**79**:1479-1487

[66] Boyapati L, Wang HL. The role of stress in periodontal disease and wound healing. Periodontology 2000. 2007;**2000**(44):195-210

[67] Hardman MJ, Ashcroft GS. Estrogen, not intrinsic aging, is the major regulator of delayed human wound healing in the elderly. Genome Biology. 2008;**9**:R80

[68] Vincent AM, Russell JW, Low P, Feldman EL. Oxidative stress in the pathogenesis of diabetic neuropathy. Endocrine Reviews. 2004;**25**:612-628

[69] Woo K, Ayello EA, Sibbald RG. The edge effect: Current therapeutic options to advance the wound edge. Advances in Skin & Wound Care. 2007;**20**:99-117

[70] Loots MA, Lamme EN, Zeegelaar J, Mekkes JR, Bos JD, Middelkoop E. Differences in cellular infiltrate and extracellular matrix of chronic diabetic and venous ulcers versus acute wounds. The Journal of Investigative Dermatology. 1998;**111**:850-857

[71] Galkowska H, Olszewski WL, Wojewodzka U, Rosinski G, Karnafel W. Neurogenic factors in the impaired healing of diabetic foot ulcers. The Journal of Surgical Research. 2006;**134**:252-258

[72] Greco JA 3rd, Castaldo ET, Nanney LB, Wendel JJ, Summitt JB, Kelly KJ, et al. The effect of weight loss surgery and body mass index on wound complications after abdominal contouring operations. Annals of Plastic Surgery. 2008;**61**:235-242

[73] Wilson JA, Clark JJ. Obesity: Impediment to postsurgical wound healing. Advances in Skin & Wound Care. 2004;**17**:426-435

[74] Wagner AE, Huck G, Stiehl DP, Jelkmann W, Hellwig-Bürgel T. Dexamethasone impairs hypoxia-inducible factor-1 function. Biochemical and Biophysical Research Communications. 2008;**372**:336-340

[75] Franz MG, Steed DL, Robson MC. Optimizing healing of the acute wound by minimizing complications. Current Problems in Surgery. 2007;**44**:691-763

[76] Campos AC, Groth AK, Branco AB. Assessment and nutritional aspects of wound healing. Current Opinion in Clinical Nutrition and Metabolic Care. 2008;**11**:281-288

Chapter 2

Approaching the Complex Abdominal Wall Hernia: General Principles of Component Separation Techniques

Fotios Seretis, Paraskevi Dedopoulou, Nikiforos Rodis, Konstantina Soukouli, Nikolaos Bogiatzopoulos, Charalampos Seretis and Georgios Zacharis

Abstract

Abdominal wall hernias represent a clinical spectrum ranging from a small defect in the abdominal wall causing minimal interruption to patients up to massive defects with severe impairment in abdominal wall function and physiology. Principles of successful hernia repair rely on re-approximation of fascial defect edges to achieve primary closure in a tension free manner and subsequent reenforcement of the repair with a mesh. In the case of large defects, especially in the incisional hernia scenario, advanced fascial release techniques with separation of components is often required to recreate normal anatomy. Relevant techniques are anterior component separation with or without sparing of periumbilical vascular perforators and posterior component separation with transverse abdominis release, representing an expansion of the retrorectus Rives-Stoppa repair. With regards to surgical planning, preoperative imaging, standardization of techniques according to patient and hernia defect characteristics as well as prehabilitation of the abdominal wall with botulinum toxin ("chemical component separation") represent significant weapons in the armamentarium of the complex abdominal wall reconstruction surgeon. The scope of this chapter is to attempt to unify pathophysiologic concepts of hernias with anatomic-based advanced repairs.

Keywords: hernia, abdominal wall reconstruction, incisional hernia, retrorectus repair, rives-Stoppa repair, posterior component separation, anterior component separation, mesh

1. Introduction

The definition of complex abdominal wall hernia comprises a hernia in the abdominal wall that requires advanced techniques for its repair. The vast majority of complex hernias develop in the area of a postoperative scar and are thus a subgroup of incisional hernias, according to the most recent European Hernia Society Classification of Hernias [1]. Complex hernias, although not defined per se, represent a constellation of unfavorable factors preventing simple repair of the defect, both patient- and disease-related. A recent consensus used as criteria for complex hernias size and location, contamination and soft tissue condition, patient history and risk factors as well as clinical scenario [2]. Surgical treatment of this subgroup of patients requires a detailed understanding not only of the techniques involved in advanced abdominal wall reconstruction, but also of the underlying pathophysiologic processes in this disease entity, in order for surgery to have a role of restoring normal anatomy as means to restore normal function [3].

2. General principles of component separation techniques

2.1 Pathophysiology of hernias

Abdominal wall hernias occur with loss of architecture in the load-bearing areas of muscle, fascial and tendinous tissues. Focusing on our task to enlighten the pathophysiological processes in the complex abdominal wall hernia setting, it seems prudent to attempt to establish a correlation between the macroscopic and the microscopic level of abdominal wall healing in the postoperative setting, as the majority of complex hernias are incisional in nature. Abnormal collagen metabolism with either a genetic basis, namely genetically acquired collagen disorders, or acquired, secondary to nutrition or smoking, seems to be one critical precipitating factor, leading to both primary and incisional hernias [4]. More importantly, however, and of probably greater interest for the cause of the present review, is fascial pathology secondary to acute laparotomy wound failure. Early laparotomy wound failure, as demonstrated in an animal model, seems to be a key event driving the subsequent development of incisional hernias [5]. Using radiopaque metal clips, the authors in the aforementioned paper followed laparotomy wound failure sequentially in time and showed that early laparotomy wound failure resulted in the formation of an incisional hernia, with authors assuming in their critical discussion part of the paper that early laparotomy wound failure resulted in distortion of normal wound healing architecture, thus creating a selecting process for abnormal population of wound repair fibroblasts deposing abnormal collagen [6–8]. It is this loss of normal healing architecture that creates an alteration in load forces that produces effects at the wound fibroblast and extracellular matrix level through mechanisms of mechanotransmission, in accordance with previous studies to play a significant role in tissue remodeling and repair. Apart from genetic factors in wound healing key mediators, wound ischemia of any cause also impairs normal processes [9]. Early wound laparotomy failure, unfortunately, is a clinical senescent process initially, and its incidence is, therefore, significantly underestimated before manifesting as a clinically evident incisional hernia at a later time [10]. Although useful for the purposes of academic research, dichotomising the pathophysiologic processes into mechanical and molecular in nature, these should be viewed as interweaving and overlapping.

Previous studies have shown that loss of insertion of the lateral abdominal wall musculature into the linea alba, as is the case in an incisional hernia, causes distinct changes in abdominal wall physiology [11, 12], because the normal force across the composite myofascial structure ceases to exist, thus decreasing the loads transferred onto lateral muscles. Lateral abdominal wall muscles present with shortening and oblique muscles develop exempt a histopathologic pattern similar to disuse atrophy that chronically unloaded skeletal muscles develop. Stiffening of oblique muscles decreases abdominal wall compliance and increases the mechanical loads exerted on the midline, which per se could be a deleterious event for the "healing" midline in the early postoperative period, in which wound tensile strength grossly depends on sutures to withstand opposing mechanical forces, while allowing sufficient time for the normal healing processes to take place [13]. This process creates a perpetuating cycle of lateral muscle retraction away from the midline, thereby further enlarging the hernia defect [14]. These pathophysiologic processes seem to be reversed with hernia repair, though not up to the full tensile strength of the uninjured abdominal wall [15]. Interestingly, function of rectus abdomini muscle complex is preserved in the incisional hernia setting, implying that it is the reconstitution of the abdominal wall muscle complex as functional unit that should be the goal of abdominal wall reconstruction surgery [16]. Mesh repair of incisional hernias has been established as superior to suture only repair of incisional hernias even for small-sized hernia defects [17]. Augmentation of primary fascial closure with mesh seems to yield better results in terms of hernia recurrence rates and postoperative complications compared to bridging the fascial defect with mesh [18]. In an attempt to unify "reconstitution of anatomy" with restoration of physiology, it seems prudent to assume that the most effective strategy for repair of complex hernia defects would be achievement of primary fascial closure with sutures and reenforcement of a tension-free repair with mesh. Contrary to this rationale is a study including both a prospective cohort of patients in addition to a retrospective one, both undergoing laparoscopic repair in the primary hernia- and incisional hernia- setting [19]. In this study, closure of the defect did not result in fewer hernia recurrences, but rather increased postoperative complications.

2.2 Relevant surgical anatomy and techniques

In accordance with the pathophysiologically-oriented discussion in the previous section, that fascial approximation should be pursued for in incisional hernia repair. Complex hernias present in that sense unique challenges because they require advanced techniques and elaborate preoperative planning in order to mobilize fasciae in the correct planes and achieve the goal of tension-free midline reconstitution while minimizing morbidity. The idea to mobilize the fascial layers of rectus abdominis sheath, thus gaining increased fascial length to overlap a wide defect gave birth to anterior component separation techniques and to the Rives-Stoppa initially and posterior component separation with transverse abdominis release.

Anterior component separation [20] entails extensive separation of lipocutaneous flap over the rectus abdominis complex with lateral extension past linea semilunaris over the lateral abdominal wall muscles. A longitudinal incision of the external oblique aponeurosis along with some of its muscle fibers is performed 1–2 cm laterally to the linea semilunairis, extending from the coastal margins cranially to the ipsilateral inguinal ligament caudally. A potential plane is thus created between the external oblique muscle and the internal oblique muscle, which enables midline fascial approximation by 5 centimeters (cm) on each side at the level of the epigastrium, 10 cm around the umbilical area and 3 cm suprapubically. Midline tension-reconstitution is reinforced with mesh to achieve a wide overlap over the original hernia defect fascial edges [21]. Major morbidity of the anterior component separation technique [22] arises mainly from the disruption of the periumbilical perforators and the extensive mobilization of lipocutaneous flaps, thus dysruptic normal perfusion of suprafascial tissues and giving rise to hematomas and seromas. In an attempt to avoid creation of large lipocutaneous flaps, a perforator-sparing approach [23, 24] has been described, a tunnel is created longitudinally over the subsequent external oblique aponeurosis fasciotomy, while staying 4 cm laterally to the midline, which is the area corresponding to the vascular distribution of periumbilical perforators. Preservation of blood supply has been repeatedly shown to decrease perioperative complications [25]. Perforator-sparing anterior component separation techniques are increasingly performed using laparo-endoscopic techniques, resulting in decreased perioperative morbidity with equivalent rates of hernia recurrence compared to original component separation techniques [26, 27].

Focusing on the posterior lamella of the rectus sheath gave rise to innovative ideas in complex hernia repair initially with the Rives-Stoppa technique and its subsequent extension, namely the posterior component separation technique with tranverse abdominis release. Rationale for the Rives-Stoppa technique was to create a potential space in the retrorectus plane for mesh placement in a well vascularised position, protected from the underlying viscera, while intrabdominal pressures exert forces that aid in the process of mesh integration into the relevant anatomic planes [28]. An incision is made in the posterior sheath 0.5 cm laterally to the linea alba and the retrorectus plane is developed towards the linea semilunaris, while preserving the inferior epigastric vessels that run over the posterior sheath as well as the insertion of intercostal nerves as they enter into the rectus sheath approximately 1 cm medial to the linea semilunaris. The retrorectus plane is subsequently developed on the contralateral side finishing on the natural lateral extension of the Rives-Stoppa technique, that is the linea semilunaris. Dissection on each side extends until 5–8 cm past the superior and inferior edge of the hernia defect on each side to achieve wide overlap of it. The two respective dissection planes are joined by entering the suprapubic space of Retzius caudally and by releasing the posterior rectus sheath from its insertion in the xiphoid process. With regards to the pelvic dissection, due to the fact that below the arcuate line, the posterior rectus sheath is comprised only of peritoneum and transversalis fascia the dissection plane in essence extends into the preperitoneal space laterally all the way towards the pubic bone, Cooper ligament on each side as well as the medial edge of psoas muscle. The same applies for the subxiphoid dissection, where the original retrorectus plane continues essentially into the preperitoneal plane. With the aforementioned strategy, a new visceral sac is recreated achieving tension free reconstitution of the midline with primary repair and allowing placement of a mesh with wide overlap of the hernia defect. Intrinsic in the nature of Rives-Stoppa repair is the limit set by the linea semilunaris as the far most lateral border of dissection, resulting in maximum coverage of defects up to 10 cm wide [28–30]. Posterior component separation [31] technique aims to overcome the lateral limit of Rives-Stoppa dissection plane, thus enabling repair of hernias with widths greater than 10 cm or hernias in sites other than midline, such as flank hernias, lumbar hernias or complex hernias encompassing more than one areas and/or being huge in size. Advancing in lateral direction from the retrorectus plane past linea semilunaris can be accomplished by either switching towards the preperitoneal plane of dissection or by incising the muscle fibers of the transverse abdominis muscle, popularized as transversus abdominis release (TAR). It is important to notice at this point that transversus abdominis muscle fibers do not contribute to linea semilunaris, but rather reside medial to it and behind the rectus abdominis muscle in the upper 1/3 of the abdominal wall. Entering the TAR dissection plane is initiated approximately 0.5 cm medially to the linea semilunaris, where the muscle fibers are divided, thus opening an avascular plane behind the transverse abdominis muscle, that can be bluntly extended up to the costal margins, diaphragm, retropubic space, inguinal orifices and psoas muscles bilaterally. A new visceral sac is subsequently developed and a synthetic mesh is usually positioned in the sublay position. A key technical point is that the point of initiation of the TAR dissection is just medial to insertion of the neural bundles in the rectus sheath and therefore by traversing "one level' below them as the plane is developed naturally, intercostal nerves are essentially protected, thus preventing denervation and subsequent atrophy of the rectus abdominus muscle complex. Of notice, intercostal nerves course below internal oblique and above transverse abdominis muscles and enter the rectus sheath medially to the linea semilunaris as noted above. As is the cause with Rives-Stoppa repair, retrorectus planes bilaterally are unified. In the subxiphoid area, if needed, the insertion of the posterior sheath into the xiphoid process can be divided, thus exposing the subxiphoid fatty triangle, and in extreme cases or in the case of subxiphoid hernias the dissection can be extended preperitoneally all the way to the tendinous portion of the diaphragm. Due to variable anatomic relation and overlap between the rectus abdominis sheath and transverse abdominis muscle at different anatomic levels [32], it is best to initiate TAR dissection plane above the umbilicus, in order to maintain the development of the correct plane. Of notice, advancing from the retrorectus plane towards division the transversus abdominus muscle fibers, by definition, involves, at an intermediate stage, division of the posterior lamella of the internal oblique, which has been shown to contribute crucially towards the subsequent medial advancement of the rectus myofascial complex [33]. Posterior component separation technique with transversus abdominis release and insertion of wide synthetic mesh in the sublay position has been established as an effective means of treating even wide hernia defects with minimal complications and excellent results in terms of hernia recurrence rates [34]. From the physiological standpoint, posterior component separation with TAR induces rectus abdominis muscle hypertrophy and is, furthermore, associated with hypertrophy of the lateral abdominal wall musculature, thus leading to restoration of function of the abdominal wall, in contrast to bridging the hernia defect with a synthetic mesh, which has no effects on abdominal wall muscles [35]. Posterior component separation has been shown to achieve significant medialization of the anterior and posterior lamella of the rectus sheath, thus enabling primary fascial closure in defects up to 20 cm wide [36].

Comparing anterior and posterior component separation techniques, both yield equivalent and excellent results regarding hernia recurrence, while the latter is associated with fewer wound complications. It is of notice, that both component separation techniques with primary fascial closure and use of mesh have better safety profiles in terms of surgical site occurrences when compared with bridged repair (spanning the hernia defect with a mesh) [37].

2.3 Outcomes

When comparing medial advancement achieved with Rives-Stoppa, anterior component separation and posterior component separation, it is noted that the anterior lamella of the rectus sheath is advanced by 1.2, 2.6 and 1.9 cm on each side for each respective technique, while the posterior lamella advancement reached 2.2,

3.0 and 5.2 cm respectively, favoring on the whole posterior component separation technique with regards to the ability to reconstitute large defects [38]. Both myofascial release techniques yield equivalent results in terms of hernia recurrence rates, while anterior component separation techniques comparatively have more surgical site occurrences with no long term sequelae of those, however [39]. An exhaustive review comparing anterior and posterior component separation is outside the scope of the current chapter, while clear-cut comparisons between posterior component separation with TAR, anterior component separation and/or perforator-sparing anterior component separation are lacking in the existing literature [36]. What is more clear, however, at the current time, is that abdominal wall reconstruction is associated with improvement in physiology and function of truncal muscles, yielding improved quality of life for patients [26, 40, 41]. A combination of anterior and posterior component separation techniques for extreme cases has been reported, although it is a strategy associated with increased morbidity mainly due to respiratory complications and issues of truncal stability due to the associated sacrifice of key core muscle stabilizers [42, 43], and is therefore a strategy that should be viewed with caution. From the anatomic standpoint, anterior component separation causes significant lateral displacement of the external oblique muscle, while transversus abdominis muscle is shifts very little after posterior component separation [44]. Anatomy and physiology of abdominal wall muscles are preserved by the muscles' overlapping function and their ability to undergo compensatory trophism after reconstitution of midline, which results in reloading of the aforementioned muscles due to redistribution of mechanical loads. Anterior component separation creates, therefore, an autologous flap that moves across the abdomen to cover a hernia defect on the contralateral side. Different to that, is the presumed mechanism of action of posterior component separation. TAR essentially unloads tensions off neo-midline creation by means of disruption of a continuous hoop tension system spanning over the entire thoracoabdominal fascia. It is exactly this differential mechanism of action of the two myofascial release techniques, as well as the preservation of overlap of abdominal wall muscles that allows for rationalization and careful presurgical planning with potential combination of the two operative strategies [44].

2.4 Preoperative planning - Abdominal wall prehabilitation

Careful preoperative planning is required for successful treatment of complex hernias. Complex hernias can be large in size and a large proportion of abdominal viscera can be contained in the hernia sac relative to the viscera remained in the native abdominal cavity, thus predicting traumatic reduction of hernia contents and increased postoperative complications such as abdominal compartment syndrome [45]. This disease entity is often termed "loss of domain hernia", although established diagnostic criteria are currently lacking [46]. What appears to closely describe loss of domain hernias, is the ratio of hernia sac volume/total abdominal contents, or the ratio of hernia sac volume/native abdominal cavity volume [47, 48]. Using these defect quantification strategies, preoperative use of cross-sectional imaging usually with computed tomography (CT) can be employed to study relevant anatomy in complex hernias and predict the need for utilization of advanced myofascial release techniques [49]. Advanced imaging interpretation algorithms aiding in detailed complex hernia characterization and preoperative planning [50] can be employed, thus underlying the need for standardized terminology in complex hernias and multidisciplinary planning and treatment [51].

A new strategy for abdominal wall prehabilitation is use of botulinum toxin in the preoperative setting to achieve chemical paralysis of lateral abdominal wall musculature, often termed as "chemical component separation" [52]. Botulinum toxin can be injected in a standardized manner at points of insertion of lateral abdominal wall muscles into the rectus sheath, thus causing an elongation of the aforementioned muscles [53] which not only unloads tension off the future reconstituted midline at the early postoperative period. Relieving tension off the future neo-midline postoperatively by negating lateral abdominal muscle pulling forces, essentially, allows for wound healing and remodeling for a predicted time frame (corresponding to the duration of action of botulinum toxin), which is in line with the principles of successful abdominal wall reconstruction. Chemical component separation has been consistently shown to augment gain of length of medialisation of the lateral myofascial complexes, thus enabling primary fascial approximation even for large hernia defects, especially when combined with the aforementioned myofascial release techniques [54, 55]. Additionally, a hernia defect initially presumed to require complex repair techniques for achievement of primary fascial closure, may after chemical components separation be downgraded to a more simple repair [56]. Progressive preoperative pneumoperitoneum to augment hernia sac volume and native abdominal cavity volume can be added to chemical component separation, thus further enhancing the ability to tackle complex hernias [57]. Of notice, chemical component separation, which induces temporary paralysis of abdominal wall muscles only, can have a differential effect on hernia sac versus the native abdominal cavity, thus creating a selective effect of progressive preoperative pneumoperitoneum on abdominal wall prehabilitation, essentially, canceling its otherwise non-selective nature of action on both the hernia sac volume and native abdominal cavity volume, which theoretically leaves the aforementioned ratio of them unaltered [58].

3. Conclusions

Complex hernias comprise a disease entity, which requires a firm grasp of the related anatomy and pathophysiology before embarking on reconstitutional surgery. The goal of surgery should be reconstruction of anatomy to achieve reconstruction of function of the abdominal wall, translating into better outcomes for patients both in terms of quality of life as well as immediate postoperative complications and hernia recurrence rates. We have tried to create a unifying pathophysiologically- oriented approach to this complex problem and we have purposefully attempted to position new techniques, such as preoperative planning, chemical component separation with or without preoperative progressive pneumoperitoneum, into this frame. In order not to deviate from this strategy, we have not discussed topics such as component separation in the setting of contaminated fields or in the setting of open abdomen, both being a dynamic field of application of these strategies.

Complex hernias should be planned and dealt with in multidisciplinary and individualized fashion. Further studies with more strict diagnostic and patient selection criteria shall, in our opinion, be of great clinical benefit, along with generation of good quality data comparing the different reconstruction techniques. Standardization of procedures and creation of robust therapeutic algorithms for an ever-changing landscape of clinical problems, shall both aid in spreading knowledge of advanced abdominal wall reconstruction techniques among the surgical community.

Acknowledgements

None to be declared by the authors.

Conflict of interest statement

The authors report no conflict of interest.

Author details

Fotios Seretis[1], Paraskevi Dedopoulou[2], Nikiforos Rodis[2], Konstantina Soukouli[2], Nikolaos Bogiatzopoulos[2], Charalampos Seretis[2*] and Georgios Zacharis[2]

1 Department of General Surgery, "Konstantopoulio" General Hospital, Athens, Greece

2 Department of General Surgery, "Agios Andreas" General Hospital of Patras, Greece

*Address all correspondence to: babismed@gmail.com

References

[1] Muysoms FE, Miserez M, Berrevoet F, et al. Classification of primary and incisional abdominal wall hernias. Hernia. 2009;**13**(4):407-414. DOI: 10.1007/s10029-009-0518-x

[2] Slater NJ, Montgomery A, Berrevoet F, et al. Criteria for definition of a complex abdominal wall hernia. Hernia. 2014;**18**(1):7-17. DOI: 10.1007/s10029-013-1168-6

[3] Rangwani SM, Kraft CT, Schneeberger SJ, Khansa I, Janis JE. Strategies for mesh fixation in Abdominal Wall reconstruction: Concepts and techniques. Plastic and Reconstructive Surgery. 2021;**147**(2):484-491. DOI: 10.1097/PRS.0000000000007584

[4] Reilly MJ, Larsen NK, Agrawal S, Thankam FG, Agrawal DK, Fitzgibbons RJ. Selected conditions associated with an increased incidence of incisional hernia: A review of molecular biology. American Journal of Surgery. 2021;**221**(5):942-949. DOI: 10.1016/j.amjsurg.2020.09.004

[5] Xing L, Culbertson EJ, Wen Y, Franz MG. Early laparotomy wound failure as the mechanism for incisional hernia formation. The Journal of Surgical Research. 2013;**182**(1):e35-e42. DOI: 10.1016/j.jss.2012.09.009

[6] Schmidt C, Pommerenke H, Dürr F, Nebe B, Rychly J. Mechanical stressing of integrin receptors induces enhanced tyrosine phosphorylation of cytoskeletally anchored proteins. The Journal of Biological Chemistry. 1998;**273**(9):5081-5085. DOI: 10.1074/jbc.273.9.5081

[7] Benjamin M, Hillen B. Mechanical influences on cells, tissues and organs - 'Mechanical Morphogenesis'. European Journal of Morphology. 2003;**41**(1):3-7. DOI: 10.1076/ejom.41.1.3.28102

[8] DuBay DA, Wang X, Adamson B, Kuzon WM Jr, Dennis RG, Franz MG. Progressive fascial wound failure impairs subsequent abdominal wall repairs: A new animal model of incisional hernia formation. Surgery. 2005;**137**(4):463-471. DOI: 10.1016/j.surg.2004.12.016

[9] Mudge M, Hughes LE. Incisional hernia: A 10 year prospective study of incidence and attitudes. The British Journal of Surgery. 1985;**72**(1):70-71. DOI: 10.1002/bjs.1800720127

[10] Burger JW, Lange JF, Halm JA, Kleinrensink GJ, Jeekel H. Incisional hernia: Early complication of abdominal surgery. World Journal of Surgery. 2005;**29**(12):1608-1613. DOI: 10.1007/s00268-005-7929-3

[11] DuBay DA, Choi W, Urbanchek MG, et al. Incisional herniation induces decreased abdominal wall compliance via oblique muscle atrophy and fibrosis. Annals of Surgery. 2007;**245**(1):140-146. DOI: 10.1097/01.sla.0000251267.11012.85

[12] Jensen KK, Arnesen RB, Christensen JK, Bisgaard T, Jørgensen LN. Large incisional hernias increase in size [published correction appears in J Surg Res. 2022 Jan;269:142-143]. The Journal of Surgical Research;**2019**(244):160-165. DOI: 10.1016/j.jss.2019.06.016

[13] Franz MG. The biology of hernia formation. The Surgical Clinics of North America. 2008;**88**(1):1-vii. DOI: 10.1016/j.suc.2007.10.007

[14] Lien SC, Hu Y, Wollstein A, et al. Contraction of abdominal wall

muscles influences size and occurrence of incisional hernia. Surgery. 2015;**158**(1):278-288. DOI: 10.1016/j.surg.2015.01.023

[15] Culbertson EJ, Xing L, Wen Y, Franz MG. Reversibility of abdominal wall atrophy and fibrosis after primary or mesh herniorrhaphy. Annals of Surgery. 2013;**257**(1):142-149. DOI: 10.1097/SLA.0b013e31825ffd02

[16] Jensen KK, Oma E, Kjaer M, Jørgensen LN, Andersen JL. Histology and function of the rectus abdominis muscle in patients with incisional hernia. The Journal of Surgical Research. 2020;**253**:245-251. DOI: 10.1016/j.jss.2020.03.033

[17] Burger JW, Luijendijk RW, Hop WC, Halm JA, Verdaasdonk EG, Jeekel J. Long-term follow-up of a randomized controlled trial of suture versus mesh repair of incisional hernia. Annals of Surgery. 2004;**240**(4):578-585. DOI: 10.1097/01.sla.0000141193.08524.e7

[18] Booth JH, Garvey PB, Baumann DP, et al. Primary fascial closure with mesh reinforcement is superior to bridged mesh repair for abdominal wall reconstruction. Journal of the American College of Surgeons. 2013;**217**(6):999-1009. DOI: 10.1016/j.jamcollsurg.2013.08.015

[19] Lambrecht JR, Vaktskjold A, Trondsen E, Øyen OM, Reiertsen O. Laparoscopic ventral hernia repair: Outcomes in primary versus incisional hernias: no effect of defect closure. Hernia. 2015;**19**(3):479-486. DOI: 10.1007/s10029-015-1345-x

[20] Heller L, McNichols CH, Ramirez OM. Component separations. Seminars in Plastic Surgery. 2012;**26**(1):25-28. DOI: 10.1055/s-0032-1302462

[21] Majumder A, Martin-Del-Campo LA, Miller HJ, Podolsky D, Soltanian H, Novitsky YW. Evaluation of anterior versus posterior component separation for hernia repair in a cadaveric model. Surgical Endoscopy. 2020;**34**(6):2682-2689. DOI: 10.1007/s00464-019-07046-9

[22] de Vries Reilingh TS, van Goor H, Rosman C, et al. "components separation technique" for the repair of large abdominal wall hernias. Journal of the American College of Surgeons. 2003;**196**(1):32-37. DOI: 10.1016/s1072-7515(02)01478-3

[23] Elhage SA, Marturano MN, Prasad T, et al. Impact of perforator sparing on anterior component separation outcomes in open abdominal wall reconstruction. Surgical Endoscopy. 2021;**35**(8):4624-4631. DOI: 10.1007/s00464-020-07888-8

[24] Daes J, Morrell D, Pauli EM. Changes in the lateral abdominal wall following endoscopic subcutaneous anterior component separation. Hernia. 2021;**25**(1):85-90. DOI: 10.1007/s10029-020-02303-6

[25] Saulis AS, Dumanian GA. Periumbilical rectus abdominis perforator preservation significantly reduces superficial wound complications in "separation of parts" hernia repairs. Plastic and Reconstructive Surgery. 2002 Jun;**109**(7):2275-2280 discussion 2281-2

[26] Philipp M, Leuchter M, Klar E. Quality of life after complex Abdominal Wall reconstruction. Visceral Medicine. 2020;**36**(4):326-332. DOI: 10.1159/000505247

[27] Harth KC, Rosen MJ. Endoscopic versus open component separation in complex abdominal wall reconstruction. American Journal of Surgery. 2010;**199**(3):342-346 discussion 346-7

[28] Tastaldi L, Alkhatib H. Incisional hernia repair: Open Retromuscular approaches. The Surgical Clinics of North America. 2018;**98**(3):511-535. DOI: 10.1016/j.suc.2018.02.006

[29] McLanahan D, King LT, Weems C, et al. Retrorectus prosthetic mesh repair of midline abdominal hernia. American Journal of Surgery. 1997;**173**(5):445-449

[30] Ferranti F, Triveri P, Mancini P, et al. The treatment of large midline incisional hersnias using a retromuscular prosthetic mesh (Stoppa-rives technique). Chirurgia Italiana. 2003;**55**(1):129-136

[31] Pauli EM, Rosen MJ. Open ventral hernia repair with component separation. The Surgical Clinics of North America. 2013;**93**(5):1111-1133. DOI: 10.1016/j.suc.2013.06.010

[32] Punekar IRA, Khouri JS, Catanzaro M, Shaikh AL, Langstein HN. Redefining the rectus sheath: Implications for Abdominal Wall repair. Plastic and Reconstructive Surgery. 2018;**141**(2):473-479. DOI: 10.1097/PRS.0000000000004043

[33] Moores N, Conway H, Donato D, Gociman B, Pannucci CJ, Agarwal J. Is release of the posterior lamella enough? A cadaveric exploration of posterior component separation techniques. American Journal of Surgery. 2019;**218**(3):533-536. DOI: 10.1016/j.amjsurg.2018.12.011

[34] Novitsky YW, Fayezizadeh M, Majumder A, Neupane R, Elliott HL, Orenstein SB. Outcomes of posterior component separation with transversus abdominis muscle release and synthetic mesh sublay reinforcement. Annals of Surgery. 2016;**264**(2):226-232. DOI: 10.1097/SLA.0000000000001673

[35] De Silva GS, Krpata DM, Hicks CW, et al. Comparative radiographic analysis of changes in the abdominal wall musculature morphology after open posterior component separation or bridging laparoscopic ventral hernia repair. Journal of the American College of Surgeons. 2014;**218**(3):353-357. DOI: 10.1016/j.jamcollsurg.2013.11.014

[36] Kumar S, Edmunds RW, Dowdy C, Chang YW, King R, Roth JS. Anterior versus posterior component separation: Which is better? Plastic and Reconstructive Surgery. 2018;**142**(3 Suppl):47S-53S. DOI: 10.1097/PRS.0000000000004852

[37] Holihan JL, Askenasy EP, Greenberg JA, et al. Component separation vs. bridged repair for large ventral hernias: A multi-institutional risk-adjusted comparison, systematic review, and meta-analysis. Surgical Infections (Larchmt). 2016;**17**(1):17-26. DOI: 10.1089/sur.2015.124

[38] Sneiders D, Yurtkap Y, Kroese LF, et al. Anatomical study comparing medialization after rives-Stoppa, anterior component separation, and posterior component separation. Surgery. 2019;**165**(5):996-1002. DOI: 10.1016/j.surg.2018.11.013

[39] Bilezikian JA, Tenzel PL, Faulkner JD, Bilezikian MJ, Powers WF, Hope WW. Comparing the outcomes of external oblique and transversus abdominus release using the AHSQC database. Hernia. 2021;**25**(2):365-373. DOI: 10.1007/s10029-020-02310-7

[40] Jensen KK, Munim K, Kjaer M, Jorgensen LN. Abdominal Wall reconstruction for incisional hernia optimizes truncal function and quality of life: A prospective controlled study. Annals of Surgery. 2017;**265**(6):1235-1240. DOI: 10.1097/SLA.0000000000001827. PMID: 27280505

[41] Criss CN, Petro CC, Krpata DM, et al. Functional abdominal wall reconstruction improves core physiology and quality-of-life. Surgery. 2014;**156**(1):176-182. DOI: 10.1016/j.surg.2014.04.010

[42] Zuvela M, Galun D, Bogdanovic A, et al. The combination of the three modifications of the component separation technique in the management of complex subcostal abdominal wall hernia. Hernia. 2022;**26**(5):1369-1379. DOI: 10.1007/s10029-022-02622-w

[43] Lopez-Monclus J, Muñoz-Rodríguez J, San Miguel C, et al. Combining anterior and posterior component separation for extreme cases of abdominal wall reconstruction [published correction appears in hernia. 2021;25(1):251]. Hernia. 2020;**24**(2):369-379. DOI: 10.1007/s10029-020-02152-3

[44] Daes J, Winder JS, Pauli EM. Concomitant anterior and posterior component separations: Absolutely contraindicated? Surgical Innovation. 2020;**27**(4):328-332. DOI: 10.1177/1553350620914195

[45] Parker SG, Halligan S, Liang MK, et al. Definitions for loss of domain: An international Delphi consensus of expert surgeons. World Journal of Surgery. 2020;**44**(4):1070-1078. DOI: 10.1007/s00268-019-05317-z

[46] Parker SG, Halligan S, Blackburn S, et al. What exactly is meant by "loss of domain" for ventral hernia? Systematic review of definitions. World Journal of Surgery. 2019;**43**(2):396-404. DOI: 10.1007/s00268-018-4783-7

[47] Tanaka EY, Yoo JH, Rodrigues AJ Jr, Utiyama EM, Birolini D, Rasslan S. A computerized tomography scan method for calculating the hernia sac and abdominal cavity volume in complex large incisional hernia with loss of domain. Hernia. 2010;**14**(1):63-69. DOI: 10.1007/s10029-009-0560-8

[48] Sabbagh C, Dumont F, Robert B, Badaoui R, Verhaeghe P, Regimbeau JM. Peritoneal volume is predictive of tension-free fascia closure of large incisional hernias with loss of domain: A prospective study. Hernia. 2011;**15**(5):559-565

[49] Blair LJ, Ross SW, Huntington CR, et al. Computed tomographic measurements predict component separation in ventral hernia repair. The Journal of Surgical Research. 2015;**199**(2):420-427. DOI: 10.1016/j.jss.2015.06.033

[50] Elhage SA, Deerenberg EB, Ayuso SA, et al. Development and validation of image-based deep learning models to predict surgical complexity and complications in Abdominal Wall reconstruction. JAMA Surgery. 2021;**156**(10):933-940. DOI: 10.1001/jamasurg.2021.3012

[51] Grove TN, Kontovounisios C, Montgomery A, et al. Perioperative optimization in complex abdominal wall hernias: Delphi consensus statement. BJS Open. 2021;**5**(5):zrab082. DOI: 10.1093/bjsopen/zrab082

[52] Motz BM, Schlosser KA, Heniford BT. Chemical components separation: Concepts, evidence, and outcomes. Plastic and Reconstructive Surgery. 2018;**142**(3 Suppl.):58S-63S. DOI: 10.1097/PRS.0000000000004856

[53] Farooque F, Jacombs AS, Roussos E, et al. Preoperative abdominal muscle elongation with botulinum toxin a for complex incisional ventral hernia repair. ANZ Journal of Surgery. 2016;**86**(1-2):79-83. DOI: 10.1111/ans.13258

[54] Deerenberg EB, Elhage SA, Shao JM, et al. The effects of preoperative botulinum toxin a injection on Abdominal Wall reconstruction. The Journal of Surgical Research. 2021;**260**:251-258. DOI: 10.1016/j.jss.2020.10.028

[55] Timmer AS, Claessen JJM, Atema JJ, Rutten MVH, Hompes R, Boermeester MA. A systematic review and meta-analysis of technical aspects and clinical outcomes of botulinum toxin prior to abdominal wall reconstruction. Hernia. 2021;**25**(6):1413-1425. DOI: 10.1007/s10029-021-02499-1

[56] Bueno-Lledó J, Martinez-Hoed J, Torregrosa-Gallud A, Menéndez-Jiménez M, Pous-Serrano S. Botulinum toxin to avoid component separation in midline large hernias. Surgery. 2020;**168**(3):543-549. DOI: 10.1016/j.surg.2020.04.050

[57] Tashkandi A, Bueno-Lledó J, Durtette-Guzylack J, et al. Adjunct botox to preoperative progressive pneumoperitoneum for incisional hernia with loss of domain: no additional effect but may improve outcomes. Hernia. 2021;**25**(6):1507-1517. DOI: 10.1007/s10029-021-02387-8

[58] Seretis F, Chrysikos D, Samolis A, Troupis T. Botulinum toxin in the surgical treatment of complex abdominal hernias: A surgical anatomy approach, current evidence and outcomes. In Vivo. 2021;**35**(4):1913-1920. DOI: 10.21873/invivo.12457

Chapter 3

Clinical Features, Diagnosis, Prevention, and Management of Incisional Hernias

Suat Benek, İlhan Bali, Seyfi Emir and Selim Sözen

Abstract

The incidence of incisional hernia after intra-abdominal surgery is approximately 10–15%. Midline incisions are riskier than other incisions. Smoking, surgical site infections, conditions that impair wound healing, and incorrect surgical technique are among the risk factors, especially obesity. It typically presents as swelling on or near the incision. Computed tomography or ultrasonography can be performed for incisional hernias that cannot be detected by physical examination. Preoperative CT scan is important for the surgical strategy, especially for ventral hernias larger than 10 cm and with loss of space. The surgical strategy may vary depending on the size of the hernia. Tension-free repair is accepted as the standard approach by many authors, and suture repair alone is rarely used. The technique of separating into anterior or posterior components can be used in hernias larger than 10 cm with loss of space. Reconstruction using prosthesis material placed preperitoneally (underlay or sublay) is the most commonly used method today.

Keywords: incisional hernia, rives–Stoppa repair, classification, laparoscopic repair, component seperation technique

1. Introduction

An incisional hernia is defined as a swelling or abdominal wall cavity in the postoperative incision area that can be detected by physical examination or radiological imaging [1]. Incisional hernia occurs in approximately 10 to 15 percent of patients with a previous abdominal incision [2]. It may develop after midline, mc burney, paramedian, or other abdominal incisions [3, 4]. Its incidence varies according to the incision that has been made. In general, the risk of hernia formation in midline incisions is higher than the other incision types [5–7]. In addition, the risk of incisional hernia formation is higher in upper abdominal incisions compared to lower abdominal incisions [8–11]. Both patient-related and technical factors play a role in the development of incisional hernias.

1.1 Patient related factors

Age, obesity, smoking, connective tissue diseases, use of immunosuppressive drugs, malnutrition, diabetes, vascular, and other comorbid diseases are factors that increase the risk of having an incisional hernia. Numerous studies have shown that obesity, in particular, increases the risk of having an incisional hernia, and the rate of postoperative complications and recurrence [12–18].

1.2 Technical factors

Wound infection, excessive wound tension, and not following the abdominal closure principles predispose to the formation of incisional hernia [19]. The incidence of incisional hernia increases in open bariatric surgery and interventions for repairing abdominal aortic aneurysm.

Abdominal closure should be done effectively, neither tension nor ischemia. In order to achieve this, it is necessary to comply with the appropriate suture material and stitch size. The suture should be the smallest, it can be to be strong enough to hold the wound intact [20]. Suture diameter and its type (monofilament, multifilament, or synthetic) is an effective factor on the amount of foreign matter and bacterial accumulation in the wound. It has been proved that nonabsorbable sutures reduce the risk of wound separation and developing a hernia compared to absorbable sutures. Synthetic nonabsorbable monofilament sutures (polypropylene, etc.) are more resistant to infections than multifilament sutures and natural fibers. Therefore, suture composition and structure affect the rate of bacterial absorption and proliferation [20]. Some studies have reported that sutures coated with antimicrobial compounds can reduce surgical site infection rates [21–29]. However, in other studies, whether the suture was covered or uncoated with antimicrobial compounds did not differ in terms of surgical site infection [25].

The method of closing the abdominal wall is another factor that affects developing an incisional hernia. While stratified closure is defined as the closure of individual components of the abdominal wall (peritoneum, muscular and aponeurotic structures, subcutaneous adipose tissue), mass closure is the closure of other abdominal wall layers as a single structure excluding the skin [30–32]. Studies have shown that mass closure is associated with a lower incidence of developing an incisional hernia [28, 29, 33]. Other than this, it has been shown that intermittent and uninterrupted closures have different effects on the tension of the wound and perfusion of the tissue. The amount of the suture used depends on the size of each suture (depends on the distance from fascial edge) and gap between sutures. For continuous closure, the total length of the suture should be about four times the incision length [31, 32]. In a randomized study, hernia recurrence was shown to be decreased if the ratio of 1/4 was adhered to [34]. The suture should be placed approximately about 1 cm from the edge of the fascia. The 2015 guidelines of the European Hernia Society recommend reducing the suture width from 10 mm to about 5 to 8 mm [31–36]. In a randomized study, it was shown that longer suture width increases the risk of developing both incisional hernia and surgical site infection [32]. Studies have shown that the most appropriate method for abdominal wall closure is continuous mass closure using slowly absorbable sutures with a 4:1 ratio of suture length to wound length [37–39].

2. Classification

Incisional hernias can be classified as anatomically and clinically.

Anatomical classification is made according to the location of the hernia on the abdominal wall. The European Hernia Society (EHS) divides the abdomen into medial and lateral zones for incisional hernias. The medial zone includes the region between the lateral edges of the rectus muscle. This region is divided into five subregions as subxiphoid, epigastric, umbilical, infraumbilical, and suprapubic. The lateral region is divided into four subregions as costal, lateral, iliac, and lumbar regions (**Figure 1**).

According to size, incisional hernias are classified into three categories: <1 cm, 1 to 10 cm, and > 10 cm [40]. Hernias larger than 10 cm in width are defined as complex or giant ventral hernias. These require additional preparation [41].

Clinical classification – Depending on the clinical picture, incisional hernias can be asymptomatic, reductible, incarcerated, or strangulated.

An incarcerated hernia is a hernia that its contents cannot be reduced to the abdomen due to a narrow opening in the abdominal wall facial defect or adhesions between the contents and the hernia sac [42]. An incarcerated hernia containing an intestinal loop can cause intestinal obstruction [43]. In a population study of more than 23,000 patients followed without surgery, a cumulative rate of incarceration of incisional hernias was reported 1.24% in 1 year and 2.59% in 5 years [44].

Diagnosis – In most patients without obesity, incisional hernia can be diagnosed by physical examination. It is usually recognized by palpation of a bulge on or around the abdominal incision.

Diagnostic evaluation – About the patients we cannot rely on our physical examination, we need a computed tomography (CT) scan or ultrasound of the abdomen and/or pelvis to confirm the presence of the hernia and to identify the contents of the hernia sac. Contrast is not usually required for a CT scan. Ultrasound is less sensitive than CT.

CT imaging – Preoperative CT imaging is recommended for complex ventral hernias with large size and significant loss of space. Repair of such hernias usually requires advanced abdominal wall reconstructive techniques such as disassembly. The volume of the hernial sac and abdominopelvic cavity can be estimated on a CT scan by multiplying the length, width, and depth of each cavity by a factor to estimate the ellipsoid volume [41].

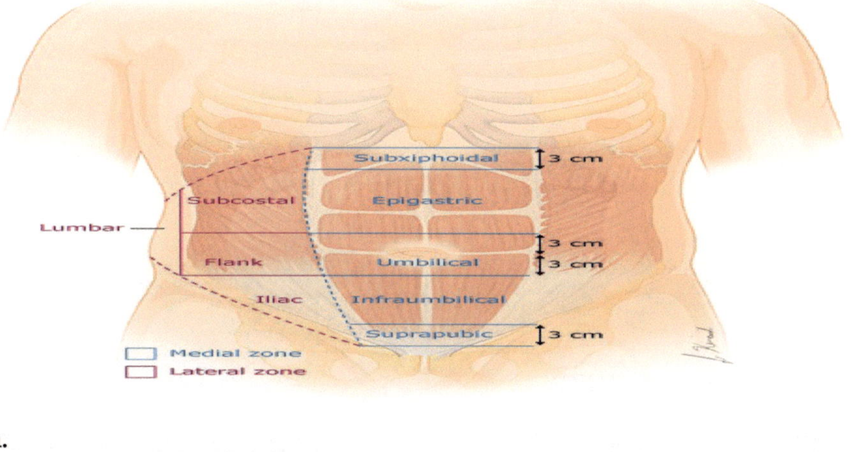

Figure 1.
The European hernia society (EHS) classification for incisional abdominal wall hernias divides the abdomen into a medial zone and a lateral zone. The medial zone, defined as medial to the lateral margin of the rectus sheath, is subdivided into five subzones (subxiphoid, epigastric, umbilical, infraumbilical, and suprapubic). The lateral zone is subdivided into four subzones (subcostal, flank, iliac, and lumbar).

The degree of domain loss has been calculated differently by various authors. When the ratio of hernia sac volume to residual abdominopelvic cavity volume is calculated and if it is 25% and above, preoperative abdominal expansion is required [45]. When the ratio of the hernia sac volume to the entire peritoneal volume is calculated and if it is higher than 20%, it predicts how hard the closure will be [46]. Hernia reduction may lead to serious complications such as persistent hypertension in the abdominopelvic cavity, abdominal compartment syndrome due to visceral edema and postoperative fluid resuscitation.

3. Management

3.1 Acute incarcerated or strangulated hernias

Acute incarcerated or strangulated incisional hernias require immediate surgical repair (**Figure 2**). The aim of emergency surgery is to resolve the acute problem (intestinal necrosis or obstruction) and to perform a safe and durable repair. The optimal technique of hernia repair depends on the patient's anatomy, stability, comorbidities, and the degree of operative site contamination. Once the source of the contamination is controlled, surgical repair of the hernia can be done only with suture repair, mesh repair, or incremental repair (placement of absorbable mesh and leaving the hernia to be repaired electively). There is no consensus because the clinical situation is heterogeneous [47].

The best practice for a ventral hernia in a contaminated area is safe and, whenever possible, suture-only or incremental repair. Hernia repair with synthetic mesh

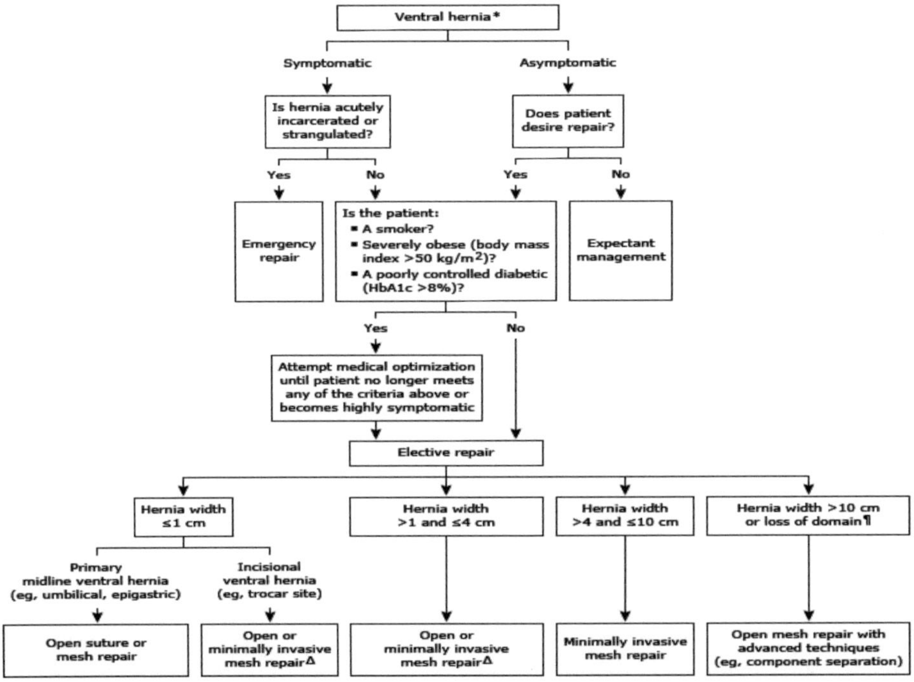

Figure 2.
Management of ventral hernias.

has been proved to be safe and effective in the hands of powerful surgeons in these complex cases [48]. The role of biological and biosynthetic networks has not yet been defined.

Asymptomatic incisional hernias – Patients with asymptomatic or minimally symptomatic ventral hernias can be followed nonoperatively if they are hesitate to have a surgery [49, 50]. However, these patients should be informed that the lifetime risk of acute presentation can be high and for most patients, nonsurgical follow will fail after the first 2 years [49, 51, 52].

Symptomatic incisional hernias – Surgical repair is recommended for patients with symptomatic ventral hernias. However, in patients with comorbidities such as smoking, diabetes, obesity, and obstructive pulmonary diseases, surgery can be temporarily delayed. Such restrictions are relative contraindications and can be relieved by preoperative optimization [53].

3.2 Surgical treatment of incisional hernias

Incisional ventral hernia < 1 cm – Usually occurs at laparoscopic trocar sites. Mesh repair is recommended for all ventral incisional hernias, including those less than 1 cm. Repairing such hernias with stitches will likely result with a recurrent hernia.

Ventral hernias from 1 to 10 cm – The most common incisional hernias in daily practice fall into this category. Mesh reinforcement is required for these hernias. The surgical approach and mesh selection depend on the clinical situation and the surgeon's preference. Open or minimally invasive mesh repair can be performed for incisional hernias which are 1 to 4 cms. While open repair is preferred in frail patients, minimally invasive repair is preferred in patients who are at risk of developing obesity or other wound infections. Minimally invasive mesh repair is performed for ventral hernias which are 4 to 10 cm [54].

Large (>10 cm in width) or complex hernias – Large or complex incisional hernias are difficult to repair [55]. These hernias can be repaired using minimally invasive underlay, open inlay, or component separation techniques.

Underlay meshes are used on standard laparoscopic repairs. Although it has advantages such as less pain, healing fast, and having lower infection rate, swelling continues at the defect site when intra-abdominal pressure increases. Repair of large defects with mesh has been shown not to reduce abdominal and back pain and respiratory problems when compared to component separation, which restores the dynamic muscle component to the abdominal wall.

In patients with large incisional hernias and patients with space gap, we recommend using advanced techniques such as component separation to achieve primary fascial closure prior to mesh augmentation, rather than using inlay mesh to bridge a facial defect.

The decomposition, pioneered by Ramirez [56], is used to repair the large and complex midline abdominal wall defects and has the advantage of restoring abdominal wall function. Component separation involves dividing the anterior or posterior rectus sheaths and/or portions of the lateral oblique muscle to allow the rectus abdominis muscle to advance by about 10 cm from each side to allow a fascial closure under physiological tension [56–58].

The decision to separate its components is made based on physical examination and cross-sectional imaging. Depending on the width of the hernia and the surgeon's experience and preference, any dissection technique can be chosen.

Typically, hernias less than 7 cm do not require a component separation (**Figure 3**) and can usually be repaired with an open, laparoscopic, or robotic approach with intraperitoneal mesh, or with an open or robotic approach with retrorectus mesh, as described by Rives and Stoppa. Such hernias can also be repaired using open techniques with onlay mesh [58].

Hernias that are 7 to 10 cm typically do not require a component separation for the midline facial approach and can be repaired laparoscopically with a large piece of intraperitoneal mesh or with an open retromuscular approach. If necessary, an open or robotic TAR can be added to ensure closure of the posterior rectus sheath. A ratio of rectus width to hernia width > 2 reliably predicts that the fascia can be closed with a Rives–Stoppa repair alone, with no further myofascial loosening in nearly 90% of cases [59].

Hernias larger than 10 cm might require separation of the anterior or posterior component for both the rectus approach (midline closure) and posterior facial

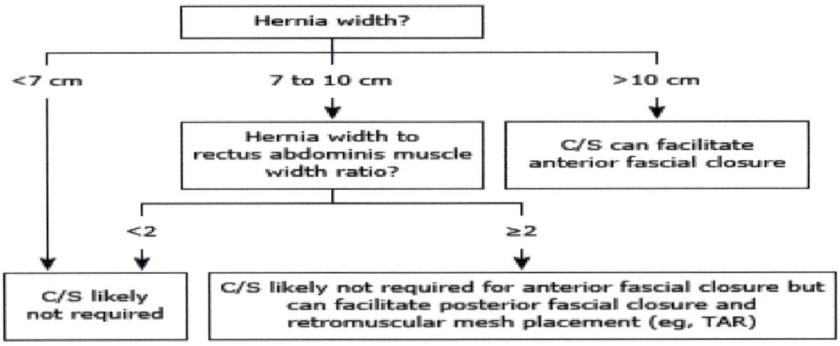

Figure 3.
Determining the need for component separation in ventral hernia repair.

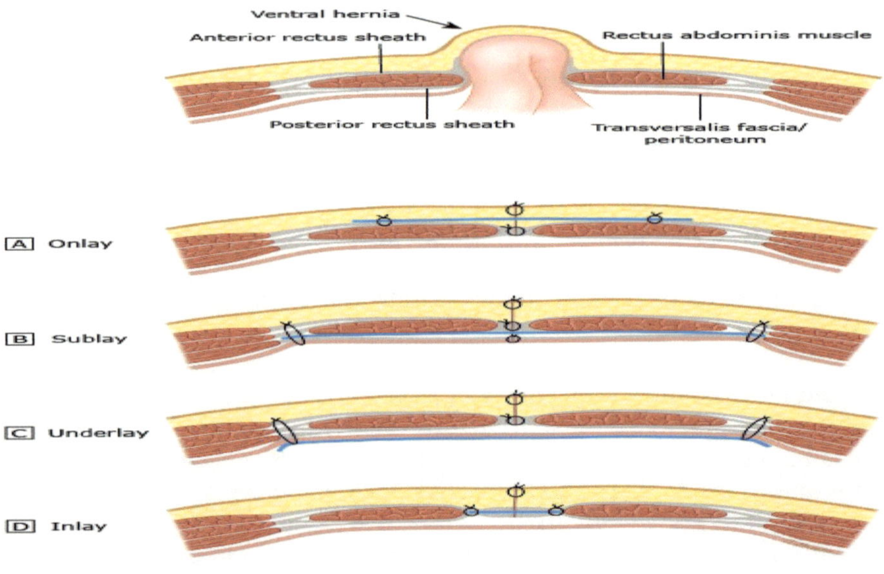

Figure 4.
Mesh locations: (A) onlay, (B) sublay, (C) underlay, and (D) inlay. The blue line depicts mesh location.

approach, depending on the compliance of the abdominal wall. This can be accomplished with open anterior component separation or open or robotic TAR.

Location of the mesh – Mesh can be placed over the fascia (onlay), between the rectus muscles and the peritoneum/posterior rectus sheath (sublay), under the peritoneum (underlay or intraperitonealonlay), or between the fascial margins (inlay) [60] (**Figure 4**). While onlay and sublay techniques use an open or robotic surgical approach, an underlay technique can be performed open, laparoscopically, or robotically. The mesh bridging inlay technique is used only when the facial defect is too large to be primarily closed with any other technique.

Randomized studies have proved that both recurrence and complication rates were higher with onlay andinlay meshes than with sublay and underlay meshes [61].

Mesh sizes – The mesh used for ventral hernia repair should cover >5 cm from each side for open repair of ventral incisional hernias and > 5 cm for all laparoscopic repairs. For laparoscopic repair, other guidelines suggest that the radius of the mesh should be four times the radius of the fascial defect being addressed [62].

4. Open anterior component separation technique

Posterior rectus sheath is cut 1 to 2 cm from lateral to the medial border of the rectus muscle, starting from the costal margin and continuing below the arcuate line

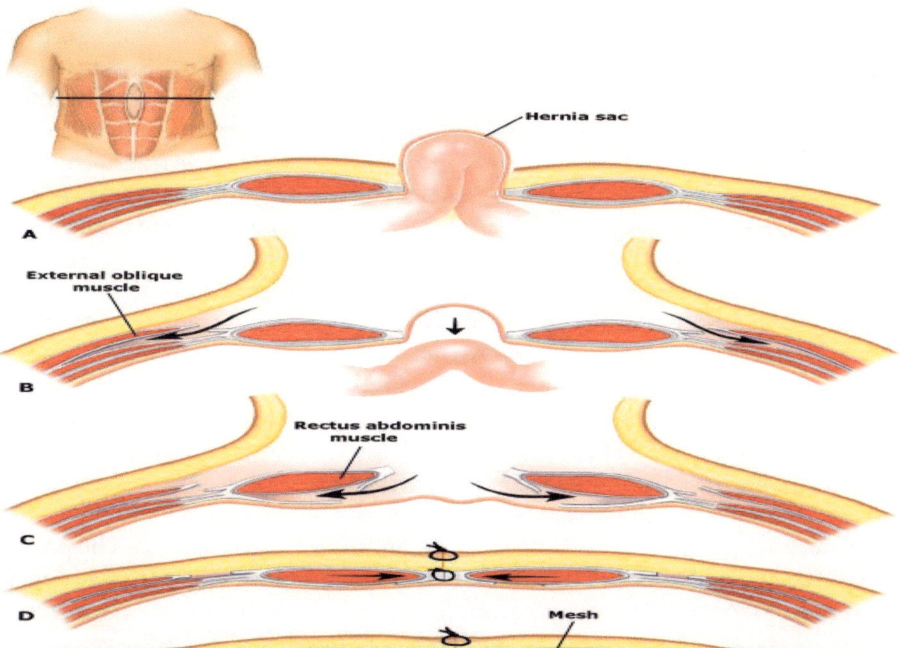

Figure 5.
Component seperation technique: A(Hernia sac), B(external oblig muscles be divided), C(Posterior rectus sheath is cut 1 to 2 cms from lateral to the medial border of the rectus muscle), D(After adequate myofascial relaxation is achieved, the fascia should be closed with a slowly absorbable monofilament suture), E(mesh location).

where the posterior sheath becomes continuous with the peritoneum and transversalis fascia. Next, the external oblig muscles should be divided. It is made through an incision about 1 to 2 cm length from lateral of the linea semilunaris. The external oblig muscle is not always divided in its entire length; instead, the length of the cleavage can be adjusted according to the location of the facial defect in the midline.

Releasing the underlying internal oblig/transversus abdominis muscle apparatus from the divided external oblig muscle reveals an avascular plane. The midline facial approach should be attempted after each myofascial relaxation, not after the division of both the posterior rectus sheaths and the EO muscles. Further myofascial relaxation should be avoided after a tension-free midline approach that has been achieved. After adequate myofascial relaxation is achieved, the fascia should be closed with a slowly absorbable monofilament suture. After a sufficiently large mesh is fixed to the external oblig muscle edge, an absorbent drain is placed on the mesh and the skin is closed (**Figure 5**).

5. Separation technique to open posterior components (rives: stoppa retrorectus dissection and transverse abdominis release (TAR))

The operation begins with a large midline laparotomy that includes the patient's previous scar. During myofascial dissection, intra-abdominal adhesions are completely dissolved and the internal organs are released from the abdominal wall and a wide towel is laid on the intestine. After the towel is placed, the edges of the facial defect are determined and the length/width is measured.

Five Kocher clamps are then placed on the medial edge of a rectus. Using a toothed forceps, the posterior rectus sheath is retracted and cut just beside the rectus margin to expose the underlying muscle hub. The entire medial edge of the posterior rectus sheath should be separated and the medial edge of the rectus muscle should be exposed. The retrorectus area is developed using firm but gentle traction on the anterior and posterior rectus sheaths and cautery to control small epigastric perforators. The lateral extension of this space is marked by large neurovascular bundles and deep lower epigastric vessels, especially in the upper and lower directions of this dissection, before the vessels progress toward the rectus muscle hub. Typically, there is one large medial neurovascular perforator that can be sacrificed in the superior third of the retrorectus space, but the remainder should be preserved if possible. Neurovascular bundles define the lateral extension of the retrorectus space, and their preservation prevents accidental division of the lineasemilunaris, a devastating complication of this technique. At this point, if the posterior rectus sheath is sufficiently medialized to the midline and the contralateral dissection allows isolation of the internal organs, then the Rives–Stoppa dissection alone is sufficient. If the release is not sufficient until this stage, transverse abdominis release is started. The posterior lamella of the internal oblique (IO) and transversus abdominis (TA) muscle departs just from medial to the neurovascular bundles marking the lineasemilunaris. After the transversusabdominis muscle is completely separated from the transversus fascia from cranial to caudal, the posterior rectus sheath is reapproximated and the mesh is placed on it and fixed. After the anterior rectus is approached in the sheath, a drain is placed and the skin is closed (**Figure 6**).

Anterior component separations should not be performed in conjunction with posterior component separation (e.g., TAR) as this might significantly destabilize the abdominal wall and cause permanent disability.

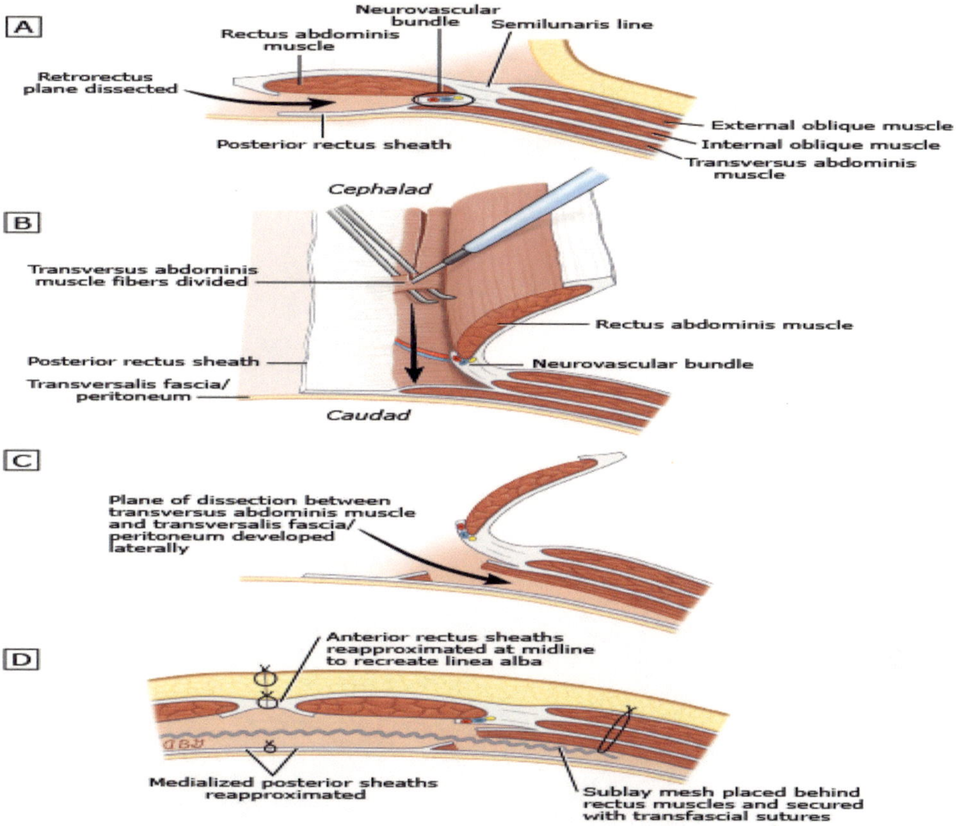

Figure 6.
Transversus abdominis release (TAR): A(Retrorectus plane dissected), B(Transversus Abdominis muscle fibers divided), C(Plane of dissection), D(Sublay mesh placed).

Separation into both anterior and posterior components can also be done laparoscopically or robotically.

6. Presurgery assistants

Preoperative adjuvants (such as botulinum toxin injection or tissue expansion) were used to facilitate fascial and/or abdominal wall closure when the ratio of hernia volume to peritoneal volume was above 20–25%.

Botulinum toxin – Botulinum neurotoxin type A (BoNT-A) can be used preoperatively to relax the lateral abdominal wall muscles [63].

There is no consensus on which patients would benefit from BoNT-A injections prior to ventral hernia repair. However, many authors indicate that preoperative BoNT-A can be used in patients with a hernia volume to peritoneal volume ratio > 20 to 25% [64]. This should be done at least 2 weeks before attempting ventral hernia repair.

Tissue expanders – Tissue expansion is done by placing a silicone balloon under subcutaneous tissue or fascia followed by an injection of saline to inflate the balloon to expand the local tissue in preparation for local reconstruction. It should begin at least 6–12 weeks before hernia repair. Complications such as device infections or flap necrosis may occur in 15% of patients [65, 66].

Author details

Suat Benek[1*], İlhan Bali[1], Seyfi Emir[2] and Selim Sözen[3]

1 Faculty of Medicine, Department of General Surgery, Tekirdağ Namık Kemal University, Tekirdağ, Türkiye

2 Department of General Surgery, Private Reyap Hospital, Tekirdağ, Türkiye

3 Department of General Surgery, Sözen Surgery Clinic, Tekirdağ, Türkiye

*Address all correspondence to: cerrahsbenek@gmail.com

References

[1] Korenkov M, Paul A, Sauerland S, et al. Classification and surgical treatment of incisional hernia. Langenbeck's Archives of Surgery. 2001;**386**:65-73

[2] Nachiappan S, Markar S, Karthikesaligam A, et al. Prophylactic mesh placement in high-risk patients undergoing elective laparotomy: A systematic review. World Journal of Surgery. 2013;**37**:1861-1871

[3] Mudge M, Hughes LE. Incisional hernia: A 10 year prospective study of incidence and attitudes. British Journal of Surgery. 1985;**72**(1):70-71

[4] Kingsnorth A, LeBlanc K. Hernias: Inguinal and incisional. The Lancet. 2003;**362**(9395):1561-1571

[5] Bucknall TE, Cox PJ, Ellis H. Burst abdomen and incisional hernia: A prospective study of 1129 major laparotomy. British Medical Journal (Clinical Research Ed.). 1982;**284**(6320):931-933

[6] SSanders DL, Kingsnorth AN. The modern management of incisional hernias. BMJ. 9 May 2012;**344**:e2843. DOI: 10.1136/bmj.e2843. PMID: 22573647

[7] Bickenbach KA et al. Up and down or side to side? A systematic review and meta-analysis examining the impact of incision on outcomes after abdominal surgery. The American Journal of Surgery. 2013;**206**(3):400-409

[8] Fassiadis N et al. Randomized clinical trial of vertical or transverse laparotomy for abdominal aortic aneurysm repair. Journal of British Surgery. 2005;**92**(10):1208-1211

[9] Inaba T et al. Prospective randomized study of two laparotomy incisions for gastrectomy: Midline incision versus transverse incision. Gastric Cancer. 2004;**7**:167-171

[10] Levrant SG, Bieber E, Barnes R. Risk of anterior abdominal wall adhesions increases with number and type of previous laparotomy. The Journal of the American Association of Gynecologic Laparoscopists. 1994;**1.4**(Part 2):S19-S19

[11] Brown SR, Goodfellow PB. Transverse verses midline incisions for abdominal surgery. Cochrane Database Syst Rev. 19 Oct 2005;**2005**(4):CD005199. DOI: 10.1002/14651858.CD005199.pub2. PMID: 16235395; PMCID: PMC8866010

[12] Itatsu K, Yokoyama Y, Sugawara G, et al. Incidence of and risk factors for incisional hernia after abdominal surgery. The British Journal of Surgery. 2014;**101**:1439

[13] George CD, Ellis H. The results of incisional hernia repair: A twelve year review. Ann R Coll Surg Engl. Jul 1986;**68**(4):185-187. PMID: 3789602; PMCID: PMC2498374

[14] Bosanquet DC, Ansell J, Abdelrahman T, et al. Systematic review and meta-regression of factors affecting midline incisional hernia rates: Analysis of 14,618 patients. PLoS One. 2015;**10**:e0138745

[15] Lau B, Kim H, Haigh PI, Tejirian T. Obesity increases the odds of acquiring and incarcerating noninguinal abdominal wall hernias. The American surgeon. 2012;**78**:1118

[16] Holihan JL, Alawadi Z, Martindale RG, et al. Adverse events after ventral hernia repair: The vicious cycle of complications. Journal of the American College of Surgeons. 2015;**221**:478

[17] Berger RL, Li LT, Hicks SC, et al. Development and validation of a risk-stratification score for surgical site occurrence and surgical site infection after open ventral hernia repair. Journal of the American College of Surgeons. 2013;**217**:974

[18] Liang MK, Goodenough CJ, Martindale RG, et al. External validation of the ventral hernia risk score for prediction of surgical site infections. Surgical Infections. 2015;**16**:36

[19] Seiler CM, Deckert A, Diener MK, et al. Midline versus transverse incision in major abdominal surgery: A randomized, double-blind equivalence trial (POVATI: ISRCTN60734227). Annals of Surgery. 2009;**249**:913

[20] Yaltirik M, Dedeoglu K, Bilgic B, et al. Comparison of four different suture materials in soft tissues of rats. Oral Diseases. 2003;**9**:284

[21] McGeehan D, Hunt D, Chaudhuri A, Rutter P. An experimental study of the relationship between synergistic wound sepsis and suture materials. The British Journal of Surgery. 1980;**67**:636

[22] Alexander JW, Kaplan JZ, Altemeier WA. Role of suture materials in the development of wound infection. Annals of Surgery. 1967;**165**:192

[23] Justinger C, Moussavian MR, Schlueter C, et al. Antibacterial [corrected] coating of abdominal closure sutures and wound infection. Surgery. 2009;**145**:330

[24] Nakamura T, Kashimura N, Noji T, et al. Triclosan-coated sutures reduce the incidence of wound infections and the costs after colorectal surgery: A randomized controlled trial. Surgery. 2013;**153**:576

[25] Diener MK, Knebel P, Kieser M, et al. Effectiveness of triclosan-coated PDS plus versus uncoated PDS II sutures for prevention of surgical site infection after abdominal wall closure: The randomized controlled PROUD trial. Lancet. 2014;**384**:142

[26] Nordkam RA, Bluyssen SJ, van Goor H. Randomized clinical trial comparing blunt tapered and standard needles in closing abdominal fascia. World Journal of Surgery. 2005;**29**:441

[27] Iwase K, Higaki J, Tanaka Y, et al. Running closure of clean and contaminated abdominal wounds using a syntheticfilament absorbable looped suture. Surgery Today. 1999;**29**:874

[28] Rucinski J, Margolis M, Panagopoulos G, Wise L. Closure of the abdominal midline fascia: Meta-analysis delineates the optimal technique. The American Surgeon. 2001;**67**:421

[29] Ceydeli A, Rucinski J, Wise L. Finding the best abdominal closure: An evidence-based review of the literature. Current Surgery. 2005;**62**:220

[30] Gislason H, Grønbech JE, Søreide O. Burst abdomen and incisional hernia after major gastrointestinal operations--comparison of three closure techniques. The European Journal of Surgery= Actachirurgica. 1995;**161**(5):349-354

[31] Muysoms FE, Antoniou SA, Bury K, et al. European hernia society guidelines on the closure of abdominal wall incisions. Hernia. 2015;**19**:1

[32] Millbourn D, Cengiz Y, Israelsson LA. Effect of stitch length on wound complications after closure of midline incisions: A randomized controlled trial. Archives of Surgery. 2009;**144**:1056

[33] van't Riet M, Steyerberg EW, Nellensteyn J, et al. Meta-analysis of techniques for closure of midline abdominal incisions. The British Journal of Surgery. 2002;**89**:1350

[34] Israelsson LA, Jonsson T. Closure of midline laparotomy incisions with polydioxanone and nylon: The importance of suture technique. The British Journal of Surgery. 1994;**81**:1606

[35] Cengiz Y, Gislason H, Svanes K, Israelsson LA. Mass closure technique: An experimental study on separation of wound edge. The European Journal of Surgery. 2001;**167**:60

[36] Deerenberg EB, Harlaar JJ, Steyerberg EW, et al. Small bites versus large bites for closure of abdominal midline incisions (STITCH): A double-blind, multicentre, randomized controlled trial. Lancet. 2015;**386**:1254

[37] Seid MH, McDaniel-Owens LM, Poole GV Jr, Meeks GR. A randomized trial of abdominal incision suture technique and wound strength in rats. Archives of Surgery. 1995;**130**:394

[38] Meeks GR, Nelson KC, Byars RW. Wound strength in abdominal incisions: A comparison of two continuous mass closure techniques in rats. American Journal of Obstetrics and Gynecology. 1995;**173**:1676

[39] Colombo M, Maggioni A, Parma G, et al. A randomized comparison of continuous versus interrupted mass closure of midline incisions in patients with gynecologic cancer. Obstetrics and Gynecology. 1997;**89**:684

[40] Muysoms FE, Miserez M, Berrevoet F, et al. Classification of primary and incisional abdominal wall hernias. Hernia. 2009;**13**:407

[41] Halligan S, Parker SG, Plumb AA, Windsor ACJ. Imaging complex ventral hernias, their surgical repair, and their complications. European Radiology. 2018;**28**:3560

[42] Birendelli A, Sartelli M, Di Saverio S, et al. 2017 update of the WSES guidelines for emergency repair of complicated abdominal wall hernias. World Journal of Emergency Surgery. 2017;**12**:37

[43] Courtney CA, Lee AC, Wilson C, O'Dwyer PJ. Ventral hernia repair: A study of current practice. Hernia. 2003;**7**:44

[44] Dadashzadeh ER, Huckaby LV, Handzel R, et al. The risk of incarceration during nonoperative Management of Incisional Hernias: A population-based analysis of 30,998 patients. Annals of Surgery. 2022;**275**:e488

[45] Tanaka EY, Yoo JH, Rodrigues AJ Jr, et al. A computerized tomography scan method for calculating the hernia sac and abdominal cavity volume in complex large incisional hernia with loss of domain. Hernia. 2010;**14**:63

[46] Sabbagh C, Dumont F, Robert B, et al. Peritoneal volume is predictive of tension-free fascia closure of large incisional hernias with loss of domain: A prospective study. Hernia. 2011;**15**:559

[47] Bondre IL, Holihan JL, Askenasy EP, et al. Suture, synthetic, or biologic in contaminated ventral hernia repair. The Journal of Surgical Research. 2016;**200**:488

[48] Harris HW, Primus F, Young C, et al. Preventing recurrence in clean and contaminated hernias using biologic versus synthetic mesh in ventral hernia repair: The PRICE randomized clinical trial. Annals of Surgery. 2021;**273**:648

[49] Liang MK, Holihan JL, Itani K, Alawadi ZM, Gonzalez JR, Askenasy EP, et al. Ventral Hernia Management: Expert Consensus Guided by Systematic Review. Ann Surg. Jan 2017;**265**(1):80-89. DOI: 10.1097/SLA.0000000000001701. PMID: 28009730

[50] Kokotovic D, Sjølander H, Gögenur I, Helgstrand F. Watchful waiting as a

treatment strategy for patients with a ventral hernia appears to be safe. Hernia. 2016;**20**:281

[51] Holihan JL, Alawadi ZM, Harris JW, et al. Ventral hernia: Patient selection, treatment, and management. Current Problems in Surgery. 2016;**53**:307

[52] Martin AC, Lyons NB, Bernardi K, et al. Expectant Management of Patients with ventral hernias: 3 years of follow-up. World Journal of Surgery. 2020;**44**:2572

[53] Delaney LD, Howard R, Palazzolo K, et al. Outcomes of a Presurgical optimization program for elective hernia repairs among high-risk patients. JAMA Network Open. 2021;**4**:e2130016

[54] Frey S, Jurczak F, Fromont G, et al. Are the relative benefits of open versus laparoscopic intraperitoneal mesh repair of umbilical hernias dependent on the diameter of the defect? Surgery. 2022;**171**:419

[55] Bikhchandani J, Fitzgibbons RJ Jr. Repair of giant ventral hernias. Advances in Surgery. 2013;**47**:1

[56] Ramirez OM, Ruas E, Dellon AL. "Components separation" method for closure of abdominal-wall defects: An anatomical and clinical study. Journal of Plastic, Reconstructive & Aesthetic Surgery. 1990;**86**:519

[57] de VriesReilingh TS, van Goor H, Rosman C, et al. "Components separation technique" for the repair of large abdominal wall hernias. Journal of the American College of Surgeons. 2003;**196**:32

[58] Rosen MJ, Williams C, Jin J, et al. Laparoscopic versus open-component separation: A comparative analysis in a porcine model. American Journal of Surgery. 2007;**194**:385

[59] Love MW, Warren JA, Davis S, et al. Computed tomography imaging in ventral hernia repair: Can we predict the need for myofascial release? Hernia. 2021;**25**:471

[60] Parker SG, Halligan S, Liang MK, et al. International classification of abdominal wall planes (ICAP) to describe mesh insertion for ventral hernia repair. The British Journal of Surgery. 2020;**107**:209

[61] Albino FP, Patel KM, Nahabedian MY, et al. Does mesh location matter in abdominal wall reconstruction? A systematic review of the literature and a summary of recommendations. Plastic and Reconstructive Surgery. 2013;**132**:1295

[62] Bittner R, Bingener-Casey J, Dietz U, et al. Guidelines for laparoscopic treatment of ventral and incisional abdominal wall hernias (International Endohernia Society [IEHS])—Part 2. Surgical Endoscopy. 2014;**28**:353

[63] Ibarra-Hurtado TR, Nuño-Guzmán CM, Echeagaray-Herrera JE, et al. Use of botulinum toxin type a before abdominal wall hernia reconstruction. World Journal of Surgery. 2009;**33**:2553

[64] Afaque MY. Assessing the complexity of ventral hernia by methods of Tanaka, Sabbagh, Carbonell, and Love. Hernia. 2021;**25**:557

[65] Altubaiti G, Butler CE. Abdominal wall and chest wall reconstruction. Plastic and Reconstructive Surgery. 2014;**133**:688e

[66] Paletta CE, Huang DB, Dehghan K, Kelly C. The use of tissue expanders in staged abdominal wall reconstruction. Annals of Plastic Surgery. 1999;**42**:259

Chapter 4

Controversies in Laparoscopic Ventral Hernia Repair

Mohamed Alfatih Hamza, Mekki Hassan and Sean Johnston

Abstract

Ventral hernia is one of the common anterior abdominal wall hernias after groin hernias. These hernias can be classified into primary hernias and secondary (incisional) hernias. Ventral hernia repair is a very common procedure performed in everyday surgical practice. Ventral/Incisional hernias are a frequent long-term complication of abdominal surgery. Roughly half of the incisional hernias develop within the first 2 years after abdominal surgery, and more than 70% manifest within 3 years. The recurrence rate of these hernias after primary suture repair exceeds 50%. However, after the prosthetic materials (meshes) were introduced in the repair procedure, this rate was reduced to 10–20%. The optimal approach with the best short- and long-term outcomes remains controversial. An increasing interest in laparoscopic surgery and its accessibility as well as the availability of innovative techniques have influenced the choice of repair. This chapter provides an overview of ventral hernias, their causes, risk factors, symptomatology, diagnosis, and different approaches to ventral hernia management, focusing mainly on laparoscopic surgery. Additionally, several controversies related to the technique will be discussed, such as mesh fixation, whether the hernia defect should be fixed or not, and mesh overlap. Pre- and post-operative care will also be covered.

Keywords: hernia, ventral, incisional, abdominal wall hernia, laparoscopic techniques, mesh

1. Introduction

Ventral hernias are common conditions encountered by general surgeons, characterized by abdominal contents protruding through a weakness in the anterior abdominal wall. If left untreated, they can lead to discomfort, pain, and life-threatening complications. This chapter provides an overview of ventral hernias, covering their causes, diagnosis, and surgical management, as well as the latest advances in surgical techniques for repairing them.

Ventral hernias can manifest into two main categories: primary hernias, which include epigastric, umbilical, paraumbilical, and Spigelian hernias, and secondary hernias resulting from prior surgical procedures (known as incisional hernias).

The European Registry for abdominal wall hernias (EuraHS) released a classification system in 2012 [1] that categorizes ventral hernias based on their size:

- Small-sized hernia: This category encompasses hernias with a defect size of less than 1 cm.
- Medium-sized hernia: Hernias falling into this group have defects ranging from 1 cm to 4 cm in size.
- Large-sized hernia: This classification pertains to hernias with defects larger than 4 cm in size.

2. Anatomy of the abdominal wall

A good understanding of the abdominal wall's anatomy is crucial for effectively managing hernia repair.

Rectus abdominis muscles form the central core of the abdomen. They are flanked laterally by the Linea semilunaris and separated medially by the Linea alba. These muscles originate from the xyphoid and the costal margin at the upper end, and they connect to the pubic symphysis at the lower end.

The anterior and posterior rectus sheaths are created by the ongoing extension of the external and internal oblique muscles.

There are three abdominal muscles that make up the lateral bulk of the abdominal wall: the transversus abdominis, the internal oblique, and the external oblique.

Upon coming together at the lateral margin of the rectus abdominis muscle, they give rise to the linea semilunaris and rectus sheath.

Transversus abdominis muscle fibers are responsible for forming the posterior rectus sheath in the upper one-third of the abdomen, while in the lower two-thirds, these fibers terminate on the lateral side of the rectus muscle, and the posterior rectus sheath is exclusively constituted by the transversalis fascia (**Figures 1** and **2**).

The fibers of the internal oblique muscle possess an oblique orientation and culminate at the linea semilunaris. Within the upper part of the abdomen, the anterior and posterior rectus sheath is formed by the anterior and posterior layers of the internal oblique muscle, while in the lower third of the abdomen below the arcuate

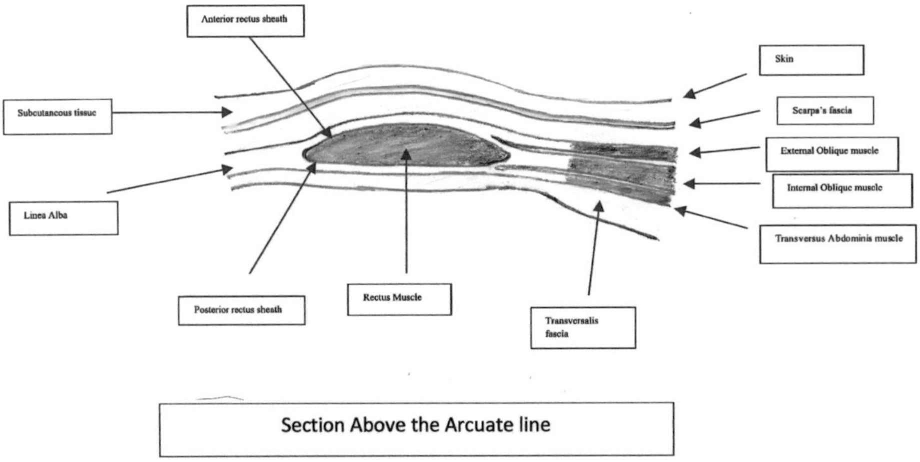

Figure 1.
Anatomy of the anterior Abdominal Wall. Axial view of the Abdominal Wall above the arcuate line.

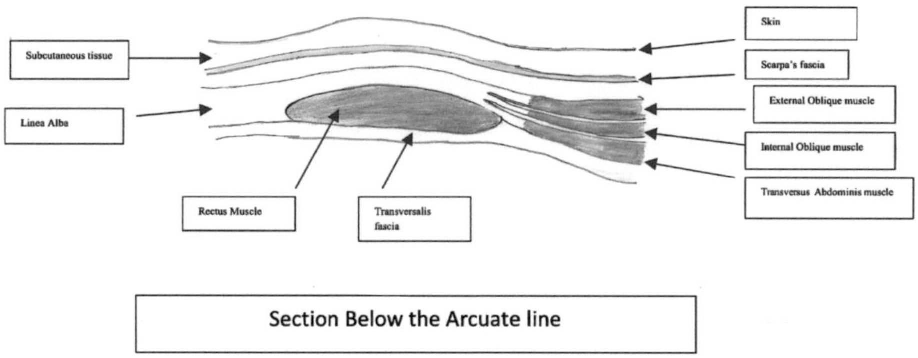

Figure 2.
Anatomy of the anterior Abdominal Wall. Axial view of the Abdominal Wall below the arcuate line.

line, the transversalis fascial layer the exclusive component of the posterior rectus sheath, as the posterior component of the internal oblique shifts anterior to the rectus abdominis muscle.

The external oblique muscle fibers are oriented at a right angle to the internal oblique fibers, and they assume a comparable anatomical arrangement in relation to the rectus sheath.

Based on the blood supply, the abdominal wall is divided into zones as follows.

Zone 1

- Located in the central upper abdomen.
- Blood supply from the descending superior epigastric artery, a derivative of the internal mammary artery in the upper direction, and the ascending inferior epigastric artery, arising from the external iliac artery in the lower direction, delivering blood to the periumbilical perforator vessels.

Zone 2

- Located below the arcuate line.
- Blood supply is derived from branches of the inferior epigastric artery medially, and superficial circumflex iliac artery laterally.

Zone 3

- Located lateral to the Linea semilunaris and above the arcuate line.
- Blood supply is derived from the musculophrenic artery superiorly, and the deep circumflex iliac artery inferiorly.

The abdominal wall nerves run between the transversus abdominis and internal oblique muscles. The top nerves arise from spinal roots T6-T12, while the L1 nerve root innervates the lower area via the ilioinguinal and iliohypogastric nerves.

3. Causes of ventral hernia

Several factors play a role in the formation of hernias. Hernias can be linked to various medical conditions, including connective tissue disorders, as well as collagen-related abnormalities.

The majority of hernias are associated with disorder of a collagen metabolism, where the type I to III collagen ratio plays a key role. A lower ratio, around 5 on average, increases the likelihood of hernia development [2].

Common risk factors include:

- Weakness in the abdominal wall: aging, or previous abdominal surgeries.
- Pregnancy can strain and weaken abdominal muscles, making women more susceptible.
- Obesity: Excess weight stresses abdominal muscles.
- Chronic cough: increases intra-abdominal pressure.
- Straining during bowel movements.
- Trauma or abdominal wall injury.
- Smoking: Impaired body healing and increased hernia risk are linked to smoking.

3.1 Symptoms

The symptoms of ventral hernias can differ, and some individuals may not exhibit any symptoms:

- A bulge or lump in the abdominal region, especially while standing or straining.
- Discomfort or pain in the affected area.
- In certain instances, the hernia may become incarcerated, resulting in the entrapment of abdominal contents. This situation can lead to intense pain, nausea, and vomiting, necessitating urgent medical attention.

3.2 Diagnosis

The identification of an abdominal lump during a physical examination typically validates the diagnosis. For obese patients, feeling the lump by palpation might be challenging, and using ultrasound (US) or computed tomography (CT) can be useful for confirming the diagnosis.

4. CT Imaging in ventral hernia

CT serves as a valuable tool for the preoperative assessment of most patients, providing information about the size and position of the hernia defect, its relation to nearby surrounding structures, involvement of the bowel, and loss of domain. It is a relatively lower cost compared to magnetic resonance imaging (MRI) [3].

This imaging technique is especially crucial for atypical ventral hernias situated away from the midline, such as parastomal and spigelian hernias.

Some studies have explored the use of ultrasound for diagnosing and monitoring incisional hernias, yielding positive outcomes. Ultrasound is an appealing imaging option due to its cost-effectiveness and reduced radiation exposure for patients who often undergo multiple irradiation procedures.

However, ultrasound has limitations such as being highly dependent on the user's expertise, inability to accurately assess the size of larger hernias, and limited capabilities in evaluating other factors like mesh location, bowel patterns, and occult hernias [4].

Preoperative considerations:

- *Patient selection:*

- Indications:

Symptomatic hernia, risk of incarceration: narrow-necked large hernias containing bowel on CT [5].

- Relative contraindications [5]

Hernia size: large >10 CM OR small <3 cm,

High BMI, multiple previous scars,

Hernia in unusual locations [6]: e.g. subxiphoid [5], flank, suprapubic [7] in which high-grade experience is required to place and fix mesh subfascial and avoid injuring vital structures or posterolateral hernias where is difficult to anatomically obtain mesh landing zone,

Strangulation/incarceration. These are considered as relative contraindications.

- Special circumstances [5, 8] in which it is difficult to obtain safe laparoscopic repair:

  1. Loss of domain.

  2. Presence of skin graft or abdominal wall flaps (e.g. TRAM flap).

  3. Presence of enterocutaneous fistula.

  4. Loss of abdominal wall muscles like in gunshots.

  5. Recurrent hernia that require large mesh removal are considered as absolute contraindications of laparoscopic ventral hernia repair.

- Medical comorbidities [5, 8]:

Severe COPD, congestive Heart failure and child C Liver Cirrhosis are absolute contraindications of laparoscopic ventral hernia repair.

- *Patient Optimization* [8]*:*

- Weight reduction
  - Stop smoking.
  - Treat constipation

Techniques [8, 9]*:*

- General anesthesia
- Antibiotics during induction according to the local hospital policy.
- Supine position and abdominal prep +/− incise drape (e.g. Ioban)
- Ports positioning:
  - Commonly three ports are placed at the left side of the abdomen +/- assistant port at the right side of the abdomen
- Camera and mesh insertion port: 10–12 mm port at left upper quadrant midclavicular line below the tip of 11th rib mainly inserted in open Hasson technique fashion. Other options include Veress needle and optical port.
- Another 2 x 5 mm ports were inserted under vision in the anterior axillary line.
- Surgical field/space:
  - Intraabdominal (in IPOM), most commonly.
  - Preperitoneal space (in TAPP) [10]: peritoneum incised 7–8 cm distance from linea alba parallel to the midline and 12–15 cm long craniocaudally, preperitoneal space developed around the hernia and to the contralateral side prior to hernia reduction.
  - Retro rectus space (in eTEP) [6]: 15 mm subcostal incision, balloon space used to create retro rectus space to pubic bone medial to linea semilunaris to preserve neurovascular bundles, brief intraperitoneal entry to dissect and inspect the hernia contents, retro rectus space creation continued to the contralateral side.
  - Oblique muscle complex (in endoscopic component separation) [11]: create space between external and internal oblique, perforator sparing technique used to release external oblique from its origin obliquely, mainly used as adjunct for open ventral/incisional hernia repair but can also be used for laparoscopic repair.
- Adhesiolysis and hernia reduction: Care not to injure the bowel and also meticulous hemostasis (consideration of open conversion largely depend on the operative experience but generally significant bowel injury or bleeding that is difficult to control laparoscopically should be an indication of early conversion).

- Hernia defect measurement and closure: Hernia defect can be measured laparoscopically using tape or externally sometimes with the aid of a spinal needle passed close to the edge of the fascial defect. Hernia defect is then closed either laparoscopically or transfacially using a fascial closure instrument or endo close.
- Mesh placement and fixation:
    - Allowing 4–5 cm overlap around the hernia defect.
    - Fixation: tacks +/- anchoring sutures. Tacks can be absorbable or non-absorbable. The general consensus is to use absorbable tacks although there is no strong evidence to support it [12]
- Location of the mesh:
    - Intraperitoneal Onlay Mesh (IPOM): It is the commonest mesh placement technique. Easier but higher mesh complications rate. Other techniques: reduce mesh complications rate but technically difficult).
    - Transabdominal preperitoneal (TAPP) [10]: It is suitable for medium-sized hernia (2–4 cm according to European Hernia Society [13].
    - Extended totally extra peritoneal (eTEP) [6] which can be done as Rives Stoppa.
    - Preperitoneal mesh placement procedure or accompanied with posterior component separation (i.e. Transversus abdominis release).

Types of mesh:
Three main types of Mesh:

1. Composite
    - Polypropylene collagen (Parietene, Sofradim, Trevoux, France).
    - Polypropylene polytetrafluoroethylene (Composix, CR Bard, Cranston, NJ, USA)
    - Monofilament polyester collagen (Sympotex, Medtronic, UK)
2. Expanded polytetrafluoroethylene (Dual mesh, Gore-Tex, Gore Medical, Flagstaff, AZ, USA)
3. Polypropylene covered with oxidized regenerated cellulose (Proceed (Ethicon).

Complications [5, 8]*:*

1. Bowel injury (enterotomy) 2–6%: Intra op management depend on the degree of injury or contamination. Option will be:
    - Repair the injury (lap or open) + repair the hernia with or without mesh.

- Repair the injury (lap or Open) + delayed hernia repair either less than 1 week or after 6–8 weeks.

- Delayed enterotomy usually as result of delayed diathermy injury or tacks injury and should be managed by laparotomy, repair /excise or divert the injury + mesh removal.

2. Seroma formation: more than 90% of patients develop seroma which is likely to spontaneously resolve. Therefore treatment is reserved to symptomatic seroma (1–24%) or persistent seroma for more than 8 weeks (3–4%) which can be managed with sterile aspiration or drainage, rarely chronic seromas might require mesh removal.

3. Post-Operative Ileus (1–3%): usually managed expectantly, reduced bowel manipulation may reduce the incidence of post-op adynamic ileus.

4. Infections:

   - Surgical site infections: 2.8% can be treated with dressing and antibiotics.

   - Skin Cellulitis: 2–4% could be as a result of an inflammatory reaction caused by the mesh or infected mesh, treated with antibiotics. Low evidence of prophylactic antibiotic use.

   - Mesh Infection: 0.6% difficult to treat and may require mesh excision, the following strategies can be adopted:

     - Antimicrobial therapy + image-guided drainage of abscesses.

     - Mesh salvage, debridement + vac therapy with antimicrobial therapy, especially of mesh is well incorporated.

     - Mesh removal, for septic patients or when the above measures failed.

   - Fistula formation [14]:0.1% usually as a result of chronic mesh erosion, unrecognized enterotomy or anchoring suture injury. Treated with mesh removal and surgical repair.

5. Chronic pain more than 6 weeks post-operative, 1.3–3.3%, usually as the result of tacks or anchoring stitch, rarely as a result of neuroma development. It can be managed with, NSAID, nerve blocks, local anesthetic or steroid injections. Surgical removal of anchoring stitches or tacks.

Post-operative care [8]*:*

- Adequate analgesia: range from simple analgesia to PCA.

- DVT prophylaxis should be initiated within 24 hours.

- Patient education: lifestyle adjustments to reduce hernia recurrence, recognize signs of infection or hernia recurrence

5. In summary

The abdominal wall's anatomy is crucial for effective hernia repair.

Blood supply zones in the abdominal wall are defined based on location and vascular sources.

Diagnosis involves physical examination, ultrasound, or computed tomography (CT) imaging.

CT imaging is cost-effective and useful for assessing hernia size, location, and relation to nearby structures. Ultrasound is another option but has limitations. Understanding ventral hernias and their diagnosis is essential for effective management and surgical repair.

Preop considerations for hernia surgery include patient selection, indications, hernia size, high BMI, previous scars, and hernia in unusual locations. Special circumstances include loss of domain, skin graft or abdominal wall flaps, enterocutaneous fistula, loss of abdominal wall muscles, and recurrent hernias requiring large mesh removal. Patient optimization includes weight reduction, stopping smoking, and treating constipation.

Operatively Surgical fields include intraabdominal (IPOM), preperitoneal space (TAPP), retro rectus space (eTEP), and oblique muscle complex (endoscopic component separation). Hernia defect measurement and closure are done laparoscopically or externally, and the hernia defect is closed either laparoscopically or transfacially.

Mesh placement and fixation are performed using intraperitoneal Onlay Mesh (IPOM), transabdominal preperitoneal (TAPP) and extended totally extraperitoneal (eTEP). Mesh types include polypropylene + collagen, polypropylene+polytetrafluor oethylene, monofilament. Polyester+collagen, expanded polytetrafluoroethylene, and polypropylene covered with oxidized regenerated cellulose.

Complications include bowel injury (enterotomy). The option 0f treatment depends on the degree of injury or contamination.

In conclusion, laparoscopic ventral hernia repair is a challenging process that requires careful patient selection and optimisation together with the availability of surgical experience. Therefore, complex laparoscopic ventral/incisional hernia repair should be reserved to centers where high volume of these surgeries are conducted in regular bases.

Author details

Mohamed Alfatih Hamza*, Mekki Hassan and Sean Johnston
St James's University Hospital, Midland Regional Hospital Tullamore, Tullamore, County Offaly, Ireland

*Address all correspondence to: mohamed.alfatih86@gmail.com

References

[1] Muysoms F, Campanelli G, Champault G, DeBeaux AC, Dietz UA, Jeekel J, et al. Eura HS: The development of an international online platform for registration and outcome measurement of ventral abdominal wall hernia repair. DOI: 10.1007/s10029-012-0912-7

[2] Korutha S, Chettyb YVN. Hernias-Is it a primary defect or a systemic disorder? Role of collagen III in all hernias - A case control study. DOI: 10.1016/j.amsu.2017.05.012

[3] Tonolini M. Multidetector CT of expected findings and complications after contemporary inguinal hernia repair surgery. Diagnostic and Interventional Radiology. 2016;**22**(5):422-429

[4] Baucom RB, Beck WC, Phillips SE, Holzman MD, Sharp KW, Nealon WH, et al. Comparative evaluation of dynamic abdominal sonography for hernia and computed tomography for characterization of incisional hernia. JAMA Surgery. 2014;**149**(6):591-596

[5] Earle D, Roth JS, Saber A, Haggerty S, Bradley JF, Fanelli R, et al. SAGES guidelines for laparoscopic ventral hernia repair. Surgical Endoscopy. 2016;**30**:3163-3183

[6] Baig SJ, Priya P. Extended totally extra peritoneal repair (eTEP) for ventral hernias: Short-term results from a single Centre. Journal of Minimal Access Surgery. 2019;**15**(3):198

[7] Sikar HE, Çetin K, Eyvaz K, Kaptanoglu L, Küçük HF. Laparoscopic repair of large suprapubic hernias. Videosurgery and Other Mini-invasive Techniques. 2017;**12**(3):245-250

[8] Park Y, Chung M. Laparoscopic ventral hernia repair. Journal of Minimally Invasive Surgery. 2017;**20**(3):93-100

[9] Misiakos EP, Machairas A, Patapis P, Liakakos T. Laparoscopic ventral hernia repair: Pros and cons compared with open hernia repair. Journal of the Society of Laparoendoscopic Surgeons. 2008;**12**(2):117

[10] Skolimowska-Rzewuska M, Romańczuk M, Mitura B, Wyrzykowska D, Mitura K. Laparoscopic transabdominal preperitoneal repair (umbilical TAPP) versus open ventral patch repair for medium size umbilical hernias in overweight and obese patients. Videosurgery and Other Miniinvasive Techniques. 2022;**17**(1):170-178

[11] Novitsky YW. Hernia Surgery: Current Principles. Switzerland: Springer International Publishing; 2016. DOI: 10.1007/978-3-319-27470-6. ISBN: 978-3-319-27468-3. ISBN: 978-3-319-27470-6 (eBook). Library of Congress Control Number: 2016935505

[12] Khan RMA, Bughio M, Ali B, Hajibandeh S, Hajibandeh S. Absorbable versus non-absorbable tacks for mesh fixation in laparoscopic ventral hernia repair: A systematic review and meta-analysis. International Journal of Surgery. 2018;**53**:184-192

[13] Muysoms FE, Antoniou S, Bury K, Campanelli G, Conze J, Cuccurullo D, et al. European hernia society guidelines on the closure of abdominal wall incisions. Hernia. 2015;**19**:1-24

[14] Ghanem OM, Zahiri HR, Devlin S, Sibia U, Park A, Belyansky I. Laparoscopic subxiphoid hernia repair with intracorporeal suturing of mesh to the diaphragm as a means to decrease recurrence. Journal of Laparoendoscopic & Advanced Surgical Techniques. 2016;**26**(2):129-132

Chapter 5

Management of Ventral Hernia in Obese Patients: Before or After Bariatric Surgery?

Bachir Elias, Carine El Hajj and Caline Zeaiter

Abstract

Obesity is a known risk factor for ventral hernias and their recurrences. The timing of ventral hernia repair in obese patients who are candidates for bariatric surgery is still a debatable topic. To this date, there is no consensus, neither for the timing nor for the surgical repair technic. In this chapter, we will review briefly what was already discussed about this dilemma and explore our experience with our retrospective study. If asymptomatic, the ventral hernia should be repaired after bariatric surgery when there is stabilization of the weight loss. Laparoscopic approach is recommended to allow an exploration of the trocars sites and a second look after obesity surgery. An algorithm for ventral hernia management in obese patients is proposed.

Keywords: ventral hernia, ventral hernia repair, bariatric surgery, technique of hernia repair, management of hernias in obese patients

1. Introduction

Obesity is a risk factor increasing the occurrence of primary and secondary ventral hernia; as well as the risk of complications when operating hernia, especially the risk of recurrence. On the other hand, when ventral hernia becomes symptomatic in obese patients with incarceration or strangulation, there is an increased risk of major complications or delayed diagnosis because obese patients can have little or no major clinical symptoms. Concerning bariatric surgery, hernia of the abdominal wall can make the operation more complicated while increasing also the operative time.

In order to manage ventral hernia in the bariatric population while having the lowest risk, it is mandatory to choose the best time to operate a hernia during the management of the obesity of this group. After studying 47 ventral hernias diagnosed during the preparation of 643 patients for their bariatric surgery and after a review of the literature that is relatively poor concerning this subject, we concluded that many factors are to consider during the management of ventral hernia in bariatric population; but, in general, if asymptomatic, ventral hernia should be repaired after bariatric surgery when here is the stabilization of the weight loss; and laparoscopic approach is recommended to allow an exploration of the trocars sites and a second look after obesity surgery.

2. Ventral hernia repair in obese patients

There are many techniques for ventral hernia repair and many approaches. Whether to combine it or not with bariatric surgery, the repair is most of the time inevitable. Since obesity is a risk factor for an increased incidence and recurrences of ventral hernia, the timing of repair is essential to balance out between a late repair with an increased risk of hernia-related complication, an early repair with its increased risk of recurrence, and a concomitant repair with higher morbidity.

2.1 Definition of obesity

To be able to discuss bariatric surgery we need to start by defining obesity. Even though this is a common pathology, the medical expert failed to define obesity properly in the 10th edition of the International Classification of Diseases relating it to its definition of "excess of calories" which was considered as a demeaning description. However, they managed to change that in the 11th edition and defined this chronic pathology as [1]:

"Abnormal or excessive fat store secondary to different causes including energy imbalance, drugs, and genetic disorders."

According to the WHO, 4 million deaths per year resulted in 2017 from being obese or overweight. Its prevalence has increased globally, especially for children and adolescents. In 2016, more than 650,000,000 adults over 18 years old were obese (WHO). Globally, this preventable and treatable disease kills more than malnutrition. Moreover, this disease is no longer a high-income region problem with rates increasing even in the urban areas of low- and middle-income countries therefore it is now considered a global epidemic.

BMI or body mass index approximates the total body fat and it is equivalent to the weight divided by the square of the height in meters [2, 3].

This index is easy to calculate and consistent. It can correlate to the total fatness in the body but is not an accurate measure of body fat. For instance, muscular patients who are overweight will have a lower degree of adiposity compared to the same patients in the same category. Older adults will have a lower percentage of muscles and a higher percentage of fat in the same BMI category [3].

This Index is used to group patients into mainly 4 categories: Underweight (<18.5 kg/m^2), normal range (18.5 to 24.9 kg/m^2), overweight (25 to 29.9 kg/m^2), and obese (≥ 30 kg/m^2).

2.2 Abdominal wall hernia: definition, incidence, risk factor, classifications, and prognosis

2.2.1 Definition and incidence

An abnormal protrusion of abdominal contents through a weakness in the anterior abdominal wall is referred to as a ventral hernia. Abdominal wall hernias are quite prevalent, with a prevalence of 1.7% for people of all ages and 4% for people over the age of 45. It is estimated that more than 20 million hernias are treated annually throughout the world. About 75% of abdominal wall hernias are inguinal hernias, which have a lifetime risk of 27% in men and 3% in women. Inguinal hernias are the most prevalent type of ventral hernias. Umbilical, paraumbilical, epigastric, incisional, and rarer hernias including Spigelian and traumatic hernias are further forms of ventral hernias. In the postoperative setting, patients have approximately 10%

risk of developing hernia following a midline laparotomy, 5% following a transverse muscle splitting incision, and less than 1% following laparoscopic repair.

2.2.2 Classification and risk factors

Ventral hernias can be mainly classified as primary or secondary: umbilical, epigastric, and hypogastric hernias are classified as primary while secondary ventral hernias occur following surgery, and are referred to as incisional hernias.

Inguinal and femoral groin hernias are not included in the classification of anterior abdominal wall hernias as primary or incisional hernias used by the European Hernia Society. The midline umbilical and epigastric hernias, as well as lateral spigelian hernias, are subclasses of primary hernias (or "ventral" hernias). Parastomal hernias are a specific type of ventral hernia with a variety of treatment options, despite the fact that they are incisional by definition. Before this consensus definition, the literature on abdominal wall hernias had been hindered by inconsistent nomenclature, and despite distinct etiology, epidemiology, and surgical outcomes, incisional and primary ventral hernias continue to be combined in studies [4]. Congenital or acquired causes of ventral hernias can be distinguished with acquired hernias being more frequent, and frequently brought on by previous surgery, trauma, or repetitive stress on vulnerable areas of the abdominal wall.

A big contributing cause of acquired ventral hernias is obesity, which weakens the abdomen's fascia by stretching it.

In a study published in 2021 and entitled "Abdominal Wall Hernias: An Epidemiological Profile and Surgical Experience from a Rural Medical College in Central India," predisposing factors in a majority of the patients were:

- Chronic cough (55%)
- Prostatic problems (23%)
- Chronic constipation (20%)
- Previous surgeries (10%)
- Obesity (1.2%)
- Ascites (1.1%)
- Multiparity (6.1%)
- Transabdominal gynecological surgeries (4.0%)
- Excessive crying (25% of the pediatric population)
- Chronic respiratory infections (23% of the pediatric population) [5]

2.2.3 Prognosis

The type, size, and potential for reducing risk factors that contribute to the development of a hernia are only a few of the variables that affect the prognosis of a certain hernia. The prognosis is usually favorable with prompt diagnosis and treatment. However, if the hernia is not identified or if problems develop while treating the condition, morbidity may result.

An incarcerated, obstructed, or even strangulated intestine with a poor blood supply is a potential hernia consequence. Missing this could lead to peritonitis and bowel perforation, both of which are potentially fatal. Therefore, surgical intervention is necessary to stop additional complications such as sepsis and perforation.

It is crucial to remember that surgery to repair a hernia can put the patient at risk for adhesions or infection. Hernias can also recur in the same place even after surgical correction [6].

Medical illiteracy, financial constraints, and societal inhibitions might cause delayed presentations and higher postoperative morbidity and mortality in rural parts of developing nations. To guarantee that early diagnosis and the finest procedures are available to various social strata, efforts must be made to conduct area-wise surveys, educate the populace, and reduce costs [7].

2.3 Indications for bariatric surgery

Bariatric surgery includes several procedures to target weight loss. They may target intestinal absorption or restrict the meal volume or do both. Before proceeding with any bariatric procedure, a multidisciplinary team will evaluate the patient's nutritional status, psychological state, and lifestyle. Like any surgical procedure, it comes with multiple post-operative morbidities and mortality risk.

Bariatric surgery is indicated when [3]:

- BMI > 40
- 35 < BMI < 39.9 with an obesity-related comorbidity (Table 1: HTA DM GI reflux osteoarthritis.)
- BMI > 30 with an uncontrollable DM II or dysmetabolic syndrome X.

More than 300,000 procedures were performed in 2011 [3]. In the USA, 2000000 patients had a bariatric procedure between 1993 and 2016. Within that period, the evolution of bariatric surgery started, and there was a switch from open procedures to laparoscopic procedures. Due to technological advances and the escalation of the surgical experience, the postoperative morbidity and mortality rates decreased by around 10% from 1998 to 2016 (11.7–0.04). It is debatable whether these procedures should be offered before the start of the subordinate health impairments or limited to those who already suffer from comorbidities. However, all agree that these procedures should not be considered cosmetic interventions [8].

2.4 Review of different approaches to bariatric surgery

Currently, we have four common bariatric procedures that work on reducing the gastric space and or limiting the intestinal length:

- Gastric banding reduces food intake. It consists of banding the upper part of the stomach and connecting it to a subcutaneous port. Filling this port with saline will control the stricture of this band. This reversible and minimal invasive technique had its side effects like vomiting and solid food intolerance.

- Sleeve gastrectomy [3, 8] popularity has increased because of its feasibility and satisfying results. It consists of removing the lateral part of the stomach and fundus keeping just a small portion of the lesser curve and the antrum. It reduces the stomach's capacity by almost 90% and preserves the pylorus and the totality of the intestines. It is simple to perform laparoscopically and eliminates the risk of many postoperative complications. Since the intestines are intact the risk of internal herniations is totally absent.

- Gastric bypass is a popular alternative developed 40 years ago that maintained its popularity since Wittgrove managed to perform this procedure laparoscopically [3, 8]. In the long run, this procedure can generate life-threatening complications such as ulcers or internal hernias and many nutritional deficiencies. The Roux en Y gastric bypass consists of creating a small gastric pouch by resecting the stomach horizontally than vertically. Then two anastomoses are made a gastro jejunal and a jejuno-jejunal anastomosis to create two limbs a biliary and an alimentary limb. The omega loop bypass or mini bypass consists of creating a mini gastric pouch and then a gastrojejunal anastomosis at the 200 cm mark from the Treitz angle.

- The duodenal switch was created by Hess [8] and it combines a gastric sleeve with a small bowel bypass. The sleeve gastrectomy is performed then the duodenum is transected away from the pylorus. The small bowel at 2.5 to 3 m from the ileocecal valve is transected then a 1.5 m alimentary limb is generated anastomosed to the gastric end of the duodenum. The distal part of the duodenum drains with the biliopancreatic secretion into the alimentary limb at 1.5 to 1 m from the ileocecal valve. Up to 70% of the small bowels are isolated in this procedure from the foodstream [8]. This results in a more significant reduction of fat absorption compared to other techniques, which leads to a more durable weight loss. By preserving the pylorus, this technique allows patients to eat with a lower risk of dumping [8]. Fat-soluble vitamins are required postoperatively. Since this technique is difficult to perform laparoscopically, its use is limited.

Other bariatric techniques include:

Gastric plication is a technique that resembles the gastric sleeve however without any resection. It reduces gastric volume with easier reversibility however this technique is more difficult, and it remains under investigation [8].

All these techniques should be performed, unless major contraindications, by laparoscopic approach which reduces the postoperative pain, respiratory complication, the formation of large hernia, decreases the hosiptal stay and improves esthetic outcomes.

2.5 Indications for ventral hernia repair

Among all surgical issues, abdominal wall hernias are among the most frequent. Inguinal hernia repairs account for over 770,000 of the nearly 1 million abdominal wall hernia operations performed annually in the United States. [9].

Through a thorough clinical examination and review of the patient's medical history, abdominal wall hernia can be accurately diagnosed. However, in challenging or complex cases, imaging modalities, such as CT scan, ultrasound, and MRI, can be helpful. According to one study, a clinical examination has a sensitivity of 75% and a specificity of 96% for hernia diagnosis.

Ventral hernia repair is generally indicated for a variety of reasons, but the most prevalent ones include symptom relief, cosmetic improvement, and averting morbidities, such as pain, incarceration, enlargement, and skin changes, that are linked to the defect. In low- and moderate-risk individuals, elective surgery enhances the functional status and quality of life associated with hernias, but emergency repair increases morbidity and death. Older age, female sex, and umbilical hernia defects measuring from 2 to 7 cm or incisional hernia defects measuring up to 7 cm were significant risk factors for urgent repair. For incisional and umbilical hernias, watchful waiting is safe, but it causes substantial crossover rates (11–33%) and a significantly higher incidence of intraoperative perforations, fistulas, and mortality for emergency surgery. Older patients with incisional hernias typically have poorer outcomes following incisional hernia surgery. Advanced age was a significant risk factor for both umbilical hernias and ventral/incisional hernias requiring emergency repair; and an independent risk factor for poor early outcomes (readmission, reoperation, or death within 30 days). In patients with modifiable risk factors, watchful waiting is advised for medical improvement [10].

It is advised that symptomatic hernias be surgically addressed. The laparoscopic approach (standard or robotic method) should ideally be used especially for defects with a diameter of less than 15 cm.

2.6 Review of different approaches to ventral hernia

Surgery is the most typical treatment for ventral hernias. Hernias that are asymptomatic can be treated on an elective basis, while those that are strangulated need to be operated on right away. Incarceration without strangling is not a surgical emergency. Binder, truss, or corset use for non-surgical management of abdominal wall hernias is not thought to be successful. However, if a patient is not a good surgical candidate, this might be their only option.

Hernias have been repaired using a variety of surgical methods over the years. The use of a mesh with 3 to 5 cm of overlap, careful management of the mesh, limiting surgical site infections, and adopting an approach with the closure of the fascia if possible are further considerations, with a tension-free closure being the most crucial. The most straightforward strategy is a primary open repair without mesh, which should normally only be used for fascia abnormalities smaller than 2 cm. There are various alternatives for an open repair with mesh, including the kind of mesh and the placement of the mesh [6].

When compared to open techniques, laparoscopic ventral hernia repair consistently shows lower overall complication rates, shorter hospital stays, and quicker return to work. The majority of the current literature demonstrates that the recurrence rates are marginally lower in laparoscopic repair, despite the fact that this relationship has not always been statistically significant. Laparoscopy has drawbacks, including a larger risk of visceral harm and greater technical difficulty. Due to more surgical freedom, robotic ventral hernia procedures have also gained popularity. From a technological perspective, closing the fascial defect robotically is far simpler than trying to do it using traditional laparoscopic tools. Due to the possibility of maintaining smaller incisions, the advantages of laparoscopy are maintained. At present moment, no landmark trials have shown that robotic surgery is superior to laparoscopy; instead, it is often more expensive and requires longer operating durations.

2.6.1 The rives-stoppa repair

The retrorectus dissection plane is used in the Rives-Stoppa repair, which was first reported in the 1980s. This procedure is quite durable while preventing the development of subcutaneous flaps. The procedure allows for additional mobilization by releasing the posterior rectus sheath from the rectus muscles. This is normally done by dissecting bluntly toward the semilunar line while incising the posterior rectus sheath within 0.5 cm of its medial border. Then, the mesh is frequently positioned anterior to the posterior fascial plane, in a retromuscular manner [11].

Additionally, the abdominal wall musculature is preserved during this procedure, which is important for a successful abdominal wall reconstruction because it preserves both its functional and anatomical integrity. The restricted lateral dissection performed in this procedure, however, limits its use despite its stellar track record. The Rives-Stoppa repair, however, is inherently inappropriate in some circumstances. These include nonmidline ventral hernias lateral to the linea semilunaris, insufficient medial advancement of the posterior rectus sheath and musculature, and insufficient retrorectus space required for mesh placement. These restrictions have led to the development of new operating procedures.

2.6.2 Transversus abdominis release combined with posterior component separation

The transversus abdominis release has been useful in correcting nonmidline, complicated faults that the Rives-Stoppa repair is unable to fix. In this method, mesh overlap and lateral mobilization are added to the Rives-Stoppa repair's retrorectus dissection plane. The posterior rectus sheath is incised, exposing the underlying transversus abdominis muscle, typically 0.5 cm medial to the semilunar line. After that, the underlying fascia is separated from the muscle plane, if necessary as far laterally as the psoas muscle [11].

2.6.3 Anterior component separation

A dissection anterior to the rectus muscles is used for anterior component separation. The external oblique fascia, which is located just lateral to the lateral aspect of the rectus muscles, is severed during the procedure to create a subcutaneous plane. If tension-free approximation is not initially achieved, further dissection to the anterior axillary line's margin can be done. This procedure allows for efficient midline repair while allowing for significant medial mobilization of the abdominal wall muscles [11].

3. Discussing literature about the management of hernias in obese patients

Obesity is in fact a risk factor for the occurrence and the recurrence of ventral hernias. Many hernia repair techniques failed to treat hernias in obese patients [12]. Obesity is also a risk factor for increased wound infections, increased intra-abdominal pressure, and slow healing [13]. The incidence of recurrence can reach 35%, however, laparoscopic intraperitoneal onlay mesh repair can reduce this rate to 12% [13]. Weight loss can contribute to the reduction of hernia recurrences, however, recurrences may occur faster than reaching the optimal weight loss [12, 13]. Moreover, significant weight loss means a higher risk of internal hernias and need for re-intervention. Therefore, weight loss can compromise the efficacy of an early hernia repair.

There are no guidelines for the type or timing of hernia repairs however many retrospective studies discussed these issues.

A small study done on 23 patients who had a concomitant bariatric surgery with a laparoscopic intraperitoneal onlay mesh repair showed a low rate of recurrence over 3 years of follow-up [13]. This suggested that concomitant onlay mesh repair is a good alternative to delayed repair. However, the sample size was small and 4 patients had seromas postoperatively which is 7% more risk compared to the maximal incidence of seromas cited in the literature [13, 14].

A French nationwide retrospective study conducted between 2007 and 2018 concluded that hernia repair before bariatric surgery should be avoided to avoid the higher risk of reoperation that is associated with it [15]. Operating hernias before bariatric surgery had the highest recurrence rates compared to hernia repair postbariatric surgery or concomitant to bariatric surgery [15, 16].

Hernias suture repairs concomitant to bariatric surgery did not have a high recurrence rate due to the fact that usually suture repairs are indicated for smaller hernias that are less likely to reoccur [15]. A retrospective analysis of a UK-based sample of bariatric patients showed that the reoccurrence rate of concomitant repair is sufficiently low to suggest it for non-diabetic patients who are at a higher risk of infections [17].

The biggest dilemma resides in the fact that bariatric surgery with ventral hernia is challenging but obesity is a risk factor for recurrences [18]. Also, hernia repair during bariatric surgery is technically more difficult and can increase morbidity without annulling the risk of recurrences [18]. Since bariatric surgery is considered as clean contaminated, synthetic meshes offer better results in hernia repair but put patients at risk of infections [18].

Finally, a very diplomatic answer was given by Sait MS and Al. when questioning the timing of hernia repair in morbidly obese patients [19]. As suggested in their review, a case-by-case decision should be used since out of the 179 articles reported and the 5 main articles used to answer the questions, conflicting results dominated the research. The only common fact was that hernias should be repaired to avoid occlusion, synthetic mesh usage does not increase site infection in case of concomitant repair, and that randomized controlled trials are needed to reach a consensus [19].

4. Our study sample presentation and results

4.1 Objective

The objective of the study is to determine the best moment to operate a ventral hernia in obese patients during the management of their obesity.

4.2 Materials and methods

A retrospective study was conducted over the past 4 years. About 643 patients treated for morbid obesity were included: a ventral hernia (primary and incisional) was noted at the first consultation in 47 patients. All patients were asymptomatic. The mean time from the first consultation to bariatric surgery is 9 months. Thirty five patients were operated on 1 year after bariatric surgery called the "after bariatric surgery group," five patients were operated on before bariatric surgery, four patients were in an emergency pattern for incarcerated or strangulated hernia, and three ventral hernia closed without mesh during bariatric surgery; this was "before bariatric surgery group." The laparoscopic approach was used in 30 patients. Tension-free technique was used in 42 patients.

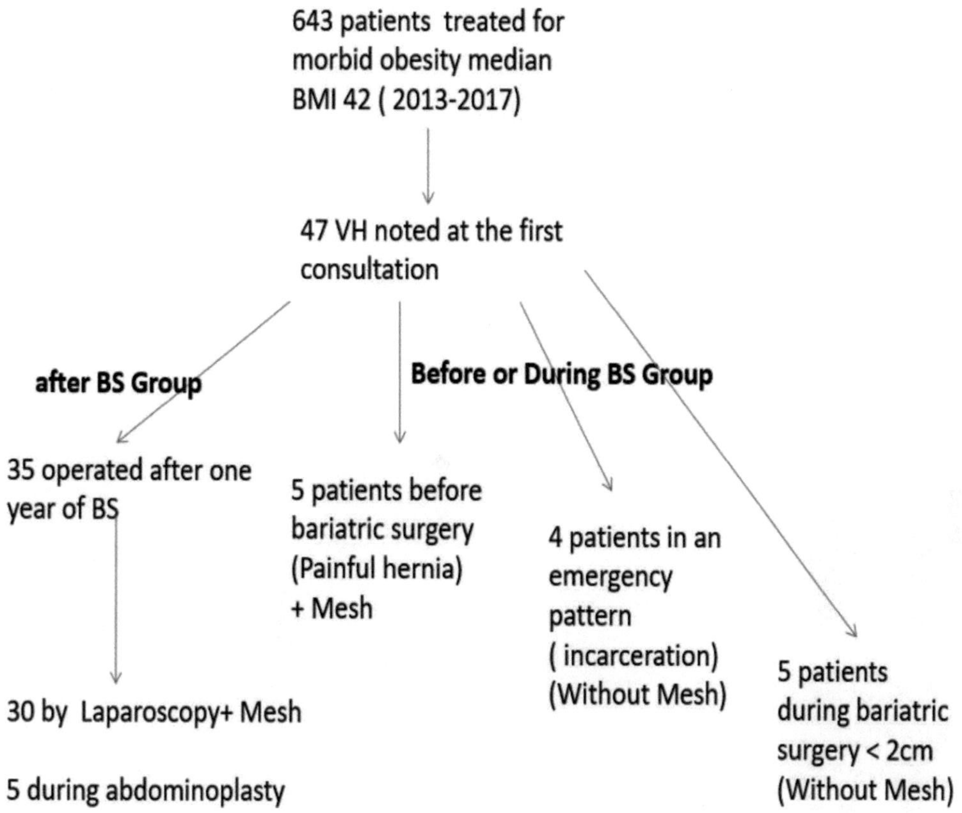

4.3 Results

Technically, it was easier to operate on patients after the weight loss.

Wound infection, hematoma, and pulmonary infection were seen in five patients, and there was no significant difference between the two groups concerning postoperative complications. No mortality was seen.

After at least 1 year of follow-up, one recurrence (2.8%) was noted in the "after bariatric surgery group" and seven recurrences (50%) in the "before bariatric surgery group." One recurrence of the 7 was noted after 2 months of the primary repair and the others occurred after the weight loss. Two asymptomatic trocars site hernias were repaired at the same time when laparoscopic approach was used.

5. Conclusion

There is a need for a large prospective study to evaluate the perfect timing with the optimal repair technique to have a golden standard solution for ventral hernias repair and obesity surgery dilemma.

According to the algorithm, we propose that, if asymptomatic, the ventral hernia should be repaired after bariatric surgery when there is stabilization of the weight loss usually after the first year. Laparoscopic approach is recommended because it allows an exploration of the trocars sites and a second look after obesity surgery.

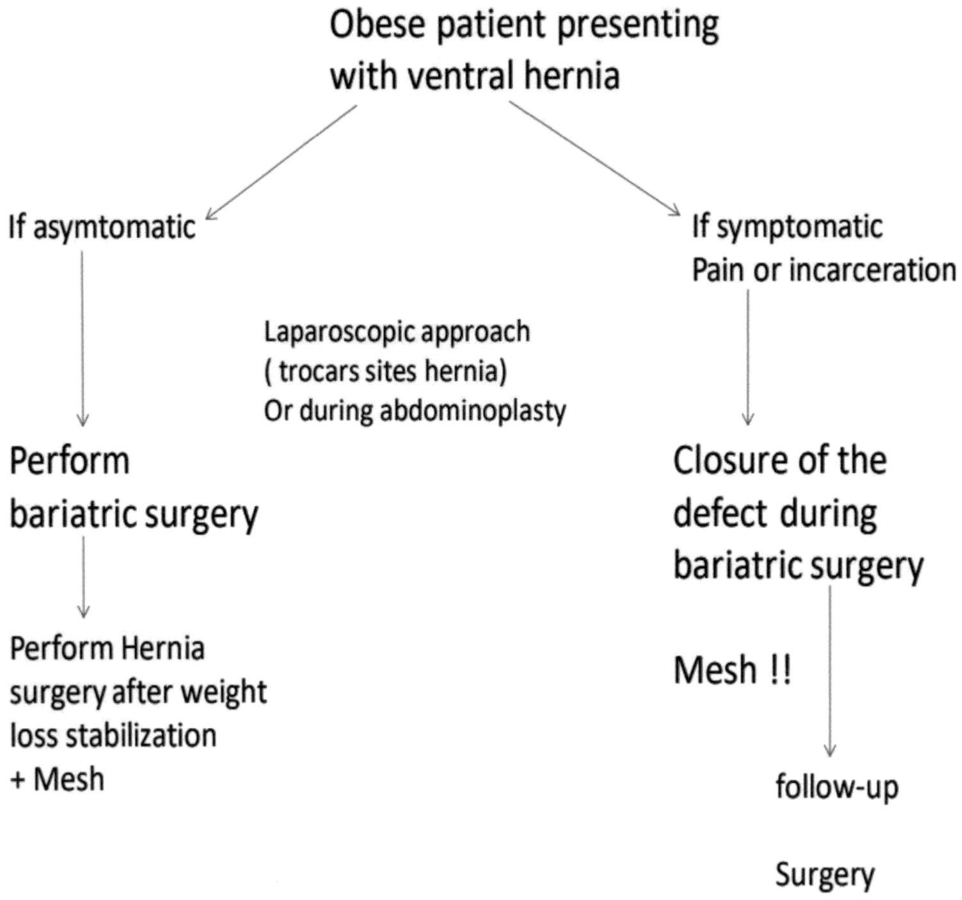

Conflict of interest

The authors declare no conflict of interest.

Author details

Bachir Elias[1,2]*, Carine El Hajj[1] and Caline Zeaiter[2]

1 General Surgery Department, Notre Dame des Secours Hospital, Holy Spirit Universty, Lebanon

2 General Surgery Department, Middle East Hospital, Balamand University, Lebanon

*Address all correspondence to: bachirelias@hotmail.fr

References

[1] Prachand VN. The evolution of minimally invasive bariatric surgery. Journal of Surgery and Research. 2011;**March**:1464-1468. DOI: 10.1007/s00268-011-1033-7

[2] Hebebrand J. Our definition of obesity and its impact on treatment. Obesity. 2020;**28**(3):22740. DOI: 10.1002/oby.22740

[3] Lim ARB. Bariatric procedures for the management of severe obesity: Descriptions. Available from: https://www-uptodate-com.ezproxy.usek.edu.lb/contents/bariatric-procedures-for-the-management-of-severe-obesity-descriptions/print?search=bar

[4] Bittner R, Bain K, Bansal VK, Berrevoet F, Bingener-Casey J, Chen D, et al. Update of guidelines for laparoscopic treatment of ventral and incisional abdominal wall hernias (international Endohernia society (IEHS))-part a. Surgical Endoscopy. 2019;**33**(10):3069-3139. DOI: 10.1007/s00464-019-06907-7 Epub 2019 Jun 27. Erratum in: Surg Endosc. 2019 Jul 12

[5] Pandya B, Huda T, Gupta D, Mehra B, Narang R. Abdominal Wall hernias: An epidemiological profile and surgical experience from a rural medical College in Central India. Surg J (N Y). 2021;**7**(1):e41-e46. DOI: 10.1055/s-0040-1722744

[6] Smith J, Parmely JD. Ventral Hernia. Treasure Island (FL): StatPearls Publishing; 2023

[7] Parker SG, Mallett S, Quinn L, Wood CPJ, Boulton RW, Jamshaid S, et al. Identifying predictors of ventral hernia recurrence: Systematic review and meta-analysis. BJS Open. 2021;**5**(2):zraa071. DOI: 10.1093/bjsopen/zraa071 Erratum in: BJS Open. 2021, 7;5(3)

[8] Carter PL. The evolution of bariatric surgery. American Journal of Surgery. 2015;**209**(5):779-782. DOI: 10.1016/j.amjsurg.2014.12.026

[9] Gillies M, Anthony L, Al-Roubaie A, Rockliff A, Phong J. Trends in incisional and ventral hernia repair: A population analysis from 2001 to 2021. Cureus. 2023;**15**(3):e35744. DOI: 10.7759/cureus.35744

[10] Evans KK, Chim H, Patel KM, Salgado CJ, Mardini S. Survey on ventral hernias: Surgeon indications, contraindications, and management of large ventral hernias. The American Surgeon. 2012;**78**(4):388-397

[11] Trujillo CN, Fowler A, Al-Temimi MH, Ali A, Johna S, Tessier D. Complex ventral hernias: A review of past to present. The Permanente Journal. 2018;**22**:17-015. DOI: 10.7812/TPP/17-015

[12] Manninen MJ, Lavonius M, Perhoniemi VJ. Results of incisional hernia repair. A retrospective study of 172 unselected hernioplasties. European Journal of Surgery Acta Chirugica. 1991;**157**(1):29-31

[13] Praveenraj P, Gomes RM, Kumar S, et al. Concomitant bariatric surgery with laparoscopic intra-peritoneal Onlay mesh repair for recurrent ventral hernias in morbidly obese patients: An evolving standard of care. Obesity Surgery. 2016;**26**(6):1191-1194. DOI: 10.1007/s11695-015-1875-4

[14] Basukala S, Tamang A, Rawal SB, et al. Comparison of outcomes of

laparoscopic hernioplasty with and without fascial repair (IPOM-plus vs IPOM) for ventral hernia: A retrospective cohort study. Annals of Medicine and Surgery. 2022;**80**:104297. DOI: 10.1016/j.amsu.2022.104297

[15] Moszkowicz D, Jacota M, Nkam L, Giovinazzo D, Grimaldi L, Lazzati A. Ventral hernia repair and obesity: Results from a Nationwide register study in France according to the timeframes of hernia repair and bariatric surgery. Obesity Surgery. 2021;**31**(12):5251-5259. DOI: 10.1007/s11695-021-05720-3

[16] Lazzati A, Nassif GB, Paolino L. Concomitant ventral hernia repair and bariatric surgery: A systematic review. Obesity Surgery. 2018;**28**:2949-2955

[17] Krivan MS, Giorga A, Barreca M, Jain VK, Al-Taan OS. Concomitant ventral hernia repair and bariatric surgery: A retrospective analysis from a UK-based bariatric center. Surgical Endoscopy. 2019;**33**(3):705-710. DOI: 10.1007/s00464-018-6492-6

[18] Vilallonga R, Beisani M, Sanchez-Cordero S, et al. Abdominal Wall hernia and metabolic bariatric surgery. Journal of Laparoendoscopic & Advanced Surgical Techniques. Part A. 2020;**30**(8):891-895. DOI: 10.1089/lap.2020.0257

[19] Sait MS, Som R, Borg CM, Chang A, Ramar S. Best evidence topic: Should ventral hernia repair be performed at the same time as bariatric surgery? Annals of Medicine and Surgery (Lond). 2016;**11**:21-25. DOI: 10.1016/j.amsu.2016.08.014

Chapter 6

Hernia as a Complication of Metabolic Bariatric Surgery

Athanasios Pantelis and Mohit Bhandari

Abstract

Metabolic Bariatric Surgery (MBS) is increasingly gaining ground, given that it constitutes the most effective treatment of obesity and associated health problems, with enduring results and a well-documented safety profile. Nevertheless, certain issues may rise in the medium and long term. Among them, there is a heterogeneous group of complications under the umbrella term "post-bariatric hernia", including internal hernias, abdominal wall hernias, and hiatal hernias. Internal hernias constitute the most studied category, but evidence on the other categories is not lacking. This chapter will attempt to cover diagnostic, treatment, and preventive aspects in the management of hernia post-MBS following a comprehensive, evidence-based approach. In brief, with regards to the prevention of internal hernias, suturing of all defects is strongly recommended for Roux-en-Y Gastric Bypass (RYGB), but the evidence is less clear when it comes to newer bypass procedures, such as One-Anastomosis/Mini Gastric Bypass (OAGB/MGB) and Single Anastomosis Duodenal-Ileal Bypass (SADI). As far as abdominal wall hernias are concerned, there is no clear evidence of the advantages of suture closure against non-closure. Finally, with respect to hiatal hernias post-MBS, the caveat rests in the documentation of *de novo* versus pre-existing hiatal hernia, which mandates meticulous preoperative evaluation of symptoms and potentially further endoscopic documentation.

Keywords: bariatric surgery, metabolic surgery, internal hernia, Petersen's defect, mesenteric defect, Brolin's space, mesocolic defect, trocar site hernia, port site hernia, incisional hernia, hiatal hernia, *de novo* hiatal hernia

1. Introduction

Metabolic bariatric surgery (MBS) is the most effective and sustainable treatment for obesity and associated health problems, such as type 2 diabetes mellitus [1–6]. Most importantly, MBS has shown a favorable safety profile over time [7], even at the extremes of age [8–10], even during pandemic periods with high epidemiological burden [11], and even for patient groups that are traditionally considered as high perioperative risk [12].

Nevertheless, there is no surgery without complications, as such bariatric operations bear an overall mortality risk of 1% and are accompanied by a number of early and late complications [13, 14]. The most studied early complications are anastomotic or staple-line leaks and hemorrhage, whereas the most referenced medium-term and late complications are malnutrition following hypoabsorptive procedures, gastro-esophageal reflux after sleeve gastrectomy, and anastomotic ulcers. Another cluster of complications following bariatric surgery falls into the umbrella term "hernia". Hernia post-MBS can take several forms but may be summarized into three cardinal categories: *internal*, *abdominal wall*, and *hiatal*.

The pathophysiology underlying post-MBS hernia remains elusive, and only extrapolations can be made about this complex issue, including but not limited to factors such as disrupted healing; nutritional deficiencies; diabetes mellitus; chronic constipation; chronic or vigorous cough; tissue subluxation and connective tissue disorders; alterations in intra-abdominal pressure; creation of visceral space defects that naturally would not exist; altered peristalsis and disrupted bowel transit; neurohormonal, immunologic, and inflammatory mediators; genetic and epigenetic influences; and so forth [15].

Most importantly, patients with hernia post-MBS may present in acute distress and their condition may mandate immediate surgical exploration, with incarcerated internal hernia being the most striking example. Consequently, the subject of hernia post-MBS expands well beyond the scope of bariatric surgery and may concern the general surgeon [16, 17].

This chapter will attempt to clarify the diagnostic challenges, treatment modalities, and prevention strategies regarding hernia post-MBS in a comprehensive and evidence-based manner.

2. Internal hernia following metabolic bariatric surgery

Internal hernias constitute the most widely studied category of hernia post-MBS. Most surgeons are familiar with the term "Petersen's defect", but this constitutes only one of many potential sites of herniation following Roux-en-Y gastric bypass (RYGB) and bariatric surgery in general.

2.1 Epidemiology and pathophysiology of internal hernia post-RYGB

Beginning with the epidemiological features of Internal Hernia (IH) post-MBS, according to the literature 42–61% of all cases of Small Bowel Obstruction (SBO) after RYGB are due to IH. This may indicate a relative increase of small bowel obstruction with the establishment of laparoscopic versus open approach in bariatric surgery, which in turn leads to the formation of less adhesions and allows for greater mobility of the small bowel. The crude incidence of IH post-RYGB is 5%, ranging 0.3–6.2%, but the true incidence is hard to assess, for reasons of short-term follow-up and/or loss to follow-up. In a large review comprising 9527 patients after RYGB and covering a period of 8 years, Koppman et al. showed that the incidence of IH ranged from 0.3% for antecolic to 2.4% for retrocolic fashioning of the Roux limb [18]. Among them, there are two seminal studies with regards to sample size and study design. The first was authored by Higa et al. in 2003 and comprised 2000 RYGB patients over the period 1998–2001 [19]. There were 63 cases and 66 IH in total (3 cases had hernia in multiple sites), with the most common site of herniation being the transverse mesocolon (67%), followed by the jejunal mesentery (21%), and Petersen's space (7.5%). The authors documented a progressive decline in the incidence of IH throughout the duration of this study. The second study by Paroz et al. included 607 patients who underwent RYGB between 1999 and 2006 [20]. There were 25 cases of IH, 2 immediate postoperative and 23 late. In contradistinction to the study of Higa et al., the authors of this study found a peak of IH incidence at 36 months and a mean time of presentation at 29 months postoperatively, followed by a progressive decline toward the end of the study at 72 months. Additionally, the most common site was the jejuno-jejunal window (56%), followed by Petersen's space (27%), and mesocolic window (17%). By contrast to both of these studies, a more recent research showed that Petersen's space is the most common site of IH (67.6%), followed by jejuno-jejunal window (24.3%), whereas multi-site hernia incidence was as high as 8.1% [21]. This indicates that not only is hernia post-MBS a heterogeneous topic, but there is inherent heterogeneity in the specific subcategories depending on each study period, which may reflect changes in surgical technique.

With regards to pathophysiology of IH, RYGB has been the most extensively studied bariatric operation because it entails a multitude of bowel loop mobilizations, dissections, and thus potential herniation sites, and also because it used to be the most commonly performed bariatric operation globally until recently [22]. The most common IH sites following RYGB include: 1) the *transmesocolic* window (when a transmesocolic Roux limb is fashioned), which is surrounded by the incised transverse mesocolon, thus allowing passage of the ascending Roux limb; 2) *Petersen's* window (or *retro-alimentary limb* space), which is defined by the transverse mesocolon posteriorly and the mesojejunum of the Roux limb anteriorly, and is located just caudally to the Roux limb's passage through the transmesocolic window (if one exists); 3) the *mesojejunal* window (or Brolin's space), which is defined by the mesojejunum of the biliopancreatic limb lying anteriorly and the mesojejunum of the Roux limb lying posteriorly; and 4) the *jejuno-jejunal* window, which is located between the Roux limb and the distal part of the biliopancreatic loop [23–26] (**Figures 1–3**). Complex hernias and hernias concomitant with volvulus and intussusception have also been described [19, 27, 28].

2.2 Prevention of internal hernia following RYGB

Considering prevention, the two major areas of debate are the construction of the Roux limb in an antecolic versus retrocolic fashion, and the closure versus non-closure of the mesenteric defects. Currently, the trend is to create the Roux limb in an antecolic fashion and close all mesenteric defects. This was first supported in a meta-analysis of 45 articles by Geubbels et al., which included a cumulative number of 31,320 post-RYGB individuals [29]. IH with the antecolic approach without defect closure yielded a 95% CI of 0.02 [0.01–0.03] in the random-effects model (I^2 91.3%), while the respective figures were 0.03 [0.02–0.05] (I^2 90.0%) for the antecolic approach with closure of only the mesojejunum, and 0.01 [0–0.03] (I^2 85.4%) for the antecolic approach with closure of all deficits. These results have recently been validated, in a comprehensive review by Vilallonga et al. [30].

The main advantages of an antecolic Roux (alimentary) limb are that there is one defect less in total and that the risk of mesocolic stenosis is non-existent. This comes at a cost of increased distance and increased tension at the gastro-jejunal anastomosis, which in turn may lead to a high incidence of leaks and strictures. However, fashioning an antecolic Roux limb may not be always technically feasible, especially in cases of short mesojejunum and thick mesocolon. In such cases, the creation of a transmesocolic window is mandatory and this essentially leads to one additional defect, which in turn potentially increases the relevant risks of IH

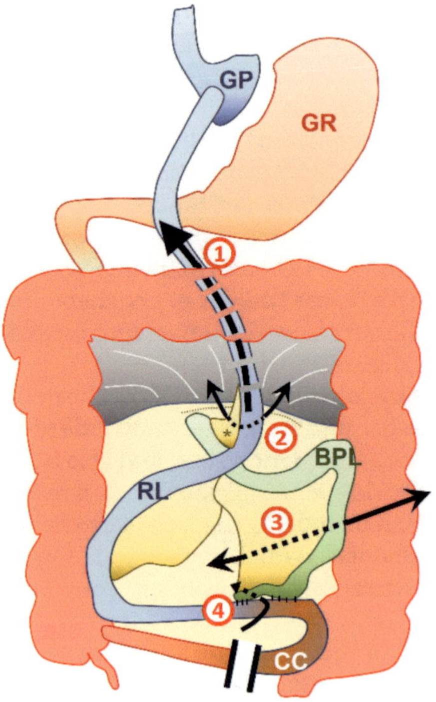

Figure 1.
Schematic representation of potential sites of internal herniation following Roux-en-Y gastric bypass. 1) Transmesocolic window. This potential site of internal herniation exists only if a transmesocolic Roux limb has been fashioned, which nowadays happens in the minority of the cases. 2) Petersen's window (or retro-alimentary limb space) defined by the transverse mesocolon posteriorly (dotted line) and the mesojejunum (asterisk) of the Roux limb anteriorly. 3) Mesojejunal window (or Brolin's space) defined by the mesojejunum of the biliopancreatic limb anteriorly and the mesojejunum of the Roux limb posteriorly. 4) Jejuno-jejunal window, between the Roux limb the biliopancreatic limb. For details, please refer to the text. GP – Gastric pouch; GR – Gastric remnant; RL – Roux limb; CC – Common channel. Vector graphic designed by Athanasios Pantelis.

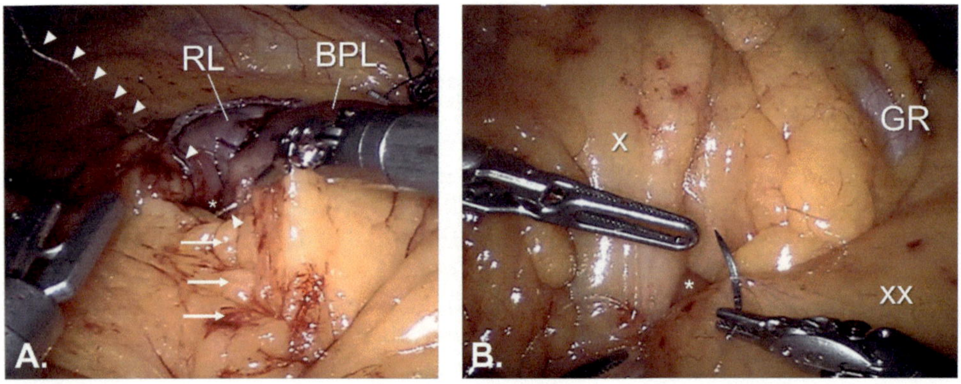

Figure 2.
Closure of internal defects in a case of robotic RYGB. A. Closure of the jejuno-jejunal defect (indicated by an asterisk), in continuity to closure of the mesojejunal defect (not clearly visible due to transparent suture material, trajectory indicated by arrows). The arrowheads indicate the course of the suture thread. RL – Roux limb; BPL – Biliopancreatic limb. B. Closure of Petersen's defect (indicated by an asterisk). The symbol "x" indicates the mesentery of the Roux limb and the symbol "xx" indicates the transverse mesocolon. GR – Gastric remnant. Images courtesy of Dr. Mohit Bhandari, archives of Mohak bariatrics and robotics, Indore, MP, India.

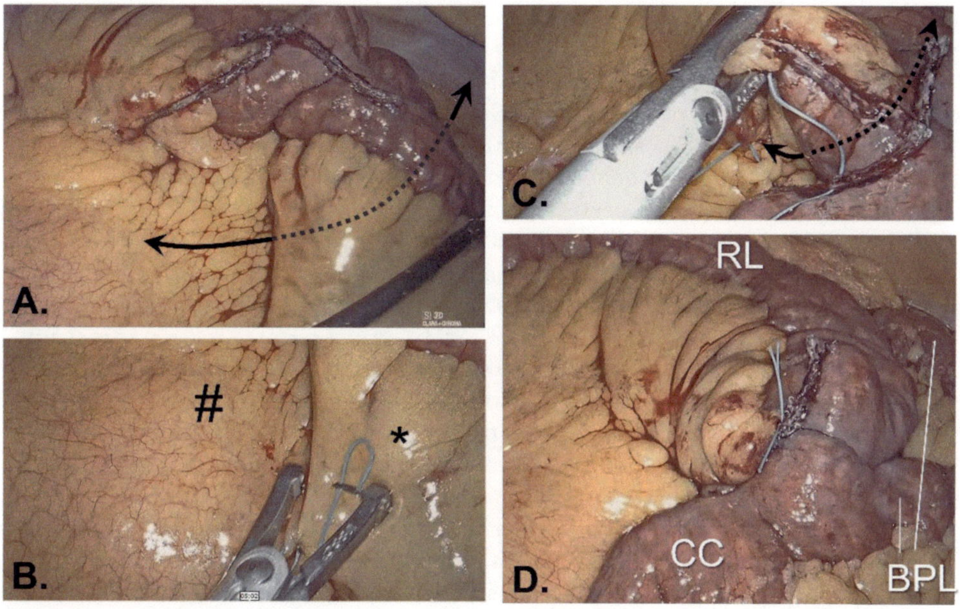

Figure 3.
The bariatric surgeon should be considerate of internal defects not only at primary operations, but also at reoperations. A case of type 1 biliopancreatic limb distalization due to weight regain following banded RYGB. A. the mesenteric defect. The principle of closing any potential site of internal herniation is common between primary and revisional bariatric surgery. B. the process of closing the defect with non-absorbable suture. The hashtag signifies the mesentery of the Roux limb, while the asterisk indicates the jejunal mesentery. C. the same suture is used in continuity in order to close the jejuno-jejunal defect created between the Roux limb and the biliopancreatic limb. D. the final picture after the closure of defects. RL – Roux limb; BPL – Biliopancreatic limb; CC – Common channel. Images courtesy of Dr. Mohit Bhandari, archives of Mohak bariatrics and robotics, Indore, MP, India.

and mesenteric stenosis [31]. Challenging this statement, in a large cohort of 1500 patients post-RYBG, Ribeiro-Parenti et al. compared antecolic versus retrocolic RYGB group and found that the latter had a significantly lower gastro-jejunal stricture rate, with no increased risk of IH, provided that the mesenteric defect was closed [32]. The risk for IH was greater for both groups in the first 4 postoperative months (maximum 4.5% in the antecolic group and < 1% in the retrocolic group), while the risk for gastro-jejunal stricture ranging approximately 25–35% for the antecolic group versus <15% in the retrocolic group, depending on the timing post-operatively. In total, there were 20 cases of IH in the antecolic group [12 without closure of defects (10.9%) and 8 with closure of all defects (1.7%)] and 11 cases in the retrocolic group (1.2%, all mesenteric defects closed in all cases). At a higher level of evidence, two meta-analyses have attempted to unravel the relationship between IH and positioning of the Roux limb. The first meta-analysis by Al Harakeh et al. included 4 studies in each group (antecolic vs. mesocolic), with 4805 vs. 2238 patients, respectively [31]. Mesenteric defects were closed in 45% of cases in each group. The antecolic group had an incidence of 1.4% regarding SBO vs. 5.2% in the retrocolic group ($p < 0.001$), whereas the respective incidences for IH were 1.3% vs. 2.3% ($p < 0.001$). The second meta-analysis by Rondelli et al. included 7 retrospective studies and 3 prospective ones [33]. In the retrospective wing, the results did not demonstrate statistical significance for any group [95% CI = 3.49 (0.71, 17.19), p 0.12] and were highly heterogeneous (I^2 88%), but the prospective wing showed a statistically significant superiority of antecolic versus retrocolic Roux limb fashioning with regards to IH prevention [95% CI = 5.95 (1.35, 26.19), p 0.02], accompanied by moderate heterogeneity (I^2 47%). In brief, it can be concluded that when performing RYGB, an antecolic Roux limb is advised when this is technically feasible, otherwise in the case of transmesocolic fashioning of the limb the mesocolic defect should be closed.

The other hot topic on IH prevention is defect closure. In a recent study of 2093 RYGB cases, Amor et al. compared a cohort of 1676 patients who underwent defect closure (period: 2005–2013) with 421 historic controls without defect closure (period: 1998–2004) [34]. The former group comprised 13 IH cases versus 7 cases in the non-closure group (0.78% vs. 1.66%, respectively; p 0.0021). In this study, both mesenteric (jejuno-jejunal) and Petersen's defects were closed. In another recent study by Blockhuys et al. of 3124 post-RYGB patients, subgroup analysis showed that closure of both defects led to a proportion of cases without hernia of >99% (incidence 1.15%), which plateaued less than 1.5 year postoperatively [35]. On the contrary, the respective proportion after closing only the mesenteric defect was 96–97% (incidence 2.58%) and the plateau took place after approximately 4 years postoperatively. Cumulatively, this strong evidence led Ianelli et al. to reasonably question whether routine closure of defects should still be a matter of debate [36], a viewpoint shared by most bariatric surgeons. Challenging this tenet, Nuytens et al. retrospectively studied post-RYGB patients, categorizing them into 3 cohorts [37]. The first included 724 without closure, the second comprised 640 patients in whom only the mesenteric defect was closed, and the third consisted of 139 patients who had both of their defects closed. Indeed, there was a decreasing incidence of IH across groups (71.4% vs. 48% vs. 42.9%, respectively), however the authors documented an inversely increasing incidence of adhesions (21.4% in group 1 vs. 48% in group 2 vs. 57.1% in group 3), a phenomenon which negated the beneficial effects of closing the defects. This article raised a heated discussion, with authors commenting that these results could be attributed to confounding factors, technical issues, and lead time or follow-up bias [38–41]. Another important factor that needs to be taken into consideration is the risk of reopening of the mesenteric defects, presumably due to rapid weight loss and loosening of the mesenteric sutures, as it has recently been stressed out by Lazaridis et al., underlining that it may affect almost half of the cases in the long run despite routine closure [42]. Thus, the question should not be whether the mesenteric defects should be closed, but what should be the optimal method of closure (loose running sutures vs. tight approximation with barbed sutures, the place of biocompatible glues, the benefits of endoscopic suturing devices etc.) [36, 41, 43].

Given the variability of outcomes regarding IH post-RYGB, which is partly attributable to the large variation in IH definition, and in an attempt to homogenize data and reporting, two main classification systems have been developed [44]. The one is AMSTERDAM classification proposed by Geubbels et al. and is based on purely clinical criteria (presence of IH, presence of other pathology, remission of complains post-laparoscopy, etiology of symptoms) [45]. The other is the SDL (space - direction - limb) classification system, and, as indicated by the acronym, the criteria include predominantly anatomical definitions: P (Petersen's) and/or B (Brolin's) regarding space; L (right-to-left) or R (left-to-right) regarding direction; and A (alimentary), B (biliopancreatic), C (common channel), and/or E (entero-enterostomy/emergency), regarding limb [46]. A detailed analysis of these classification systems is beyond the scope of this chapter, nevertheless their implementation could benefit standardization and this in turn would result in research and practices of higher quality.

2.3 Diagnostic aspects

The diagnosis of IH post-RYGB is notoriously challenging, because the symptoms may be non-specific and the patient may have been experiencing them over a long period. A high index of suspicion should be kept in any post-bariatric patient, particularly during the first 1–3 years postoperatively and in cases of massive or excessive weight loss. Imaging studies may be helpful especially during exacerbations of symptoms. Even in this case, the differential between IH and adhesions may be difficult. Moreover, in up to 20% of patients with IH, imaging studies are non-diagnostic or even normal.

In the seminal study by Higa et al., the cases of frank bowel obstruction constituted 52.3% of IH cases, followed by non-specific abdominal pain (41.3%), whereas a striking 6.3% of patients were totally asymptomatic [19]. In the other seminal study by Paroz et al., all patients with IH had experienced colicky pains, both in the elective and in the acute setting, whereas only 20% had nausea and/or vomiting in the elective setting, in contrast to 50% of patients with IH presenting acutely [20]. In a more recent study, acute abdominal pain was the first manifestation of IH for 75.7% of patients, followed by chronic abdominal pain (16.2%), and ischemic bowel necrosis (8.1%) [21]. In a recent study by Tartamella et al., the clinical features that differed significantly between IH cases (IH) and positive controls (PC) were the quality of pain (colicky: IH 31%, PC 19%, p 0.008, continuous: IH 69%, PC 12.5%, p 0.024), the intensity of pain according to the visual analogic scale (mean value for IH 8.9, mean PC 6.2, p 0.0049), and the use of analgesics (IH 100%, PC 18.7%, $p < 0.0001$) [47]. Most importantly, there was a significant correlation between excess weight loss (EWL) at 3 months postoperatively and occurrence of IH after RYGB as compared to controls (p 0.002). The difference in correlation with EWL between IH cases and controls was dampened over time.

The clinician is advised to pay attention to details, as this may facilitate the origin of IH. Internal herniation of the biliopancreatic is expected to manifest as closed-loop syndrome, with a distended gastric remnant and possibly referred left shoulder pain secondary to irritation of the diaphragm, tachycardia, or eructation [44]. Conversely, obstruction of the alimentary (Roux) limb may lead to clinical presentation more typical of SBO (nausea, vomiting, retention of gas and feces). Laboratory tests should also be critically appraised, as an elevation of amylase or lipase (in the range of hundreds instead of thousands) may falsely direct diagnostic rationale toward pathologies of pancreatic or biliary origin [44].

Imaging with CT scan may be a useful adjunct in the diagnosis of IH. There is a constellation of eponymous and characteristic imaging findings: *mesenteric swirl*, which carries great variability in terms of sensitivity (61–100%) and specificity (67–94%), and also depends on the degree of swirling ($<90^{\circ}$ practically precludes IH, whereas $>270^{\circ}$ is diagnostic in almost 100% of cases); the *mushroom* sign; the *eye of the storm*; a collapsed Roux limb anterior to a dilated loop of small bowel; an intestinal loop anterior to the superior mesenteric artery; a jejuno-jejunostomy located to the right of the midline; a tassel of intestinal loops aggregated in a specific space within the abdominal cavity; remarkable dilatation of the stomach with gastric content (in cases of IH involving the Roux limb); and so forth. In a retrospective review of 594 patients who had undergone antecolic RYGB, Al-Mansour et al. showed that mesenteric swirl was the most prevalent finding (55.6%), followed by bowel dilatation/obstruction (25%), mesenteric edema, and free abdominal fluid (11.1% each) [21]. Interestingly, in 16.7% of patients no abnormal sign could be retrieved.

Recently, a panel of experts issued a bundle of guidelines, based on the Operative management in Bariatric Acute Abdomen (OBA) Survey outcomes (the OBA guidelines) [48]. Most recommendations are based on low quality of evidence, nevertheless this is one of the first comprehensive attempts and could be utilized as a roadmap for future research and care pathways. According to the OBA guidelines, tachycardia ≥110 bpm, fever ≥38°C, hypotension, respiratory distress with tachypnea and hypoxia, and decreased urine output, altogether constitute alarming clinical signs in patients presenting with acute abdominal pain and a previous history of bariatric surgery. Additionally, persistent nausea and vomiting are alarming clinical signs for IH, volvulus, and gastrointestinal stenosis, among other entities. They also state that the most common clinical presentation of IH post-RYGB is acute onset, crampy/colicky epigastric pain. Besides, the triad of persistent epigastric pain, pregnancy, and a history of RYGB should prompt further evaluation for IH. Regarding lab investigations, there is no diagnostic biological marker, but high CRP and leukocytosis may serve as predictors of abdominal emergencies in general post-RYGB. Finally, the use of contrast-enhanced CT with oral contrast is strongly recommended, whenever possible and in suitable patients (i.e. non-pregnant, hemodynamically stable). Nevertheless, no investigation should delay surgical exploration in the presence of high index of suspicion and alarming clinical symptoms and signs, regardless of the findings of imaging studies.

2.4 Management

The cornerstones of treating IH after bariatric surgery are a high index of clinical suspicion based on a detailed history and prompt reduction of an incarcerated internal hernia before bowel ischemia settles in. It is also very important to determine which operation has been performed, because, for instance, RYGB is much more likely to be associated with IH as compared to sleeve gastrectomy.

A critical decision that the surgeon is called to make is the operative approach. In a cohort of 166 patients, Ianelli et al. reported laparoscopic access in 142 cases (85.5%) versus open in 24 cases (14.5%). Henceforth, the majority of published series of explorations for IH have implemented the laparoscopic approach. This is reflected in the recent OBA guidelines as well, which dictate exploratory laparoscopy in the first 24–48 hours in stable patients with abdominal pain and inconclusive clinical and radiological data [48]. Furthermore, exploration should proceed in a systematic distal-to-proximal fashion [ileo-cecal valve→ jejuno-jejunostomy→ mesojejunal space→ Petersen's space→ transverse mesocolon (in cases of retrocolic RYGB)→ remnant stomach] [48]. If an IH is found, the next step should be the assessment of the viability of the involved bowel. In cases of ischemic necrosis, the least possible enterectomy should be undertaken, followed by anastomosis of well-perfused bowel ends. A useful adjunct for assessing the viability of the remnant bowel could be Indocyanine (ICG) Fluorescence Angiography, although the doses, timing, and routes of administration have not been standardized yet. Closure of all mesenteric defects with non-absorbable sutures (running or interrupted) is *sine qua non*.

The flowchart in **Figure** 4 summarizes the general principles of IH management following RYGB in the form of an algorithmic flowchart.

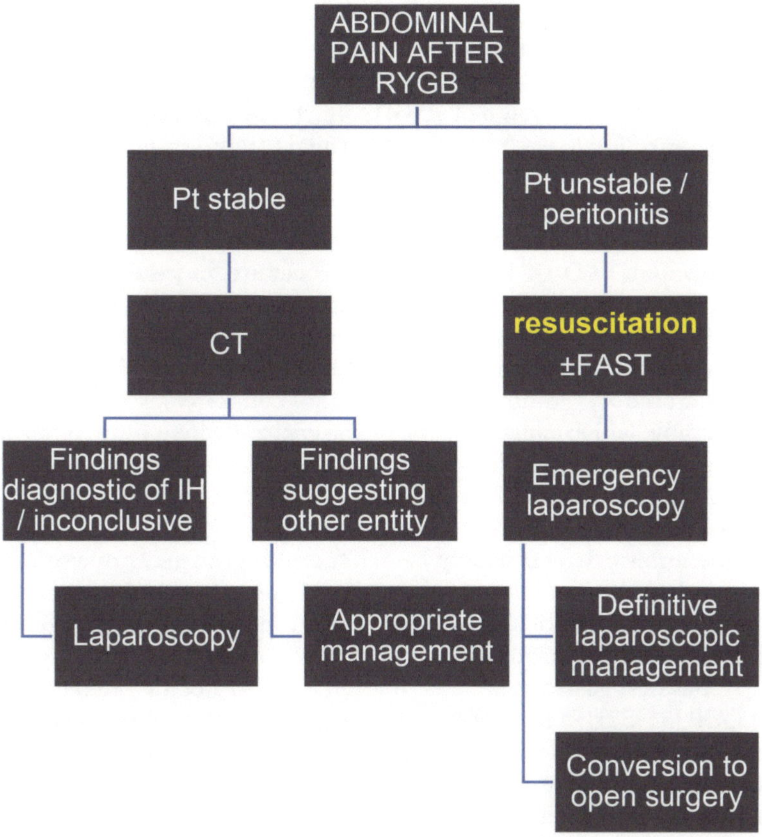

Figure 4.
A proposed algorithm outlining the principles for managing internal hernia after Roux-en-Y gastric bypass. Key: RYGB – Roux-en-Y gastric bypass; pt. – Patient; IH – Internal hernia; FAST – Focused assessment with sonography for trauma (bedside assessment for free intra-abdominal fluid).

2.5 Internal hernia following bariatric surgery other than RYGB

Although RYGB is the bariatric operation most associated with IH, it is not the only one. There have been reports of IH following Biliopancreatic Diversion with Duodenal Switch (BPD-DS), one-anastomosis/mini gastric bypass (OAGB/MGB), and single anastomosis duodeno-jejunostomy with sleeve (SADI-S). There have also been counter-intuitive associations of IH with bariatric operations such as Adjustable Gastric Band (LAGB) and Greater Curvature Plication (LGCP). Relevant reports are expected to multiply in the future, as new techniques arise and as the number of reoperations increases.

OAGB/MGB is a simplified version of RYGB, in the context of which one anastomosis (and consequently one defect) is spared. The first report of IH post-OAGB/MGB was published in 2016 [49]. In 2017, Carbajo, the inspirer of OAGB, reported an incidence of 0.26% regarding SBO and 0% regarding IH in his series of 1200 OAGB cases [50]. One year later, however, Kamal Mahawar stressed out that IH post-OAGB/MGB may be more common than previously reported [51]. Indeed, OAGB/MGB has less defects than RYGB, but Petersen's hernia may occur. More recently, the analysis of a large series of 3368 consecutive OAGB patients yielded an incidence of IH as high as 2.8% [52]. This is particularly important, in view of the fact that OAGB/MGB is continuously gaining ground over RYGB as being technically more feasible, safer, and equally effective with regards to weight loss and remission of associated disease.

If OAGB is a simplified version of RYGB, then SADI-S is a simplified version of BPD-DS. Classical BPD-DS is nowadays performed rarely, because, despite its excellent bariatric outcomes, it was accompanied by a multitude of long-term complications principally owing to malabsorption and micronutrient deficiencies. However, it is not that rare for a surgeon to come across an old case of BPD-DS, or for a bariatric surgeon to implement BPD-DS as a revisional procedure for insufficient weight loss or weight regain. Summerhays et al. presented a case of IH after revisional laparoscopic loop DS [53]. The patient presented on the 64th postoperative day with mid- and left-sided abdominal pain and the CT scan revealed non-specific findings. Upon exploratory laparoscopy, the authors noted an 180° counterclockwise twist of the duodenal ileostomy, which caused rolling of the entire afferent limb underneath the anastomosis and over the right side of the abdominal cavity. More recently, Al-Tai et al. published a series of 121 DS operations (92 standard DS and 29 SADI-S) [54]. The incidence of IH was 5% (6 patients), all cases belonging to the group of standard DS with the mesenteric defects having been left open at the index operation.

IH after non-bypass procedures is even less common, but the incidence is not null. Hamed et al. gleaned the published literature of IH secondary to tubing problems, i.e. intestinal loops tangled around the gastric band, leading to IH, strangulation, and volvulus [55]. Besides, gastro-gastric herniation is a well-documented complication following LGCP [56, 57]. In this case, there is segmental herniation of the gastric wall between plication sutures secondary to increased intraluminal pressures. The take-home message is that IH may complicate any bariatric operation that may potentially lead to the creation of anatomic spaces.

3. Abdominal wall hernia complicating metabolic bariatric surgery

The main focus of this section shall be Trocar Site Hernias (TSH – **Figure 5A**). According to a meta-analysis of 22 studies, the pooled median prevalence of TSH after laparoscopic surgery is 0.5% (range 0–5.2%, 95% CI 0.3–0.9) [58]. Obesity itself is commonly considered a predisposing factor for TSH, but the evidence is conflicting [59, 60].

TSH is a true yet underestimated complication after MBS, according to most authors. The first thing one needs to determine is the definition of TSH. Clinical symptoms may be feeble, vague, or even absent and clinical examination is notoriously misleading in post-bariatric individuals, for reasons of altered anatomical correlations, lipodystrophy of the subcutaneous adipose tissue, skin shagging, etc. In a recent study, Karampinis et al. attempted to systematize the diagnosis of TSH by means of Ultrasonography (USG), in a single-center cohort of 365 patients who had been operated over a 10-year period [61]. The incidence of TSH detected by USG in this series was 34%. Even though USG is a non-invasive, reproducible method without exposure to radiation, its implementation as a screening tool in this setting may lack cost-effectiveness and feasibility due to suboptimal adherence to follow-up on behalf of the patients. The same group of authors had performed a systematic review and meta-analysis one year earlier and found a pooled TSH incidence of 3.22% (range 0–39.2) among 68 studies that had met the inclusion criteria [62]. Overall, this evidence shows that THS may be much more common than originally thought.

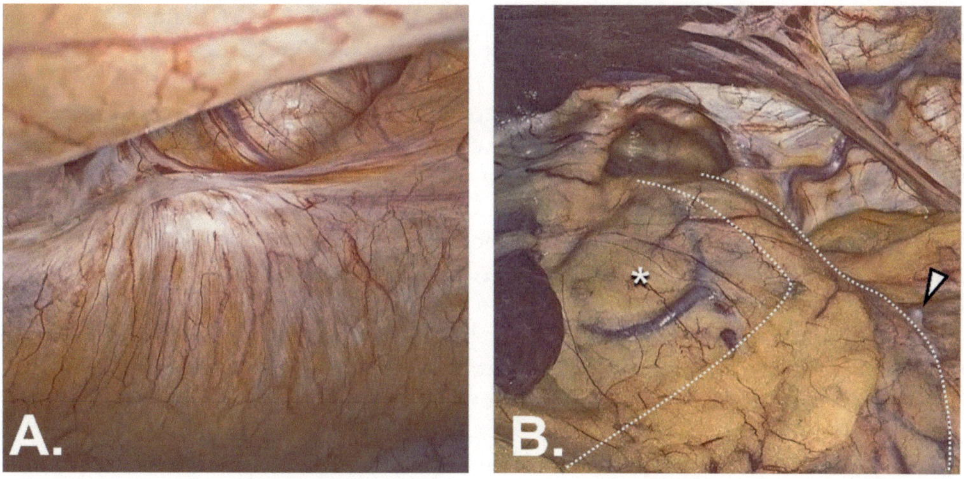

Figure 5.
A. a case of trocar site hernia (TSH) 1.5 year following single-incision sleeve gastrectomy (SILS-LSG). B. In the same patient, hiatal hernia (HH) was found incidentally during laparoscopy. This is considered a large defect of approximately 4 cm. Notably, the patient did not report any acid reflux symptoms preoperatively. Dashed lines indicate the contour of the gastric sleeve. The asterisk signifies the hepatogastric ligament, within which the course of left gastric vascular axis is clearly visible. The arrowhead points at a suture remnant that had been used to imbricate the staple line at the index operation.

Given the high incidence of TSH post-MBS and the sequelae this may potentially have, the area of debate that naturally follows is whether the trocar sites should be closed or not. Port site closure refers to fascial closure. In general, small port sizes are less likely to be associated with TSH. Conversely, according to a recent international Delphi consensus, the panel provided strong recommendation for closure of all 15 mm port sites and advised considering fascial closure for 10–12 mm ports [63]. Additionally, they recommended against drain placement through ≥10 mm sites, because this practice increases the risk of TSH after removal of the drain [63]. Beyond diameter, the type of trocars may also play its role. Bladeless trocars are thought to be associated with less risk of TSH compared to cutting ones, nevertheless there has been evidence that challenges this statement [64, 65]. Specifically regarding bariatric surgery, in a series of 624 procedures without fascial closure, Pilone et al. reported a TSH prevalence of 1.6% [66]. For LSG and BPD (totally 82 procedures) they used two 5 mm trocars and three 10–12 mm, whereas for LAGB (542 procedures) they used two 5 mm trocars, one 10–12 mm trocar, and one 15 mm trocar. Furthermore, in a meta-analysis of 36 relevant studies, the incidence for TSH after RYGB was 0.4% for fascial non-closure and 1.1% for closure ($p < 0.05$), the respective figures after LAGB were 0.4% versus 0.8% (p 0.54), and the overall TSH incidence was 0.4% vs. 1% ($p < 0.05$) [67]. More recently, in the meta-analysis of Karampinis et al., the incidence of TSH after weighting the included studies was 1.13% for fascia closure versus 0.77% for no closure, but this difference was statistically non-significant [62]. Analyzing their own series one year later, the same authors confirmed a non-significant difference in the incidence of TSH between fascial closure and non-closure (37% vs. 34%, p 0.37), with the additional disadvantage of a statistically significant elongation of operative time in the fascial closure arm [61].

Basta et al. developed a risk-stratification predictive model for TSH based upon 2161 bariatric operations with a total TSH incidence of 2.4% [68]. This study highlighted the following risk factors: open approach (hazard ratio [HR] = 10.3), malnutrition (HR = 3.10), prior abdominal surgery (HR = 2.89), and BMI >60 Kg/m^2 (HR = 2.60). The patients were stratified into low-, moderate-, and high-risk accordingly. The incidence of TSH in the low-risk group was 0.6%, whereas the respective incidence in the high-risk group was 15.2%. Such models need further clinical validation, which will confirm their usefulness for preventing TSH as adjuncts in the decision-making process.

Among the factors predisposing to hernia, obesity has been recognized as one of the most consistent ones, resulting in an increased risk for both primary and incisional hernia [69]. A detailed reference to Abdominal Wall Hernia (AWH) repair in the context of MBS is beyond the scope of this chapter, nevertheless we shall provide a general outline for the purpose of comprehensively covering the topic of hernia post-MBS. According to a recent comprehensive review by Vilallonga et al., when obesity and AWH co-exist there are 3 options regarding operative strategy [70]:

- First perform the MBS (with or without reduction of the hernia contents) and then proceed to AWH repair. Interestingly, the risk of SBO in case of reduction might be as high as 35.7% [71], whereas without reduction the respective risk is 0–5% [72].

- First perform AWH repair and then proceed to MBS. Beyond the technical difficulties that this approach may present, there is also an increased risk of surgical site infection (2–26%) and recurrence (5.5–44.4%), depending on the timing of the bariatric operation.

- Perform AWH repair and MBS simultaneously. The advantage of this single-stage approach is that the anesthetic risk is minimized. From a technical point of view, hernia repair in this context can be done in 3 different ways: If primary closure of the hernia defect is performed, the risk of SBO is 2.6%, while the risk of recurrence is as high as 25.7% [73]. If a synthetic mesh is applied, the risk of SBO minimizes to 0–0.6%, and this is also true regarding recurrence (0.6–6.6%) [74, 75]. Finally, if a biological mesh is implemented, the risk of SBO practically disappears, whereas the risk of recurrence is 14.3%.

According to a consensus joint statement issued by the American Society for Metabolic and Bariatric Surgery (ASMBS) and American Hernia Society (AHS) in 2018, management should depend on whether both obesity and AWH are amenable to laparoscopic repair [69]. If they are, then a combined approach is recommended, whereas if they are not, a staged approach is encouraged, where weight loss should take place before AWH repair, either surgically or non-operatively (very low/low-calorie diet, lifestyle modifications, pharmacotherapy, endoscopically). This will presumably render the patient fit for hernia repair surgery, while minimizing peri-operative risk and optimizing postoperative outcomes at the same time. In any case, further research is necessary, given that relevant evidence is still weak, based primarily on retrospective study designs.

4. Hiatal hernia following metabolic bariatric surgery

Hiatal Hernia (HH) after MBS is the least studied category, and the main reason is the lack of concrete definition. One must be very careful when evaluating the incidence of HH after MBS, in that it should be clear whether HH pre-existed bariatric surgery or it is a true case of *de novo* HH post-MBS. This is particularly relevant in view of the fact that obesity is an independent risk factor for HH and that the prevalence of HH in individuals living with obesity is as high as 40% [76, 77]. Preoperative diagnosis of HH is strongly recommended by experts, with routine upper gastrointestinal endoscopy plus manometry in selected patients with positive screening demonstrating a sensitivity of 100% for diagnosing HH and a negative predictive value of 95% [78, 79]. Besides, although HH and Gastroesophageal Reflux Disease (GERD) are closely interconnected, they should not be used interchangeably. Consequently, clinical symptomatology and ensuing diagnosis of HH may not be straightforward, both in the pre- and the post-MBS setting.

4.1 Hiatal hernia and sleeve migration following sleeve gastrectomy

Saba et al. attempted to map the incidence of *de novo* hiatal hernia following LSG in a cohort of 74 patients [80]. HH was defined surgically by measuring the crura after the completion of LSG. HH was present at the time of surgery in 37 patients (72.5%), whereas only 24 patients (47.1%) had been diagnosed with GERD preoperatively. GERD was documented in 56.8% of patients with HH versus 21.4% of patients without HH (p 0.01). HH post-LSG was observed in 60% of patients with a follow-up of <18 months, whereas the respective prevalence in patients with >18 months of follow-up was 80% (p 0.02). In other words, the risk of developing HH after LSG increased over time. More recently, Almutairi et al. published a series of 142 post-LSG patients who were followed up for 24 months [81]. Interestingly, the incidence of GERD was 33.1%, whereas that of de novo HH was only 3.5%. **Figure 5B** depicts one such case of *de novo* HH post-LSG.

An entity closely associated with HH, which is recognized with increasing frequency after LSG, is Intrathoracic (or trans-hiatal) Sleeve Migration (ITSM) [82–84]. Termine et al. published their experience with ITSM in a series of 1954 post-LSG patients with a minimum follow-up of 24 months [85]. The incidence of ITSM was 7% within a mean period of 24.16 ± 13.6 months. Patients with GERD due to ITSM who did not respond to conservative treatment were converted to RYGB with posterior cruroplasty (n = 15, 16%). Most importantly, surgeons are advised to keep a high index of suspicion, as this complication may present in the acute setting, in the immediate and short-term postoperative period (within 2 weeks of LSG) [84–86]. Clinical presentation may range from intolerance of oral intake, nausea, and vomiting to a dramatic symptomatology of gastric incarceration, with severe dehydration, electrolyte disturbances, and sepsis.

4.2 Hiatal hernia after Roux-en-Y gastric bypass

The evidence on HH post-RYGB is based on case reports and case series, among which the largest one includes 7 patients [87–90]. In this context, HH constitutes a late complication, with patients presenting 2–14 years following the index RYGB procedure. Several mechanisms have been proposed to contribute to this condition, including rapid weight loss after MBS which is associated with relaxation of the phrenoesophageal ligament of Laimer and widening of the hiatus, creation of a large pouch with an ensuing higher intragastric pressure, extended dissection of the cardia and the left crus, or a small pre-existing hernia that enlarges over time [90–92].

4.3 Hiatal hernia after gastric banding

In the section of internal hernia (§ 2.5), we mentioned published cases of visceral entanglement around adjustable gastric bands. Another relevant complication of gastric banding is worth mentioning in this section, that of gastric necrosis due to paraesophageal (type II) hernia [93]. In this case report, it is not clear whether the gastric band was responsible for the herniation itself or contributed only to the inability of the stomach to resume its anatomical position within the abdominal cavity. In any case, no generalizations can be made on the basis of one case report. On the other hand, a high index of suspicion should be reserved in all post-bariatric patients, regardless of the specific type of operation.

5. Conclusions

Hernia after metabolic bariatric surgery is a heterogeneous group of complications. Based on bibliographic records, internal hernias are the most common. Regarding internal hernias, the closure of all defects after Roux-en-Y gastric bypass is highly recommended. With the advent of one-anastomosis gastric bypass the risk for internal herniation is lower but not null. For trocar site hernia prevention, fascial closure has not proven its advantage over non-closure. Lastly, regarding hiatal hernia, its documentation before any bariatric operation is of paramount importance, for this is the only way to distinguish between pre-existing and *de novo* hernias.

Acknowledgements

Special thanks to Dr. Winnie Mathur for her valuable insight and for her suggestions regarding the Figures.

Special thanks to Ashish Rajvaidya for contributing substantially to this chapter with his skills in retrieval of cases and video editing.

Author details

Athanasios Pantelis* and Mohit Bhandari
Mohak Bariatrics and Robotics, Indore, Madhya Pradesh, India

*Address all correspondence to: ath.pantelis@gmail.com

References

[1] Martins C, Strømmen M, Stavne OA, Nossum R, Mårvik R, Kulseng B. Bariatric surgery versus lifestyle interventions for morbid obesity--changes in body weight, risk factors and comorbidities at 1 year. Obesity Surgery. 2011;**21**(7):841-849. DOI: 10.1007/s11695-010-0131-1

[2] Courcoulas AP et al. Three-year outcomes of bariatric surgery vs lifestyle intervention for type 2 diabetes mellitus treatment: A randomized clinical trial. JAMA Surgery. 2015;**150**(10):931-940. DOI: 10.1001/jamasurg.2015.1534

[3] Cummings DE et al. Gastric bypass surgery vs intensive lifestyle and medical intervention for type 2 diabetes: The CROSSROADS randomised controlled trial. Diabetologia. 2016;**59**(5):945-953. DOI: 10.1007/s00125-016-3903-x

[4] Schauer PR et al. Bariatric surgery versus intensive medical therapy for diabetes — 5-year outcomes. The New England Journal of Medicine. 2017;**376**(7):641-651. DOI: 10.1056/NEJMoa1600869

[5] Courcoulas AP et al. Bariatric surgery vs lifestyle intervention for diabetes treatment: 5-year outcomes from a randomized trial. The Journal of Clinical Endocrinology and Metabolism. 2020;**105**(3):866-876. DOI: 10.1210/clinem/dgaa006

[6] Kirwan JP et al. Diabetes remission in the Alliance of randomized trials of medicine versus metabolic surgery in type 2 diabetes (ARMMS-T2D). Diabetes Care. 2022;**45**(7):1574-1583. DOI: 10 .2337/dc21-2441

[7] Arterburn DE, Telem DA, Kushner RF, Courcoulas AP. Benefits and risks of bariatric surgery in adults: A review. JAMA. 2020;**324**(9):879-887. DOI: 10.1001/jama.2020.12567

[8] Goldberg I et al. Safety of bariatric surgery in patients older than 65 years. Surgery for Obesity and Related Diseases: Official Journal of the American Society for Metabolic and Bariatric Surgery. 2019;**15**(8):1380-1387. DOI: 10.1016/j.soard.2019.05.016

[9] Singhal R et al. 30-day morbidity and mortality of bariatric metabolic surgery in adolescence during the COVID-19 pandemic - the GENEVA study. Pediatric Obesity. 2021;**16**(12):e12832. DOI: 10.1111/ijpo.12832

[10] Singhal R et al. Safety of bariatric surgery in ≥ 65-year-old patients during the COVID-19 pandemic. Obesity Surgery. 2022;**32**(7):1-13. DOI: 10.1007/s11695-022-06067-z

[11] Singhal R et al. 30-day morbidity and mortality of bariatric surgery during the COVID-19 pandemic: A multinational cohort study of 7704 patients from 42 countries. Obesity Surgery. 2021;**31**(10):4272-4288. DOI: 10.1007/s11695-021-05493-9

[12] Ruzieh M et al. Safety of bariatric surgery in patients with coronary artery disease. Surgery for Obesity and Related Diseases: Official Journal of the American Society for Metabolic and Bariatric Surgery. 2020;**16**(12):2031-2037. DOI: 10.1016/j.soard.2020.07.015

[13] Kassir R et al. Complications of bariatric surgery: Presentation and emergency management. International Journal of Surgery London England. 2016;**27**:77-81. DOI: 10.1016/j.ijsu.2016.01.067

[14] Chang S-H et al. Early major complications after bariatric surgery in the United States, 2003-2014: A systematic review and meta-analysis. Obesity Reviews: Official Journal of International Association Study Obesity. 2018;**19**(4):529-537. DOI: 10.1111/obr.12647

[15] Incisional Hernia: Pathogenesis and Clinical Findings | Calgary Guide. 2019. https://calgaryguide.ucalgary.ca/incisional-hernia-pathogenesis-and-clinical-findings/ [Accessed: February 14, 2023]

[16] Healy P, Clarke C, Reynolds I, Arumugasamy M, McNamara D. 'Complications of bariatric surgery-What the general surgeon needs to know'. The Surgeon: Journal of the Royal Colleges of Surgeons of Edinburgh. 2016;**14**(2):91-98. DOI: 10.1016/j.surge.2015.08.003

[17] Contival N, Menahem B, Gautier T, Le Roux Y, Alves A. Guiding the non-bariatric surgeon through complications of bariatric surgery. Journal of Visceral Surgery. 2018;**155**(1):27-40. DOI: 10.1016/j.jviscsurg.2017.10.012

[18] Koppman JS, Li C, Gandsas A. Small bowel obstruction after laparoscopic Roux-en-Y gastric bypass: A review of 9,527 patients. Journal of the American College of Surgeons. 2008;**206**(3):571-584. DOI: 10.1016/j.jamcollsurg.2007.10.008

[19] Higa KD, Ho T, Boone KB. Internal hernias after laparoscopic Roux-en-Y gastric bypass: Incidence, treatment and prevention. Obesity Surgery. 2003;**13**(3):350-354. DOI: 10.1381/096089203765887642

[20] Paroz A, Calmes JM, Giusti V, Suter M. Internal hernia after laparoscopic Roux-en-Y gastric bypass for morbid obesity: A continuous challenge in bariatric surgery. Obesity Surgery. 2006;**16**(11):1482-1487. DOI: 10.1381/096089206778870102

[21] Al-Mansour MR, Mundy R, Canoy JM, Dulaimy K, Kuhn JN, Romanelli J. Internal hernia after laparoscopic Antecolic Roux-en-Y gastric bypass. Obesity Surgery. 2015;**25**(11):2106-2111. DOI: 10.1007/s11695-015-1672-0

[22] Welbourn R et al. Bariatric-metabolic surgery utilisation in patients with and without diabetes: Data from the IFSO global registry 2015-2018. Obesity Surgery. 2021;**31**(6):2391-2400. DOI: 10.1007/s11695-021-05280-6

[23] O'Rourke RW. Management strategies for internal hernia after gastric bypass. Journal of Gastrointestinal Surgery: Official Journal of Society Surgery Alimentary Tract. 2011;**15**(6):1049-1054. DOI: 10.1007/s11605-010-1401-x

[24] Kawkabani Marchini A et al. The four different types of internal hernia occurring after laparascopic Roux-en-Y gastric bypass performed for morbid obesity: Are there any multidetector computed tomography (MDCT) features permitting their distinction? Obesity Surgery. 2011;**21**(4):506-516. DOI: 10.1007/s11695-011-0364-7

[25] Paroz A, Calmes JM, Romy S, Giusti V, Suter M. A new type of internal hernia after laparoscopic Roux-en-Y gastric bypass. Obesity Surgery. 2009;**19**(4):527-530. DOI: 10.1007/s11695-008-9770-x

[26] Dar R, Dola T, Sakran N. Biliopancreatic limb obstruction due to an unexpected variant of internal hernia after Roux-en-Y gastric bypass. Obesity Surgery. 2020;**30**(12):5184-5185. DOI: 10.1007/s11695-020-04992-5

[27] Elkbuli A, Santarone K, Kinslow K, McKenney M, Boneva D. A rare case of internal hernia, intussusception and volvulus following gastric bypass: A case report and literature review. International Journal of Surgery Case Reports. 2020;**67**:178-182. DOI: 10.1016/j.ijscr.2020.01.060

[28] Zheng X et al. Case report: An unusual complex internal hernia after Roux-en-Y gastric bypass. Obesity Surgery. 2021;**31**(4):1833-1835. DOI: 10.1007/s11695-020-05060-8

[29] Geubbels N, Lijftogt N, Fiocco M, van Leersum NJ, Wouters MWJM, de Brauw LM. Meta-analysis of internal herniation after gastric bypass surgery. The British Journal of Surgery. 2015;**102**(5):451-460. DOI: 10.1002/bjs.9738

[30] Vilallonga R. Internal hernia after bariatric surgery: A comprehensive review. Journal of Surgery Research and Practice. 2022;**3**(3):1-7. DOI: 10.46889/JSRP.2022.3302

[31] Al Harakeh AB, Kallies KJ, Borgert AJ, Kothari SN. Bowel obstruction rates in antecolic/antegastric versus retrocolic/retrogastric Roux limb gastric bypass: A meta-analysis. Surgery for Obesity and Related Diseases: Official Journal of the American Society for Metabolic and Bariatric Surgery. 2016;**12**(1):194-198. DOI: 10.1016/j.soard.2015.02.004

[32] Ribeiro-Parenti L, Arapis K, Chosidow D, Dumont J-L, Demetriou M, Marmuse J-P. Gastrojejunostomy stricture rate: Comparison between antecolic and retrocolic laparoscopic Roux-en-Y gastric bypass. Surgery for Obesity and Related Diseases: Official Journal of the American Society for Metabolic and Bariatric Surgery. 2015;**11**(5):1076-1084. DOI: 10.1016/j.soard.2015.01.019

[33] Rondelli F et al. Antecolic or Retrocolic alimentary limb in laparoscopic Roux-en-Y gastric bypass? A meta-analysis. Obesity Surgery. 2016;**26**(1):182-195. DOI: 10.1007/s11695-015-1918-x

[34] Amor IB et al. Impact of mesenteric defect closure during laparoscopic Roux-en-Y gastric bypass (LRYGB): A retrospective study for a Total of 2093 LRYGB. Obesity Surgery. 2019;**29**(10):3342-3347. DOI: 10.1007/s11695-019-04000-5

[35] Blockhuys M, Gypen B, Heyman S, Valk J, van Sprundel F, Hendrickx L. Internal hernia after laparoscopic gastric bypass: Effect of closure of the Petersen defect - single-Center study. Obesity Surgery. 2019;**29**(1):70-75. DOI: 10.1007/s11695-018-3472-9

[36] Iannelli A, Sebastianelli L, Schneck A-S. Internal hernia and Roux-en-Y gastric bypass: Should the routine closure of defects still Be a matter of debate? Obesity Surgery. 2019;**29**(8):2614-2615. DOI: 10.1007/s11695-019-03846-z

[37] Nuytens F et al. Closure of mesenteric defects is associated with a higher incidence of small bowel obstruction due to adhesions after laparoscopic antecolic Roux-en-y gastric bypass: A retrospective cohort study. International Journal of Surgery London England. 2019;**71**:149-155. DOI: 10.1016/j.ijsu.2019.09.017

[38] Al Motlaq AA, Al Saleh K. Commentary on: "Closure of mesenteric defects is associated with a higher incidence of small bowel obstruction due to adhesions after laparoscopic ante colic Roux-en-Y gastric bypass: A retrospective cohort study". International Journal of Surgery London England. 2019;**72**:32-33. DOI: 10.1016/j.ijsu.2019.10.016

[39] Alkatary M. An invited commentary on "closure of mesenteric defects is associated with a higher incidence of small bowel obstruction due to adhesions after laparoscopic antecolic Roux-en-Y gastric bypass: A retrospective cohort study" (Int J Surg 2019; 17:149-155). International Journal of Surgery London England. 2020;**77**:119. DOI: 10.1016/j.ijsu.2020.03.011

[40] Gould L, Parmar C. A commentary on "closure of mesenteric defects is associated with a higher incidence of small bowel obstruction due to adhesions after laparoscopic antecolic Roux-en-y gastric bypass: A retrospective cohort study" (Int J Surg 2019 Oct. Epub ahead of print). International Journal of Surgery London England. 2019;**72**:55-56. DOI: 10.1016/j.ijsu.2019.10.011

[41] Sami S, Brown LR. Commentary: "Closure of mesenteric defects is associated with a higher incidence of small bowel obstruction due to adhesions after laparoscopic antecolic Roux-en-y gastric bypass". International Journal of Surgery. 2019;**71**:174. DOI: 10.1016/j.ijsu.2019.10.005

[42] Lazaridis II, Köstler T, Kübler L, Zingg U, Delko T. Risk of reopening of the mesenteric defects after routine closure in laparoscopic Roux-en-Y gastric bypass: A single-Centre experience. Obesity Surgery. 2022;**32**(9):2853-2859. DOI: 10.1007/s11695-022-06179-6

[43] Aghajani E, Jacobsen HJ, Nergaard BJ, Hedenbro JL, Leifson BG, Gislason H. Internal hernia after gastric bypass: A new and simplified technique for laparoscopic primary closure of the mesenteric defects. Journal of Gastrointestinal Surgery. 2012;**16**(3):641-645. DOI: 10.1007/s11605-011-1790-5

[44] Pokala B, Giannopoulos S, Stefanidis D. Prevention and management of internal hernias after bariatric surgery: An expert review. Mini-Invasive Surgery. 2022;**6**:23. DOI: 10.20517/2574-1225.2021.136

[45] Geubbels N, Röell EA, Acherman YIZ, Bruin SC, van de Laar AWJM, de Brauw LM. Internal herniation after laparoscopic Roux-en-Y gastric bypass surgery: Pitfalls in diagnosing and the introduction of the AMSTERDAM classification. Obesity Surgery. 2016;**26**(8):1859-1866. DOI: 10.1007/s11695-015-2028-5

[46] Karcz WK et al. 'Modification of internal hernia classification system after laparoscopic Roux-en-Y bariatric surgery', Wideochirurgia Inne tech. Maloinwazyjne Videosurgery Miniinvasive Technology. 2015;**10**(2):197-204. DOI: 10.5114/wiitm.2015.52160

[47] Tartamella F et al. Abdominal pain and internal hernias after Roux-en-Y gastric bypass: Are we dealing with the tip of an iceberg? Acta Biomedica Atenei Parmensis. 2019;**90**(2):251-258. DOI: 10.23750/abm.v90i2.7145

[48] De Simone B et al. Operative management of acute abdomen after bariatric surgery in the emergency setting: The OBA guidelines. World Journal of Emerging Surgery WJES. 2022;**17**(1):51. DOI: 10.1186/s13017-022-00452-w

[49] Kular KS et al. Petersen's hernia after mini (one anastomosis) gastric bypass. Journal of Visceral Surgery. 2016;**153**(4):321. DOI: 10.1016/j.jviscsurg.2016.05.010

[50] Carbajo MA, Luque-de-León E, Jiménez JM, Ortiz-de-Solórzano J, Pérez-Miranda M, Castro-Alija MJ. Laparoscopic one-anastomosis gastric bypass: Technique, results, and long-term follow-up

in 1200 patients. Obesity Surgery. 2017;**27**(5):1153-1167. DOI: 10.1007/s11695-016-2428-1

[51] Mahawar KK. Petersen's hernia may be commoner after OAGB/MGB than previously reported. Obesity Surgery. 2018;**28**(1):257-258. DOI: 10.1007/s11695-017-3001-2

[52] Petrucciani N et al. Internal hernia after one anastomosis gastric bypass (OAGB): Lessons learned from a retrospective series of 3368 consecutive patients undergoing OAGB with a biliopancreatic limb of 150 cm. Obesity Surgery. 2021;**31**(6):2537-2544. DOI: 10.1007/s11695-021-05269-1

[53] Summerhays C, Cottam D, Cottam A. Internal hernia after revisional laparoscopic loop duodenal switch surgery. Surgery for Obesity and Related Diseases: Official Journal of the American Society for Metabolic and Bariatric Surgery. 2016;**12**(1):e13-e15. DOI: 10.1016/j.soard.2015.08.510

[54] Al-Tai SS, Axer SS, Hoffmann L. Internal hernia after duodenal switch. Surgery for Obesity and Related Diseases. 2018;**14**(11):S120. DOI: 10.1016/j.soard.2018.09.259

[55] Hamed OH, Simpson L, Lomenzo E, Kligman MD. Internal hernia due to adjustable gastric band tubing: Review of the literature and illustrative case video. Surgical Endoscopy. 2013;**27**(11):4378-4382. DOI: 10.1007/s00464-013-3024-2

[56] Hii M, Clarke N, Hopkins G. Gastrogastric herniation: An unusual complication following greater curve plication for the treatment of morbid obesity. Annals of the Royal College of Surgeons of England. 2012;**94**(2):e76-e78. DOI: 10.1308/003588412X1317 1221588695

[57] Chang P-C, Dev A, Katakwar A, Hsin M-C, Tai C-M, Huang C-K. Management of gastric fold herniation after laparoscopic adjustable gastric banded plication: A single-center experience. Surgery for Obesity and Related Diseases: Official Journal of the American Society for Metabolic and Bariatric Surgery. 2016;**12**(4):849-855. DOI: 10.1016/j.soard.2016.02.017

[58] Swank HA, Mulder IM, la Chapelle CF, Reitsma JB, Lange JF, Bemelman WA. Systematic review of trocar-site hernia. The British Journal of Surgery. 2012;**99**(3):315-323. DOI: 10.1002/bjs.7836

[59] Hy U et al. Trocar site hernia after laparoscopic cholecystectomy. Journal of Laparoendoscopic & Advanced Surgical Techniques. Part A. 2007;**17**(5):600-603. DOI: 10.1089/ lap.2006.0182

[60] Mayol J, Garcia-Aguilar J, Ortiz-Oshiro E, De-Diego Carmona JA, Fernandez-Represa JA. Risks of the minimal access approach for laparoscopic surgery: Multivariate analysis of morbidity related to umbilical trocar insertion. World Journal of Surgery. 1997;**21**(5):529-533. DOI: 10.1007/pl00012281

[61] Karampinis I et al. Trocar site HERnias after bariatric laparoscopic surgery (HERBALS): A prospective cohort study. Obesity Surgery. 2020;**30**(5):1820-1826. DOI: 10.1007/s11695-020-04400-y

[62] Karampinis I et al. Trocar site hernias in bariatric surgery-an underestimated issue: A qualitative systematic review and meta-analysis. Obesity Surgery. 2019;**29**(3):1049-1057. DOI: 10.1007/s11695-018-03687-2

[63] Omar I et al. The first international Delphi consensus statement on

laparoscopic gastrointestinal surgery. International Journal of Surgery London England. 2022;**104**:106766. DOI: 10.1016/j.ijsu.2022.106766

[64] Chiong E, Hegarty PK, Davis JW, Kamat AM, Pisters LL, Matin SF. Port-site hernias occurring after the use of bladeless radially expanding trocars. Urology. 2010;**75**(3):574-580. DOI: 10.1016/j.urology.2009.08.025

[65] Lee J, Zheng XJ, Ng CY. Trocar site hernias from using bladeless trocars: Should fascial closure be performed? Journal of Surgical Case Reports. 2014;**2014**(5):rju044. DOI: 10.1093/jscr/rju044

[66] Pilone V et al. Trocar site hernia after bariatric surgery: Our experience without fascial closure. International Journal of Surgery London England. 2014;**12**(Suppl 1):S83-S86. DOI: 10.1016/j.ijsu.2014.05.047

[67] Coblijn UK, de Raaff CAL, van Wagensveld BA, van Tets WF, de Castro SMM. Trocar port hernias after bariatric surgery. Obesity Surgery. 2016;**26**(3):546-551. DOI: 10.1007/s11695-015-1779-3

[68] Basta MN, Mirzabeigi MN, Shubinets V, Kelz RR, Williams NN, Fischer JP. Predicting incisional hernia after bariatric surgery: A risk stratification model based upon 2161 operations. Surgery for Obesity and Related Diseases: Official Journal of the American Society for Metabolic and Bariatric Surgery. 2016;**12**(8):1466-1473. DOI: 10.1016/j.soard.2016.03.022

[69] Menzo EL, Hinojosa M, Carbonell A, Krpata D, Carter J, Rogers AM. American Society for Metabolic and Bariatric Surgery and American hernia society consensus guideline on bariatric surgery and hernia surgery. Surgery for Obesity and Related Diseases: Official Journal of the American Society for Metabolic and Bariatric Surgery. 2018;**14**(9):1221-1232. DOI: 10.1016/j.soard.2018.07.005

[70] Vilallonga R et al. Abdominal Wall hernia and metabolic bariatric surgery. Journal of Laparoendoscopic & Advanced Surgical Techniques. Part A. 2020;**30**(8):891-895. DOI: 10.1089/lap.2020.0257

[71] Eid GM et al. Repair of ventral hernias in morbidly obese patients undergoing laparoscopic gastric bypass should not be deferred. Surgical Endoscopy. 2004;**18**(2):207-210. DOI: 10.1007/s00464-003-8915-1

[72] Datta T, Eid G, Nahmias N, Dallal RM. Management of ventral hernias during laparoscopic gastric bypass. Surgery for Obesity and Related Diseases: Official Journal of the American Society for Metabolic and Bariatric Surgery. 2008;**4**(6):754-757. DOI: 10.1016/j.soard.2008.03.246

[73] Lazzati A, Nassif GB, Paolino L. Concomitant ventral hernia repair and bariatric surgery: A systematic review. Obesity Surgery. 2018;**28**(9):2949-2955. DOI: 10.1007/s11695-018-3366-x

[74] Praveen Raj P, Bhattacharya S, Saravana Kumar S, Parthasarathi R, Cumar B, Palanivelu C. Morbid obesity with ventral hernia: Is concomitant bariatric surgery with laparoscopic ventral hernia mesh repair the best approach? An experience of over 150 cases. Surgery for Obesity and Related Diseases: Official Journal of the American Society for Metabolic and Bariatric Surgery. 2019;**15**(7):1098-1103. DOI: 10.1016/j.soard.2019.04.027

[75] Marzouk AMSM, Ali HOE. Laparoscopic ventral hernia repair combined with sleeve gastrectomy

in morbidly obese patients: Early outcomes. Surgery Journal (New York, N.Y.). 2019;**5**(3):e87-e91. DOI: 10.1055/s-0039-1694979

[76] Wilson LJ, Ma W, Hirschowitz BI. Association of obesity with hiatal hernia and esophagitis. The American Journal of Gastroenterology. 1999;**94**(10):2840-2844. DOI: 10.1111/j.1572-0241.1999.01426.x

[77] Che F, Nguyen B, Cohen A, Nguyen NT. Prevalence of hiatal hernia in the morbidly obese. Surgery for Obesity and Related Diseases: Official Journal of the American Society for Metabolic and Bariatric Surgery. 2013;**9**(6):920-924. DOI: 10.1016/j.soard.2013.03.013

[78] Schneider R, Lazaridis I, Kraljević M, Beglinger C, Wölnerhanssen B, Peterli R. The impact of preoperative investigations on the management of bariatric patients; results of a cohort of more than 1200 cases. Surgery for Obesity and Related Diseases: Official Journal of the American Society for Metabolic and Bariatric Surgery. 2018;**14**(5):693-699. DOI: 10.1016/j.soard.2018.01.009

[79] Santonicola A et al. Hiatal hernia diagnosis prospectively assessed in obese patients before bariatric surgery: Accuracy of high-resolution manometry taking intraoperative diagnosis as reference standard. Surgical Endoscopy. 2020;**34**(3):1150-1156. DOI: 10.1007/s00464-019-06865-0

[80] Saba J, Bravo M, Rivas E, Fernández R, Pérez-Castilla A, Zajjur J. Incidence of de novo hiatal hernia after laparoscopic sleeve gastrectomy. Obesity Surgery. 2020;**30**(10):3730-3734. DOI: 10.1007/s11695-020-04742-7

[81] Almutairi BF, Aldulami AB, Yamani NM. Gastroesophageal reflux disease and hiatal hernia after laparoscopic sleeve gastrectomy: A retrospective cohort study. Cureus. 2022;**14**(3):e23024. DOI: 10.7759/cureus.23024

[82] Amor IB, Debs T, Kassir R, Anty R, Amor VB, Gugenheim J. De novo hiatal hernia of the gastric tube after sleeve gastrectomy. International Journal of Surgery Case Reports. 2015;**15**:78-80. DOI: 10.1016/j.ijscr.2015.08.029

[83] Alwatari Y, Roriz-Silva R, Bolckmans R, Campos GM. Intrathoracic sleeve gastrectomy migration with gastric volvulus treated with laparoscopic repair and conversion to gastric bypass. Journal of Surgical Case Reports. 2020;**2020**(8):rjaa234. DOI: 10.1093/jscr/rjaa234

[84] Meknat A, Fernandez-Ranvier G, Hariri K, Guevara DE, Beitner M, HerronDM.Intrathoracicsleevemigrations after sleeve gastrectomy: A compilation of case reports. Journal of Laparoendoscopic & Advanced Surgical Techniques. Part A. 2020;**30**(9):1013-1017. DOI: 10.1089/lap.2020.0237

[85] Termine P et al. Transhiatal migration after laparoscopic sleeve gastrectomy: Myth or reality? A Multicenter, retrospective study on the incidence and clinical impact. Obesity Surgery. 2021;**31**(8):3419-3426. DOI: 10.1007/s11695-021-05340-x

[86] Pavelko Y, Bustos R, Gruessner S, Hassan C. Acute hiatal hernia with incarcerated proximal half of recent sleeve gastrectomy: Super rare complication. Obesity Surgery. 2021;**31**(1):469-471. DOI: 10.1007/s11695-020-05101-2

[87] Iannelli A, Kassir R, Schneck A-S, Martini F, Gugenheim J. Hiatal hernia of the Roux-en-Y gastric bypass pouch

8 years after surgery. Obesity Surgery. 2014;**24**(9):1494-1496. DOI: 10.1007/s11695-014-1360-5

[88] Clapp B et al. Late-term hiatal hernia after gastric bypass: An emerging problem. Surgery for Obesity and Related Diseases: Official Journal of the American Society for Metabolic and Bariatric Surgery. 2020;**16**(4):471-475. DOI: 10.1016/j.soard.2020.01.018

[89] Guglielmetti LC, Wyss R, Biraima M, Misirlic M, Peros G. Diaphragmatic hernia after laparoscopic gastric bypass surgery. Obesity Surgery. 2020;**30**(5):2069-2070. DOI: 10.1007/s11695-020-04495-3

[90] Thomopoulos T, FitzGerald M, Mantziari S, Demartines N, Suter M. Management of a Late-Term Hiatal Hernia with intrathoracic pouch migration after Roux-en-Y gastric bypass. Obesity Surgery. 2022;**32**(3):957-958. DOI: 10.1007/s11695-021-05881-1

[91] Griffith PS, Birch DW, Sharma AM, Karmali S. Managing complications associated with laparoscopic Roux-en-Y gastric bypass for morbid obesity. Canadian Journal of Surgery Journal of Canadian Chiropractic. 2012;**55**(5):329-336. DOI: 10.1503/cjs.002011

[92] Santonicola A, Angrisani L, Cutolo P, Formisano G, Iovino P. The effect of laparoscopic sleeve gastrectomy with or without hiatal hernia repair on gastroesophageal reflux disease in obese patients. Surgery for Obesity and Related Diseases: Official Journal of the American Society for Metabolic and Bariatric Surgery. 2014;**10**(2):250-255. DOI: 10.1016/j.soard.2013.09.006

[93] Oztürk A, Necati T, Faruk AÖ. Gastric necrosis due to type II paraesophageal hernia in obese patient with gastric band: Rescue sleeve gastrectomy. Surgery for Obesity and Related Diseases: Official Journal of the American Society for Metabolic and Bariatric Surgery. 2011;**7**(3):330-331. DOI: 10.1016/j.soard.2010.08.003

Chapter 7

Hiatal Hernia Surgery

Igors Ivanovs

Abstract

Hiatal hernia is a protrusion of abdominal organs through enlarged esophageal hiatus. Hiatal hernia is a relatively common pathology but, in most cases, it remains asymptomatic. Four types of hiatal hernia exist. Type I or sliding hernia, type II or true paraesophageal hernia, type III or mixed hernia and type IV or giant hernia. Diagnosis of hiatal hernia usually is done by upper endoscopy and upper gastrointestinal (GI) barium examination. Treatment of hiatal hernia type I coincides with concomitant gastroesophageal reflux treatment, while treatment of hiatal hernia type II, III and IV is mainly surgical. The surgical approach to repair hiatal hernia could be either transabdominal or transthoracic. Currently, laparoscopy is the best method for hiatal hernia repair. Surgery consists of two main steps: hiatal hernia plasty and fundoplication. Despite modern technologies the recurrence rate in large hiatal hernia repair remains high, therefore reinforcement of the diaphragm with mesh is recommended. There are controversies about the materials and techniques used.

Keywords: hiatal hernia, paraesophageal hernia, diaphragmatic hernia, fundoplication, laparoscopic surgery

1. Introduction

Hiatal Hernia (HH) is a protrusion of abdominal organs into the thoracic cavity through an enlarged esophageal hiatus. Most HH are asymptomatic, therefore the exact incidence of HH is difficult to determine. It is estimated that HH prevalence in western populations is about 15 to 20% [1]. Risk factors for HH are obesity, elevated intra-abdominal pressure and increasing age. The pathogenesis of HH is still not very clear [2]. Four types of HH are defined by gastroesophageal junction (GEJ) and stomach localization. Type I or sliding hernia when GEJ "migrates or slides off" into the mediastinum, type II or true paraesophageal hernia—when GEJ is intra-abdominal, but stomach fundus is above diaphragm, type III is mixed hernia—the combination of the previous two types and type IV is giant hernia. Type I (sliding) of HH is the most common type, involving about 90–95%. HH type I is mostly asymptomatic. If symptoms exist, they coincide with concomitant Gastroesophageal Reflux Disease (GERD) symptoms. Treatment of HH type I is based on GERD treatment and indication for surgery depends on GERD. HH type II, III and IV are Paraesophageal Hernias (PEH) and are more dangerous than type I because of the possibility of strangulation. They are estimated to occur in only 5–10% of all HH cases [3]. Symptoms of PEH are connected not only with GERD symptoms, but also with the hernia volume effect on intrathoracic organs—the respiratory system, cardiovascular system and the esophagus. The patient could complain of dysphagia, dyspnea, or arrhythmias etc. However, many PEH are without symptoms—it is estimated that only about 50% of PEH are symptomatic [4]. Surgery is usually indicated in symptomatic PEH. Laparoscopic transabdominal access is currently the best option for HH repair. Even huge PEH can be operated laparoscopically with good results, controversies exist regarding surgical methods and materials. This chapter summarizes the latest information about surgical treatment of HH.

2. Classification

Hiatal hernias (HH) are divided into four types:

Type I (sliding HH) – characterized by displacement of the gastroesophageal junction (GEJ) > 2 cm above the diaphragm (**Figure 1**).

This type of HH is seen most in clinical practice.

Type II (true paraesophageal hernia) – is characterized by a defect in the Phrenoesophageal Membrane (PEM) where the gastric fundus migrates above the diaphragm. In this pathology, the GEJ remains in its correct intra-abdominal position (**Figure 2**).

Type III (mixed paraesophageal hernia) – is characterized by a combination of both previous types—type I and type II. In this situation, both the GEJ and the gastric fundus (or body and even antrum—depending on HH size) migrate above the diaphragm into the thoracic cavity (**Figure 3**).

Type IV (giant paraesophageal hernia) – is characterized by a large defect in the PEM, where not only is the stomach located above the diaphragm, but also other intra-abdominal organs (e.g., the colon, spleen, pancreas and small intestines etc.) (**Figure 4**).

Types II, III and IV are also named as paraesophageal hernias (PEH). HH type I and PEH differ in clinical presentation, complications and in management.

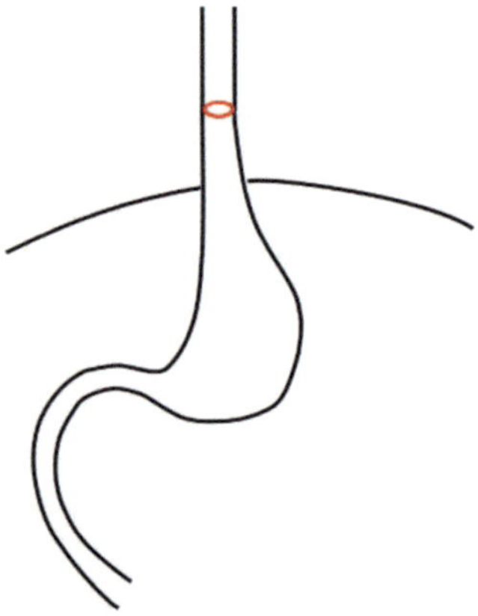

Figure 1.
Hiatal hernia type I. GEJ (red) is above the diaphragm.

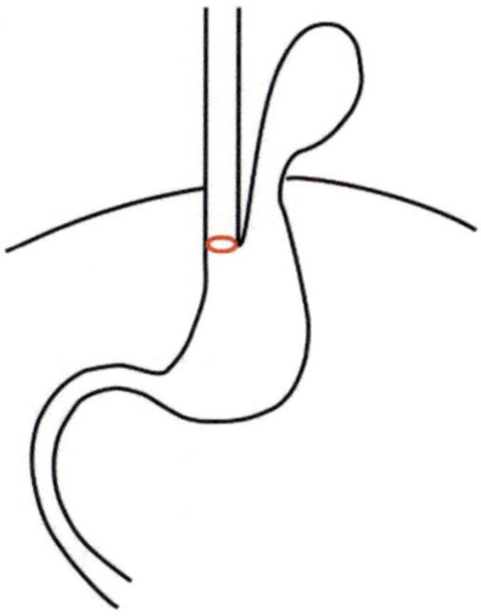

Figure 2.
Hiatal hernia type II. GEJ (red) is below the diaphragm.

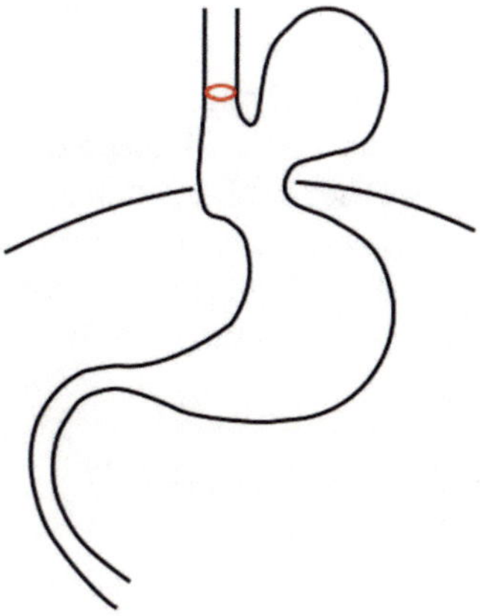

Figure 3.
Hiatal hernia type III.

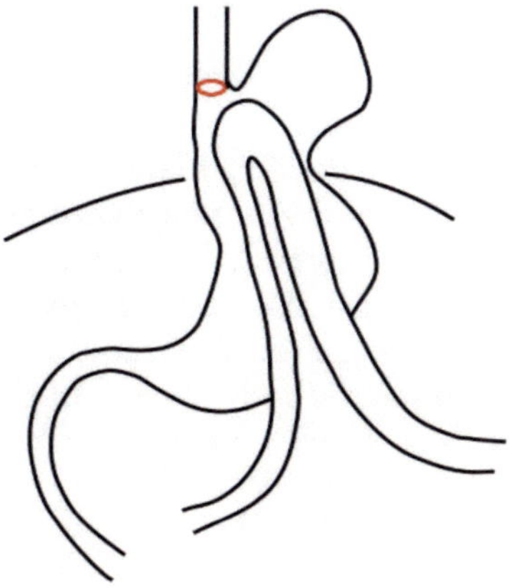

Figure 4.
Hiatal hernia type IV.

3. Clinical presentation

3.1 Sliding hiatal hernia (type I)

HH type I is often asymptomatic and found incidentally. If symptoms exist, they are associated with symptoms of GERD and could be categorized into typical and atypical symptoms.

Typical symptoms are heartburn, regurgitation, water brush, chest pain, dysphagia, belching and bloating. The most common signs are heartburn and regurgitation. Heartburn is described as a retrosternal burning sensation and refers to most specific symptoms of GERD. Regurgitation is described as food or gastric juice coming up from the stomach. GERD could cause erosions and ulcers in the esophagus. Chronic inflammation led to peptic strictures and Barrett's esophagus (when normal esophageal epithelium is replaced with metaplastic columnar cells). Patients with Barrett's esophagus have a higher risk of esophageal cancer development.

Atypical or extra-esophageal symptoms are hoarseness, throat pain, chronic cough, shortness of breath, asthma and dental erosion. The main reason for respiratory extra-esophageal symptoms is microaspiration of gastric content during reflux episodes. Dental erosions are the result of chemical irritation of the enamel by gastric acid [5]. Extra-esophageal symptoms are much more difficult to identify and diagnose because they could also have other causes, such as from pulmonary, dietary, or allergic conditions. Moreover, extra-esophageal symptoms do not often decrease with proton pump inhibitor therapy and can lead to other complications [6]. Therefore, if such symptoms cannot be explained by other pathology than GERD, it is an indication to proceed with surgical treatment.

3.2 Paraesophageal hiatal hernias (type II, III, IV)

PEH can be asymptomatic and have intermittent or constant symptoms. Most common symptoms of PEH are postprandial retrosternal pain, epigastric pain, fullness, retching, nausea, regurgitation. On the other hand, specific GERD symptoms like heartburn are less common. Compression of the mediastinum by an intrathoracic stomach can cause cardiac dysfunction—e.g., arrhythmias and respiratory dysfunction—dyspnea.

PEH can lead to acute problems due to mechanical obstruction in the stomach. The most common of such complications are:

Gastric volvulus – which occurs with large hiatal hernias, and can cause dysphagia, obstruction and even strangulation of the stomach with necrosis. Clinical signs are severe acute retrosternal or epigastric pain and vomiting [7].

Bleeding – usually from gastric erosions or ulcers caused by mechanical compression of the diaphragm. This pathology has a specific term—Cameron Lesions. A Cameron Lesion is an ulcer, localized to the gastric body mucosa in patients having PEH. It can cause acute upper GI bleeding or chronic GI bleeding with iron-deficiency anemia [8].

4. Diagnostic workup

The main option for HH diagnosis is barium swallow (**Figure 5**). This method provides the highest rate of hiatal hernia detection [9]. The method is very useful in clinical practice because of its simplicity and wide accessibility.

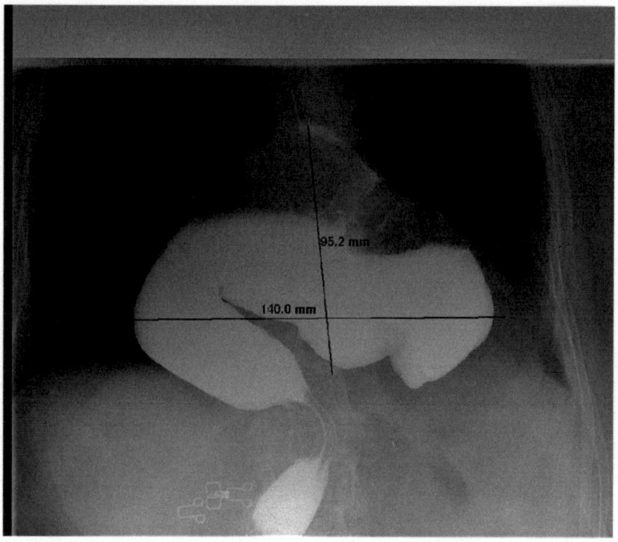

Figure 5.
Barium swallow shows large PEH with intrathoracic stomach localization.

Other diagnostic options include upper gastrointestinal (GI) endoscopy, Computed Tomography (CT), manometry and pH-metry.

Upper GI endoscopy is the obligatory diagnostic tool prior to hiatal hernia surgery. It provides visualization of mucosa in the esophagus and stomach, evaluation of possible lesions and defects. Biopsy helps to differentiate benign and malignant lesions as well as dysplasia or metaplasia. Unfortunately, recent studies show that upper endoscopy has less sensitivity for HH diagnosis and false positive results lead to overdiagnosis because of stomach distention during endoscopy [10].

Computed tomography is a good option to evaluate anatomical landmarks, size and position in PEH (**Figure 6**). CT images allow access to other pathologies outside PEH—e.g., masses in the thoracic and the abdominal cavity. CT helps to differentiate PEH from other pathologies, especially in symptomatic hernias. Although CT is not involved in standard workup, it is frequently used as an additional option prior to surgery [11]. CT may be especially useful in emergencies and for patients having suspected complications. In sliding HH, CT has limited additional information and is not routinely used.

High-Resolution Esophageal Manometry (HRM) uses a high-resolution catheter to measure intraluminal esophageal pressure. This method shows high sensitivity for HH diagnosis and helps to evaluate esophageal motility [12]. HRM plays a particularly crucial role prior to surgery in planning types of surgical treatment. HRM can be used to rule out motility disorders such as achalasia, which can mimic reflux. Unfortunately, this method is not generally available in clinical practice as HRM equipment is less accessible.

PH-metry is based on sensors placed in the esophagus. These sensors detect pH changes during a 24-hour period. This helps to detect and calculate acid refluxes in a 24-hour period, as well as to understand the connection between clinical symptoms and refluxes. PH-metry, before surgery, helps to differentiate "real" GERD from other similar conditions and avoid unnecessary operations. Recently a new method of Multichannel Intraluminal Impedance pH-metry (MII-pH) has been developed. Reflux monitoring

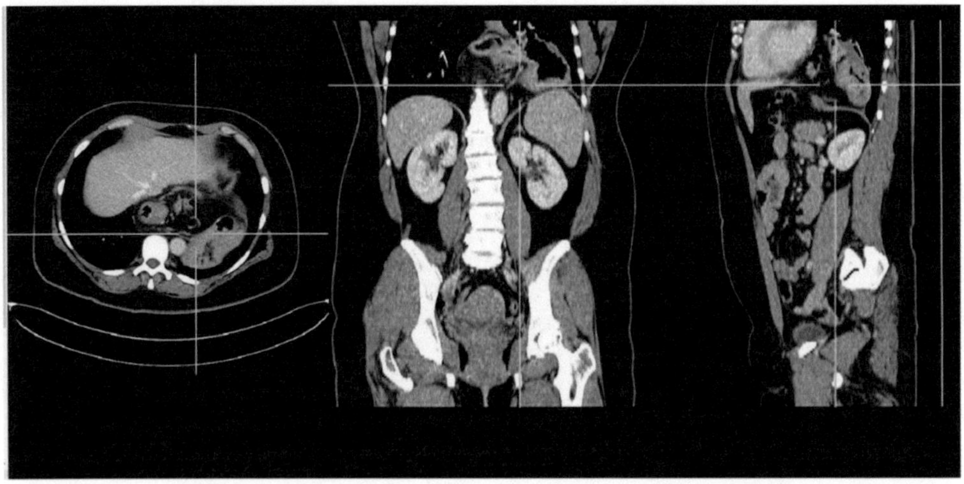

Figure 6.
Computed tomography of the PEH (3 projections). Most parts of the stomach are located above the diaphragm.

using MII-pH technology is a relatively new technique and is currently considered the "gold standard" for GERD diagnosis. The movement of intraesophageal fluids is detected by MII-pH by measuring differences in electrical conductivity. Thus MII-pH can detect both acid and non-acid refluxes [13]. As GERD is frequently combined with HH type I, this method is used for the standard diagnostic workup in HH type I. In HH type II, III, IV, reflux symptoms are less common. Consequently, the significance of MII-pH in PEH is reduced, as negative results do not change the management procedure.

5. Medical management

Treatment of GERD with sliding HH (type I) is mostly conservative and based on diet, lifestyle changes and medical therapy. The objective of this chapter is not to review principles of medical treatment. Readers are referred to other sources regarding this topic. Our goal is to review the principles of surgical therapy in HH.

6. Surgical management

6.1 Indications for surgery

6.1.1 Sliding hiatal hernia (type I)

Asymptomatic sliding HH does not require specific therapy or surgical repair [14]. Surgical therapy for HH type I should be considered for:

1. Patients who have objective diagnosis of GERD (based on preoperative evaluation) and have inadequate symptom control by medical therapy.

2. Extra-esophageal GERD complications (confirmed on preoperative evaluation and exuded other reasons).

3. Patients with GERD and severe peptic complications like recurrent esophageal ulcer, peptic stricture, Barrett's esophagus.

4. Patients with adequate control of GERD symptoms, but request surgery to avoid long-term prescription and side effects of medications.

6.1.2 Paraesophageal hiatal hernias (type II, III, IV)

Asymptomatic PEH, even large, is not an absolute indication for surgery [14]. The patient's age and comorbidities should be taken into consideration.

For such patients, the strategy called "watchful waiting" is reasonable, because the annual risk of strangulation is less than 2% [15]. However, elective procedures encounter much less mortality compared with emergency procedures which have an average mortality rate about 17% [15].

For symptomatic PEH, surgical therapy should be considered in all cases. Age should not be a barrier to repair symptomatic PEH [14].

6.2 Surgical approaches

There are three main surgical approaches for HH repair: laparoscopic (currently the best), open transabdominal, open transthoracic.

6.2.1 Laparoscopic approach

Laparoscopic HH repair has good postoperative results with low mortality and morbidity rate. Additional preferences of laparoscopy include shorter hospital stays, less postoperative pain and better cosmetic results. Nowadays laparoscopy is the preferred approach for most hiatal hernia repairs [14].

6.2.2 Open transabdominal approach

The open transabdominal approach has similar results with laparoscopy but has a higher morbidity rate and longer hospitalization. Based on this, an open approach is reserved for patients when laparoscopy is not possible or is technically challenging. Indications for open abdominal surgery include patients who have had multiple upper abdominal surgeries in the past, patients who cannot tolerate laparoscopy and for technical considerations (e.g., complicated PEH, emergency situations, lack of experience).

6.2.3 Open transthoracic approach

Open transthoracic approach involves the longest hospital stays, the greatest need for mechanical ventilation postoperatively and the greatest risk of pulmonary embolism [16]. The advantages of the transthoracic approach are better visualization and greater ease of performing esophageal mobilization and the procedure for esophageal-lengthening. Given that, the open transthoracic approach is reserved for patients with large PEH (type IV) who are not candidates for transabdominal repair. However, in experienced hands, the laparoscopic transabdominal approach has been successful also with patients having giant PEH (type IV).

6.3 Surgical techniques

Considering recommendations, the majority of HH should be treated laparoscopically. This chapter will address laparoscopic techniques. The principles of open surgery are similar.

6.3.1 Patient position and port placement

The patient is placed in a modified low lithotomy position. Attention should be taken to correct thigh position relative to patient body—thigh should be at the same level as anterior abdominal wall, not elevated above (**Figure 7**).

The surgeon stands between the patient's legs. The reversed Trendelenburg position is used to facilitate exposure of the diaphragm and to displace the stomach inferiorly. Five ports are used in standard situations: the camera port is placed 1–2 cm to the left of the midline and 8–10 cm below the sternum. The second port is placed at the midclavicular line 2–3 cm below the left costal margin. Two additional 5 mm ports are placed. The fifth port could be placed in two different positions depending on the liver retractor. For a Fan Liver Retractor, port position is at the linea axillars anterior below right costal margin. For a Nathanson Liver Retractor, a small subxiphoid incision is performed (**Figure 8**).

There are four critical steps in laparoscopic HH repair [17] (Video 1):

1. Excision of the hernia sac.

2. Sufficient mobilization of the intrathoracic esophagus to restore it intra-abdominal length.

3. Repair of the diaphragmatic crura.

4. Fundoplication.

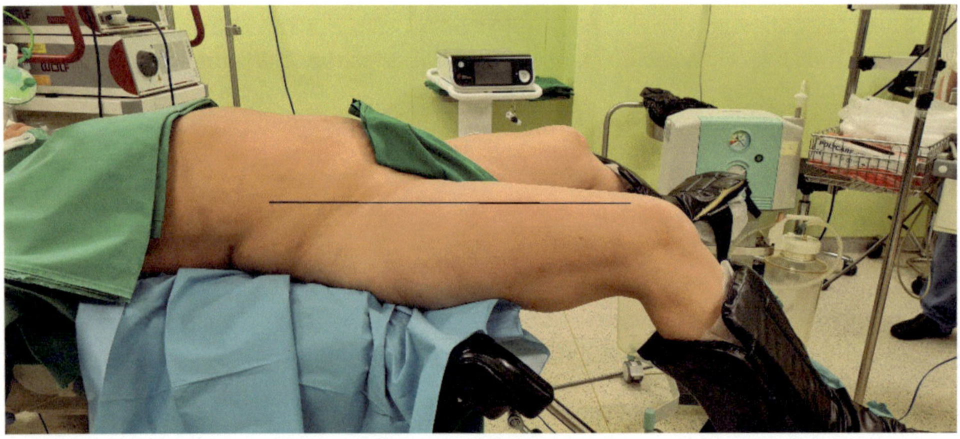

Figure 7.
The Patient's position for laparoscopic HH repair. The thigh is not elevated above the abdominal wall.

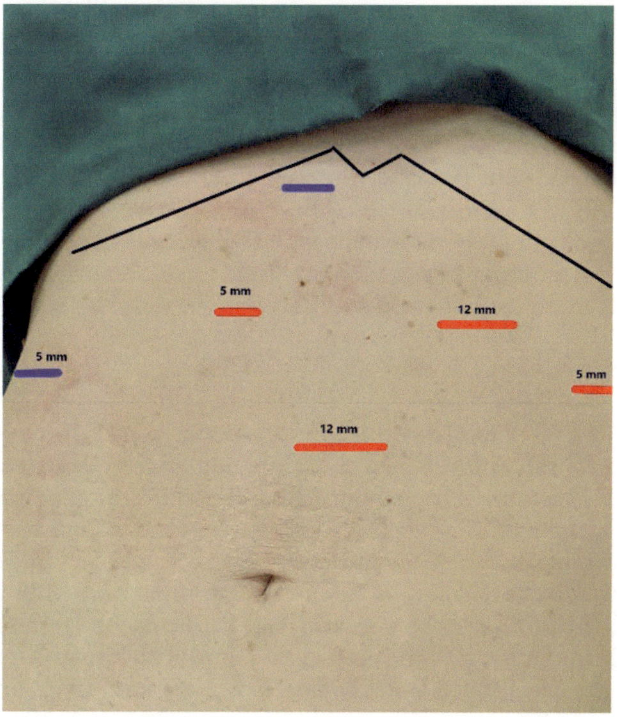

Figure 8.
Port placement (5 ports). Two ports (blue) could be placed in two different positions—Depends on liver retractor.

6.3.2 Excision of the hernia sac

Dissection is started from the left or right diaphragmatic crus by dividing the phrenogastric membrane. The dissection is continued superiorly into mediastinum and the hernia sac is divided from mediastinal tissue. Short gastric vessels are divided to facilitate right crus dissection. A retroesophageal window is created and a drain is placed around the esophagus. This helps to retract the esophagus inferiorly and facilitate mediastinal dissection. After dissection, excision of the hernia sac is performed.

6.3.3 Sufficient mobilization of the intrathoracic esophagus to restore its intra-abdominal length

Aggressive mediastinal dissection is crucial to achieve sufficient length of the intra-abdominal esophagus (at least 3 cm). During dissection, care should be taken to avoid damage to the vagal nerves. Incomplete mobilization of the esophagus can lead to constant tension in the hiatal region and recurrence of the problem. In most cases, sufficient length could be achieved by deep intrathoracic mobilization of the esophagus. The esophagus must be mobilized to the level of the inferior pulmonary veins. In rare cases, the achievement of sufficient length is not possible (short esophagus). In such situations Collis gastroplasty could be the optimal choice. This maneuver elongates the esophageal length by the creation of a tube from the cardia part of the stomach. Usually, proximal resection of the stomach is performed with staplers. The 52-French bougie is inserted in the esophagus before resection to attain an optimal neo-esophagus diameter.

6.3.4 Repair of the diaphragmatic crura

The crura are sutured together using non-absorbable sutures. It could be an interrupted suture or a continuous suture. The use of the continuous suture technique fits with principles of abdominal wall closure—the continuous small-bite technique [18]. The use of barbed continuous sutures helps to facilitate closure in large defects. Closure starts inferiorly where right and left crura join together and proceed superiorly up to the esophagus. The 52-French bougie is placed in the esophagus and should pass easily after repair. Crus closure should not be very tight, so that the closed laparoscopic instrument could freely pass between the esophagus and the crura.

6.3.5 Prosthetic mesh for crura repair

A controversy exists about the use of mesh for crura repair. From one point of view, the only suture repair of PEH has a high radiology recurrence rate—up to 59% [19]. On the other hand, mesh implantation could lead to serious complications like mesh erosion and esophageal stenosis [20]. Different types of meshes exist on the market: synthetic non-absorbable, synthetic absorbable and biologic meshes.

Synthetic non-absorbable meshes are the most popular and differ in materials, knotting structure and weight. A common feature of such meshes is that they remain as a foreign body around the esophagus, constantly causing massive fibrosis, which decreases the possibility of recurrence. However, extensive fibrosis can lead to esophageal stenosis. Mesh migration could cause mesh erosion in the esophagus, mesh infection, sepsis and mediastinitis. Mesh related complications have been reported to range from 1.3 to 20% [21]. To redo surgery in the presence of non-absorbable mesh is a very challenging procedure, even in experienced hands due to dense adhesions and fibrosis.

Biological meshes cause less extensive fibrosis, and fewer complications. No erosions in the esophagus have been reported after biological mesh implantation. This is because of complete mesh resorption after some time. In one study, a long-term follow-up of 59 months showed no biological mesh related complications [22]. Unfortunately, the biggest disadvantage of biological meshes is the high rate of radiological recurrence—up to 54%, similar to that for sutured repairs [22]. This makes implantation of biological meshes questionable.

Synthetic absorbable meshes have short-term absorption (e.g., Vicryl ™) or long-term absorption (e.g., Phasix ™). Recently, slow absorbing synthetic meshes have appeared on the market (e.g., Phasix ™). Resorption times for these meshes are long—about 12–18 months. During this period the meshes cause dense fibrotic tissue to form, which should hold the diaphragmatic crura in desirable positions. On the other hand, the meshes will completely disappear with no foreign body formation. This means that esophageal mesh erosion or infection is not possible. In recent studies [23], these meshes show promising results in large PEH repair operations.

6.3.6 Fundoplication

Fundoplication is the procedure of creating a wrap with gastric fundus around the esophagus to make a one-way valve, that allows food passage to the stomach but does not allow reflux coming up to the esophagus. Fundoplication is an important part of the operation that improves the quality of life after surgery and decreases GERD symptoms.

There are three main methods of fundoplication: posterior 360°—Nissen, posterior 270°—Toupet and anterior 180°—Dor.

Posterior 360° fundoplication (Nissen fundoplication) is the most widely used type. To achieve a complete fundoplication and wrap the fundus around the esophagus, the division of the short gastric arteries is performed. A mobilized part of the fundus is drawn posterior to the esophagus toward the right, so that it completely wraps around the esophagus and meets the left part of the fundus anteriorly. Both parts of the fundus are stitched together and also attached to the anterior wall of the esophagus with 3 permanent stitches. The length of complete fundoplication is about 2–3 cm. The 52-French bougie is placed in the esophagus during fundoplication, so that the wrap should not be too tight.

Toupet fundoplication (posterior 270°) is a partial posterior fundoplication. The initial steps of this procedure are similar to Nissen fundoplication, with the difference being that fundus fixation is performed using stitches to the right and left walls of the esophagus, leaving the anterior wall free and creating a 270° wrap. For this method, usually 6 stitches are necessary (3 on each side).

Dor fundoplication (anterior 180°) is a partial anterior fundoplication. The initial steps are similar to posterior fundoplication, but mobilized fundus is wrapped anteriorly from the esophagus and fixed with stitches to the left and right walls of the esophagus. Anterior fundoplication is less physiological than posterior, because the Hiss angle is not created.

Both posterior fundoplications (Nissen and Toupet) have better long-term GERD symptom control than anterior fundoplication (Dor) [24, 25]. Dysphagia is the most common postoperative complication after fundoplication. Usually, it is transient and resolves after 3 months. In some studies, the incidence of dysphagia after Nissen fundoplication is as high as 70% [26]. Toupet fundoplication has less postoperative dysphagia when compared to Nissen fundoplication [27]. Another common complaint after fundoplication is inability to belch or vomit, including excess flatulence and abdominal bloating. These complaints were found in up to 60% of the patients and did not depend on type of fundoplication [28].

7. Adverse outcome and failure after hiatal hernia surgery

In most cases, failure of the fundoplication depends on 3 factors: wrong indications and preoperative workup, technical issues, or wrong postoperative workup.

7.1 Wrong indication and preoperative workup

In many cases, indication for HH type I surgery is relative. Based on this, preoperative workup plays an important role in patient selection for surgery. All complications and side effects should be taken into consideration before surgery. Objective studies of GERD—pH monitoring, manometry, upper GI endoscopy and barium swallow—are important to evaluate preoperative condition and make decisions for or against surgery. Sometimes, CT provides additional information about surrounding organs and helps to make correct diagnosis. Anamnesis and previous history of medical therapy are also important.

Obesity is an important factor influencing the result of HH surgery. It has been shown that obese patients have a higher risk of HH recurrence. In such cases, a decision could be made in favor of Roux-en-Y bypass with hiatoplasty as a primary operation. This surgery could solve both problems—decrease GERD symptoms due to low acidity in redundant stomach and decrease the patient's weight.

Tobacco usage is a well-known risk factor for hernia surgery failure. It causes wound and connective tissue healing problems, as well as chronic cough which leads to constant mechanical irritation of the repaired area. Therefore, nicotine addiction should be eliminated or reduced preoperatively.

PEH surgery is more complicated, takes a longer time and has more side effects. Moreover, many patients with large PEH are elderly and have multiple comorbidities. It is good to remember that asymptomatic PEH is not an absolute indication for surgery because severe complications like volvulus are rare [14]. In some complicated or acute cases, hernia reduction with gastropexy alone (without HH repair) could be a safe alternative for high-risk patients [29].

7.2 Technical issues

Hernia sac dissection is essential to release the tethering of the esophagus and achieve sufficient length of the abdominal esophagus. It is recommended to perform sac excision. However, in large hernias, it can be difficult. It can predispose vagal injury and lead to gastroparesis. For this reason, some authors advocate sac dissection without excision or with only partial sac excision [30].

Crural reinforcement with mesh in large PEH decreases short-term recurrence. Unfortunately, there is lack of long-term data for or against the use of mesh and about type of mesh [14].

Fundoplication plays an essential role in HH surgery and should be done routinely in all cases, except for morbid patients with gastropexy only [14]. Currently, posterior fundoplication has better outcomes when compared to anterior fundoplication in terms of symptom control. Posterior fundoplication is recommended in most cases.

7.3 Postoperative workup

Early postoperative vomiting, belching, or gagging suddenly increase intra-abdominal pressure and are predisposing factors for recurrence. Aggressive treatment and prophylactic medications (e.g., ondansetron) in the early postoperative period are recommended for these factors [14].

Gastric distension and gastroparesis can lead to dangerous complications in the early postoperative period, especially after large PEH surgery. Placement of the nasogastric tube usually helps in most cases. Percutaneous endoscopic gastrostomy can be indicated sometimes. Gastric distension usually decreases spontaneously after a short time. In refractory cases, gastrojejunostomy or pyloroplasty could be the solution [31].

Early postoperative dysphagia is a common complication after HH surgery. Attention should be paid to slow diet advancement from liquids to solids. If dysphagia persists longer than 3 months and weight loss of more than 10 kg occurs, an intervention for the dysphagia should be performed.

8. Recurrent hiatal hernia

Recurrence rates after HH surgery vary. We can distinguish symptomatic recurrence and radiologic recurrence. Radiologic recurrence is confirmed by a barium esophagogram. It shows HH larger than 2 cm above the diaphragm. Some sources declare that radiologic recurrence after PEH repair is up to 59% [19]. In most cases, radiologic recurrence is asymptomatic or mild and does not require revisional surgery. However, in 5% of cases, symptoms are significant and intervention is needed [32]. In most cases, symptoms are dysphagia, regurgitation, nausea, burning, early satiety, chest pain or postprandial dyspnea. In some cases, mechanical pressure can lead to Cameron's ulcer of the mucosa and bleeding.

Gastric motility should be taken into consideration before surgery. Poor gastric emptying and hypomotility could lead to gastrostasis, bloating, nausea and severe reflux. In these cases, gastric series with barium helps the diagnosis of the problem. Endoscopy with Botulinum toxin injection in the pylorus may decrease symptoms for 3–6 months. The definitive therapy for this problem is pyloroplasty or another gastric drainage procedure (pyloric dilatation, peroral pyloromyotomy etc.) [33].

When surgical intervention is decided, thorough planning should be done. Revisional HH surgery is challenging. The surgical approach could be transabdominal or transthoracic. It depends on the surgeon's experience and preference. Laparoscopy could be safely performed in most cases, however, dissection should be done with caution. Postoperative adhesions can lead to organ damage and are found in up to 30% of cases [34]. Failure of pervious fundoplication is a common reason for recurrence. Thus, any previous fundoplication should be completely undone and then reconstructed. During reconstruction using the gastric fundus and not the gastric body is essential.

Obese patients with BMI > 35 kg/m2 should be advised for revision using the bariatric procedure. It is known that obesity is an independent risk factor for HH recurrence. On the other side, Laparoscopic Roux-en-Y Gastric Bypass (LRYGB) decreases weight and gives good control over GERD symptoms [35]. Thus, revisional surgery combination with laparoscopic Roux-en-Y gastric bypass could be a preferred option for prevention of future recurrences. In addition, it is known that HH reconstruction in combination with LRYGB does not lead to increased morbidity and mortality in comparison with LRYGB alone [36].

9. Novel techniques in hiatal hernia surgery

Linx ™, a new mechanical device for GERD treatment was recently presented and approved [37]. The Linx ™ is constructed from biocompatible titanium beads with magnetic cores hermetically sealed inside. The bead can move independently and the diameter of this device changes during esophageal movements. So, patients can swallow and eat without any resistance but for reflux to occur, the intragastric pressure should overcome the magnetic sphincter pressure. This is an alternative for the fundoplication procedure and could be used in small hiatal hernia surgery, as the only solution or as additional step after crural closure. This procedure is less invasive and less complicated than fundoplication. A study of the first 1000 implants worldwide showed 5.6% of cases needed endoscopic dilatation and 3.4% required reoperation. The main reason for removal of the devices was dysphagia and the recurrence of reflux [38]. Another study showed full thickness erosion of the esophageal wall and endoluminal penetration of the device in 1.2% of the patients, with medium-term follow-up of 48 months [39]. Based on this, the potential erosion rate could be higher in longer follow-up studies. This device implantation provides simple solution to the GERD problem in hiatal hernia surgery, but potential long-term complications of foreign body implantation limit the wider use of this device in clinical practice.

10. Conclusion

HH is a widespread problem in western populations. Treatment is multidisciplinary and requires the involvement of many specialists. While management of HH type I is mostly conservative and based on diet, lifestyle changes and medical therapy, symptomatic PEH (HH type II, III, IV) treatment is surgical. Recent advances in minimally invasive surgery (i.e., laparoscopic surgery) have significantly improved the results of surgical procedures, however, many controversies still exist in HH management (e.g., sutured repair or mesh placement). The development of new materials and procedures, the standardization of guidelines and surgical methods will continue to improve treatment results and the quality of life for patients in the future.

Acknowledgements

I wish to express my sincere gratitude to Greg MacDonald PhD. from Riseba University of Applied Sciences, Riga for his help.

I also sincerely thank Olga Berdnikova for her support and assistance.

Conflict of interest

The authors declare no conflict of interest.

Author details

Igors Ivanovs
Riga East University Hospital, University of Latvia, Riga, Latvia

*Address all correspondence to: igors.ivanovs@lu.lv

References

[1] Dunn CP, Patel TA, Bildzukewicz NA, Henning JR, Lipham JC. Which hiatal hernia's need to be fixed? Large, small or none? Annals of Laparoscopic and Endoscopic Surgery. 2020;**5**:29. DOI: 10.21037/ales.2020.04.02

[2] Menon S, Trudgill N. Risk factors in the aetiology of hiatus hernia: a meta-analysis. European Journal of Gastroenterology & Hepatology. 2011;**23**(2):133-138. DOI: 10.1097/MEG.0b013e3283426f57

[3] Dellaportas D, Papaconstantinou I, NastosC,KaramanolisG,TheodosopoulosT. Large Paraesophageal hiatus hernia: Is surgery mandatory? Chirurgia (Bucur). 2018;**113**(6):765-771. DOI: 10.21614/chirurgia.113.6.765

[4] Carrott PW, Hong J, Kuppusamy M, Koehler RP, Low DE. Clinical ramifications of giant paraesophageal hernias are underappreciated: Making the case for routine surgical repair. The Annals of Thoracic Surgery. 2012;**94**(2):421-426; discussion 426-8. DOI: 10.1016/j.athoracsur.2012.04.058 Epub 2012 Jun 27

[5] Pauwels A. Dental erosions and other extra-oesophageal symptoms of gastro-oesophageal reflux disease: Evidence, treatment response and areas of uncertainty. United European Gastroenterology Journal. 2015;**3**(2):166-170. DOI: 10.1177/2050640615575972

[6] Mainie I, Tutuian R, Shay S, Vela M, Zhang X, Sifrim D, et al. Acid and non-acid reflux in patients with persistent symptoms despite acid suppressive therapy: a multicentre study using combined ambulatory impedance-pH monitoring. Gut. 2006;**55**(10):1398-1402. DOI: 10.1136/gut.2005.087668 Epub 2006 Mar 23

[7] Lebenthal A, Waterford SD, Fisichella PM. Treatment and controversies in paraesophageal hernia repair. Frontiers in Surgery. 2015;**2**:13. DOI: 10.3389/fsurg.2015.00013

[8] Brar HS, Aloysius MM, Shah NJ. Cameron Lesions. Treasure Island (FL): StatPearls Publishing;

[9] Weitzendorfer M, Köhler G, Antoniou SA, Pallwein-Prettner L, Manzenreiter L, Schredl P, et al. Preoperative diagnosis of hiatal hernia: Barium swallow X-ray, high-resolution manometry, or endoscopy? European Surgery. 2017;**49**(5):210-217. DOI: 10.1007/s10353-017-0492-y Epub 2017 Sep 19

[10] Weijenborg PW, Van Hoeij FB, Smout AJPM, Bredenoord AJ. Accuracy of hiatal hernia detection with esophageal high resolution manometry. Neurogastroenterology and Motility. 2015;**27**:293-299

[11] Laracca GG, Spota A, Perretta S. Optimal workup for a hiatal hernia. Annals of Laparoscopic and Endoscopic Surgery. 2021;**6**:2. DOI: 10.21037/ales.2020.03.02

[12] Kahrilas PJ, Bredenoord AJ, Fox M, Gyawali CP, Roman S, Smout AJ, Pandolfino JE, International High Resolution Manometry Working Group. The Chicago classification of esophageal motility disorders, v3.0. Neurogastroenterology and Motility. 2015;**27**:160-174

[13] Gyawali CP, Kahrilas PJ, Savarino E, Zerbib F, Mion F, Smout AJPM, et al.

Modern diagnosis of GERD: The Lyon consensus. Gut. 2018;**67**(7):1351-1362. DOI: 10.1136/gutjnl-2017-314722

[14] Kohn GP, Price RR, DeMeester SR, Zehetner J, Muensterer OJ, Awad Z, et al. Fanelli RD; SAGES guidelines committee. Guidelines for the management of hiatal hernia. Surgical Endoscopy. 2013;**27**(12):4409-4428. DOI: 10.1007/s00464-013-3173-3 Epub 2013 Sep 10

[15] Stylopoulos N, Gazelle GS, Rattner DW. Paraesophageal hernias: Operation or observation? Annals of Surgery. 2002;**236**(4):492-500; discussion 500-1. DOI: 10.1097/00000658-200210000-00012

[16] Paul S, Nasar A, Port JL, Lee PC, Stiles BC, Nguyen AB, Altorki NK, Sedrakyan A. Comparative analysis of diaphragmatic hernia repair outcomes using the nationwide inpatient sample database. Arch Surg. 2012;147(7):607-612. DOI: 10.1001/archsurg.2012.127. Erratum in: Archives of Surgery 2012;147(9):804

[17] DeMeester SR. Laparoscopic paraesophageal hernia repair: Critical steps and adjunct techniques to minimize recurrence. Surgical Laparoscopy, Endoscopy & Percutaneous Techniques. 2013;**23**(5):429-435. DOI: 10.1097/SLE.0b013e3182a12716

[18] Deerenberg EB, Henriksen NA, Antoniou GA, Antoniou SA, Bramer WM, Fischer JP, et al. Updated guideline for closure of abdominal wall incisions from the European and American Hernia Societies. British Journal of Surgery. 2022;**109**(12):1239-1250. DOI: 10.1093/bjs/znac302 Erratum in: Br J Surg. 2022 Nov 10

[19] Kao AM, Otero J, Schlosser KA, Marx JE, Prasad T, Colavita PD, et al. One more time: Redo Paraesophageal hernia repair results in safe, durable outcomes compared with primary repairs. The American Surgeon. 2018;**84**(7):1138-1145

[20] Gordon AC, Gillespie C, Son J, et al. Long-term outcomes of laparoscopic large hiatus hernia repair with nonabsorbable mesh. Diseases of the Esophagus. 2018;**31**(5):156

[21] Memon MA, editor. Hiatal Hernia Surgery: An Evidence Based Approach. Switzerland: Springer International Publishing AG; 2017. pp. 134-147. DOI: 10.1007/978-3-319-64003-7

[22] Oelschlager BK, Pellegrini CA, Hunter JG, Brunt ML, Soper NJ, Sheppard BC, et al. Biologic prosthesis to prevent recurrence after laparoscopic paraesophageal hernia repair: Long-term follow-up from a multicenter, prospective, randomized trial. J Am Coll Surg. 2011;**213**(4):461-468. DOI: 10.1016/j.jamcollsurg.2011.05.017. Epub 2011 Jun 29. Erratum in: Journal of the American College of Surgeons 2011;213(6):815

[23] Jushko M, Ivanovs I. Quality of life after hiatal hernia repair with biosynthetic mesh Phasix. Proceedings of the Latvian Academy of Sciences, Section B: Natural, Exact and Applied Sciences. 2022;**76**:632-635. DOI: 10.2478/prolas-2022-0097

[24] Engström C, Lönroth H, Mardani J, Lundell L. An anterior or posterior approach to partial fundoplication? Long-term results of a randomized trial. World Journal of Surgery. 2007;**31**(6):1221-1225; discussion 1226-7. DOI: 10.1007/s00268-007-9004-8. Epub 2007 Apr 24

[25] Nijjar RS, Watson DI, Jamieson GG, Archer S, Bessell JR, Booth M, et al. International Society for the Diseases of the esophagus-Australasian section.

Five-year follow-up of a multicenter, double-blind randomized clinical trial of laparoscopic Nissen vs anterior 90 degrees partial fundoplication. Archives of Surgery. 2010;**145**(6):552-557. DOI: 10.1001/archsurg.2010.81

[26] Sato K, Awad ZT, Filipi CJ, Selima MA, Cummings JE, Fenton SJ, et al. Causes of long-term dysphagia after laparoscopic Nissen fundoplication. JSLS. 2002;**6**(1):35-40

[27] Koch OO, Kaindlstorfer A, Antoniou SA, Luketina RR, Emmanuel K, Pointner R. Comparison of results from a randomized trial 1 year after laparoscopic Nissen and Toupet fundoplications. Surgical Endoscopy. 2013;**27**(7):2383-2390. DOI: 10.1007/s00464-013-2803-0 Epub 2013 Jan 30

[28] Courtney O, Peter N. Anterior Versus Posterior Fundoplication, Are They Equal? In: Muhammed AM, editor. Hiatal Hernia Surgery: An Evidence Based Approach. Switzerland: Springer International Publishing AG; 2017. pp. 91-102. DOI: 10.1007/978-3-319-64003-7

[29] Rosenberg J, Jacobsen B, Fischer A. Fast-track giant paraoesophageal hernia repair using a simplified laparoscopic technique. Langenbeck's Archives of Surgery. 2006;**391**:38-42

[30] Trus TL, Bax T, Richardson WS, Branum GD, Mauren SJ, Swanstrom LL, et al. Complications of laparoscopic paraesophageal hernia repair. Journal of Gastrointestinal Surgery. 1997;**1**(3):221-227; discussion 228. DOI: 10.1016/s1091-255x(97)80113-8

[31] Li Z, Xie F, Zhu L, et al. Post-operative gastric outlet obstruction of giant hiatal hernia repair: a case report. BMC Gastroenterology. 2022;**22**:47. DOI: 10.1186/s12876-022-02117-z

[32] Elhefny, Amr M.M.a; Elmaleh, Haitham M.a; Hamed, Mohammed A.a; Salem, Hossam E.-D.M.b. Laparoscopic management of recurrent symptomatic hiatal hernia with and without mesh repair: a comparative prospective study. The Egyptian Journal of Surgery 40(4): p. 1064-1073, October-December 2021. DOI: 10.4103/ejs.ejs_90_21

[33] Botha AJ, Di Maggio F. Management of complications after paraesophageal hernia repair. Annals of Laparoscopic and Endoscopic Surgery. 2021;**6**:38. DOI: 10.21037/ales-19-241

[34] Juhasz A, Sundaram A, Hoshino M, Lee TH, Mittal SK. Outcomes of surgical management of symptomatic large recurrent hiatus hernia. Surgical Endoscopy. 2012;**26**(6):1501-1508. DOI: 10.1007/s00464-011-2072-8 Epub 2011 Dec 17

[35] Khan M, Mukherjee AJ. Hiatal hernia and morbid obesity-'Roux-en-Y gastric bypass' the one step solution. Journal of Surgical Case Reports. 2019;**2019**(6):rjz189. DOI: 10.1093/jscr/rjz189

[36] Kothari V, Shaligram A, Reynoso J, Schmidt E, McBride CL, Oleynikov D. Impact on perioperative outcomes of concomitant hiatal hernia repair with laparoscopic gastric bypass. Obesity Surgery. 2012;**22**(10):1607-1610. DOI: 10.1007/s11695-012-0714-0

[37] Ganz RA, Peters JH, Horgan S, Bemelman WA, Dunst CM, Edmundowicz SA, et al. Esophageal sphincter device for gastroesophageal reflux disease. The New England Journal of Medicine. 2013;**368**(8):719-727. DOI: 10.1056/NEJMoa1205544

[38] Lipham JC, Taiganides PA, Louie BE, Ganz RA, DeMeester TR. Safety analysis of first 1000 patients treated with

magnetic sphincter augmentation for gastroesophageal reflux disease. Diseases of the Esophagus. 2015;**28**(4):305-311. DOI: 10.1111/dote.12199 Epub 2014 Mar 11

[39] Asti E, Siboni S, Lazzari V, Bonitta G, Sironi A, Bonavina L. Removal of the magnetic sphincter augmentation device: Surgical technique and results of a single-center cohort study. Annals of Surgery. 2017;**265**(5):941-945. DOI: 10.1097/SLA.0000000000001785

Chapter 8

Incarcerated Inguinal Hernia in the Elderly: Surgical Implication

Fabrizio Ferranti

Abstract

Inguinal hernia is a very common clinical condition, and its incidence is higher in elderly patients. Different factors are involved in the etiology of the disease, either congenital or acquired. Most inguinal hernias are asymptomatic but may develop complications such as incarceration. Diagnosis, in uncomplicated cases, is easy and based on physical examination. Imaging studies are helpful when the diagnosis is unclear, especially if bowel strangulation is suspected. Elective surgical hernia repair is considered the treatment of choice. However, in elderly patients with a high surgical risk, a watchful-waiting approach is advisable. The choice of surgical technique depends on the experience of the surgeon and the contamination of the surgical field. The classical approach is Lichtenstein open tension-free mesh repair, although laparoscopy has been proposed. The use of mesh in incarcerated inguinal hernia is disputed because of the increased risk of postoperative wound infection. General anesthesia is usually preferred in particular if bowel ischemia is suspected and intestinal resection may be required. However, local anesthesia is expanding its indication since it provides effective anesthesia with less postoperative complications.

Keywords: inguinal hernia, incarceration, elderly patient, emergency hernia surgery, risk factors

1. Introduction

Inguinal hernia is a common clinical condition with a lifetime occurrence of 27–43% in men and 3–6% in women [1, 2]. Its incidence is higher in elderly people due to conditions frequently associated with old age such as constipation, chronic obstructive pulmonary disease (COPD), and prostatism, which are considered risk factors for hernia formation [3, 4].

Inguinal hernia is generally asymptomatic, or minimally symptomatic in most patients [5], although in 5–15% of cases may complicate with incarceration [6, 7]. Moreover, around 15% of incarcerated inguinal hernias may evolve into bowel strangulation, a life-threatening condition requiring intestine resection [8, 9].

Patients operated on for complicated hernia have poor outcomes with high postoperative complications and mortality, ranging from 6 to 43% [7, 10] and from 1 to 7%, respectively [8, 11]. Therefore early diagnosis and prompt surgical repair are critical factors in improving the prognosis of these patients [12, 13]. In typical, uncomplicated cases, diagnosis is easy and can be made by physical examination alone [14, 15]. However, if clinical features are doubtful and patients present symptoms referring to intestinal obstruction, imaging studies play an important role in clearing the diagnosis and in assessing the viability of incarcerated intestine [16–20].

Although inguinal hernia repair is one of the most common operations performed worldwide, with over 20 million operations per year [21], several methods of treatment have been proposed including conservative approach (watchful-waiting strategy), manual reduction for incarcerated hernia, and, of course, surgical repair, either open or laparoscopic [22–25].

This chapter aims to describe the diagnostic process, highlight the importance of early detection of bowel ischemia, and summarize the treatment options, especially surgery, its indications, and results.

2. Epidemiology

Groin hernia is the most common abdominal wall hernia and includes inguinal and femoral types, with the former accounting for 96% of cases [2, 26]. The incidence of inguinal hernia is higher in males than in females, with male-to-female ratio of 9:1, whereas femoral type is more common in women [27, 28].

It is estimated that one-fourth of adult men in the United States have a recognizable groin hernia that accounts for 4.7 million ambulatory visits annually [29]. Moreover, it is more common on right side and in 10% of cases is bilateral [15, 28, 30]. Inguinal hernia may evolve into incarceration with an estimated risk ranging from 0.03–3% over a person's lifetime [31–33]. Primary hernias are strangulated more than recurrent and the small ones more than the large hernias, with a ratio of 5:1 [12, 34].

Incarceration occurs more frequently during the first 3 months after the diagnosis, with no difference in gender [31]. Overall 5.8–13% of patients operated on for inguinal hernia are treated emergently [1, 32, 33], and around 10–20% of these patients will need a bowel resection [6, 34]. Interestingly, complicated hernia in elderly people shows an increased incidence of necrotic bowel compared with young adults for the same time duration of symptoms [28, 32].

The most frequent anatomical structure found in incarcerated inguinal hernia sac is the intestine, in around 75% of patients, followed by omentum in the remaining 25% [15, 35]. However, other unusual structures have been described such as ovarian in 2.9% of cases, urinary bladder in 0.36% [36], sigmoid diverticulum [37], appendix epiploica [38], Meckel's diverticulum [39], and even gallbladder [40]. The presence of a vermiform appendix is reported with an incidence of 1% [41], and, although rarely, the appendix may become inflamed (Amayand's hernia) [42].

3. Etiology

Hernia is a multifactorial condition, and several causes may play a role in its development. Risk factors are usually divided into patient and external factors [Oberg]. Patient risk factors are considered male gender, old age, and low body mass index [43–45]. Other factors such as constipation, prostate hypertrophy, and COPD are all conditions that increase intra-abdominal pressure that strains the layers of the abdominal wall and may weaken its strength [34, 46]. There is a strong correlation between the processus vaginalis and hernia formation [47]. An indirect inguinal hernia is supposed to be due to a persistent patency of processus vaginalis [48, 49]. Furthermore, an indirect hernia is more common on the right side because the right testis descends later than the left, leaving the right processus vaginalis patent for more time [50]. Patients with collagen vascular disease and connective metabolism disorders (Marfan syndrome, Ehlers-Danlos, and aneurysmal disease) are at increased risk of hernia formation [51–53]. When comparing different inguinal hernia types, direct hernia shows local collagen tissue alteration and different abdominal fascia architecture, factors that affect the elastic properties of transversalis fascia leading to hernia formation [54, 55].

Among external risk factors, smoking is supposed to increase the risk of recurrence [43], but its role in primary hernia formation is uncertain [44, 56]. Increased intra-abdominal pressure seems to be related to abdominal wall hernia formation, but its effective role is still under scrutiny [33]. Some physical activities, such as jumping, or great physical exertion, are strongly related to hernia formation [57–59]. However, in other circumstances, factors, such as leisure physical activities, lifting heavy loads, or standing for a long time, although they provoke an increase in intra-abdominal pressure, do not seem to be responsible for hernia development [60].

4. Classification

Abdominal hernia is defined as an abnormal protrusion of a peritoneal sac through the muscoloaponeurotic structures covering the abdominal wall [61]. Classification of abdominal wall hernia is generally based upon anatomic location of the bulge and includes groin, umbilical, epigastric, Spigelian, and obturatoria hernias [30, 62]. In addition, groin hernias can be classified according to etiology (congenital or acquired), anatomic location of the bulge (inguinal and femoral), defect size (small, medium, and large), and integrity of anatomic groin structure [63–66]. Some of these classifications are complex and difficult to remember; thus, surgeons, in their day-to-day practice, separate inguinal hernias essentially in two types, indirect (lateral) and direct (medial), by their relationship with the inferior epigastric vessels at surgical exploration [64, 67]. Direct hernia protrudes medially to inferior epigastric vessels, whereas indirect type laterally to the vessels [68].

Incarcerated hernia is defined as a hernia in which the sac content cannot be reduced into the abdomen due to a narrow opening orifice or because of adhesions between the sac and its content [23, 69, 70].

Hernia becomes strangulated when the blood supply of the sac content is compromised, and the tissue progresses to necrosis [71].

Unfortunately, the two terms “incarcerated” and “strangulated,” which refer to different clinical conditions, are often used interchangeably with the undesirable consequence of negatively affecting the therapeutic decision-making process [72, 73].

5. Diagnosis

The majority of uncomplicated inguinal hernias are easily diagnosed. Typically, a patient complains of pain or dull discomfort in the groin region that exacerbates during daily living activities [74, 75]. On physical examination, the hernia appears as a lump in the groin which becomes more evident when the patient performs a Valsalva maneuver or gives a cough [76]. In uncomplicated cases, the lump may go away spontaneously, when the patient is lying down, or after a gentle manual pressure over the hernia. Overall, clinical examination in the elective setting results is quite accurate and shows a sensitivity ranging from 74–92% and a specificity of 93% [14].

If the patient complains of moderate–severe groin pain, a complicated hernia should be taken into consideration [15, 23]. Incarcerated hernia may also present with symptoms of bowel obstruction such as nausea, vomiting, diffuse abdominal pain, and bloating [15, 77]. When bowel ischemia has occurred, the patient may show signs of local or general peritonitis, including abdominal tenderness, absent bowel sounds, fever, tachycardia, and systemic inflammatory response syndrome (SIS) [78]. On physical examination, incarcerated hernia will appear erythematous, indurated, swollen, painful to palpation, and irreducible [79, 80]. Therefore, early diagnosis of incarcerated hernia is paramount to improving the patients' prognosis [81, 82]. A delay in hospital admission of more than 48 hours increases postoperative morbidity and mortality by 24 and 7 times, respectively [83, 84]. Furthermore, patients hospitalized after more than 24 hours following incarceration encompass 81.8% of death cases [85]. Sometimes a delayed diagnosis, especially in elderly people, may be ascribed to inadequate awareness of the problem by the patient who does not seek medical advice [86]. However, in other circumstances, the diagnostic delay may be due to physician mistakes [87]. A study showed that strangulated hernias were misdiagnosed in 3% of patients by general physicians and in 15% by hospital registers [88].

In patients with incarcerated inguinal hernia, it is important to rule out bowel ischemia [89, 90]. Several clinical, radiological, and laboratory criteria have been analyzed in order to predict this complication. Among laboratory parameters, D-dimer level correlates well with bowel ischemia, and this parameter's high value should increase the suspicion of bowel infarction [91]. On univariate analysis, an elevated serum lactate level greater than 2.0 mmol/L [92] is strongly associated with intestine ischemia, although the test shows a low specificity [93, 94]. Moreover, lactate levels may be false normal up to 8 hours after the onset of bowel necrosis [95]. White blood count (WBC), blood fibrinogen, and serum creatinine phosphokinase (CPK) have been considered valuable predictive parameters for ischemic events occurring in different tissue of the body [96]. Fibrinogen level is increased in patients with incarcerated hernia and seems to show a positive correlation for bowel resection, need for intensive care, and higher risk of mortality [97]. Similar results have been found for CPK [96] and WBC count [80, 98]. In patients who complain of severe groin pain and show an increased level of fibrinogen and high WBC count, a prompt surgical hernia exploration is recommended [99]. Hyponatremia, defined as sodium level less than 135 mg/dl, should raise a strong suspicion of bowel necrosis [100]. Furthermore, the combination of hyponatremia and clinical features of bowel strangulation should dissuade the surgeon from any attempts to perform Taxis maneuver [101]. To conclude, procalcitonin (PTC) is considered a reliable diagnostic serum parameter in several conditions such as infections, systemic inflammatory response syndrome (SIRS), acute pancreatitis, and multiorgan dysfunction syndrome (MODS) [102]. In incarcerated inguinal hernia, PTC is significantly higher in patients with bowel ischemia compared with those without ischemia and in patients with necrosis compared with those without it. Thus, elevated levels of PTC should rise the suspicion of bowel necrosis, and repeated measurements of PTC may help the surgeon to decide if operate and the timing of surgery [89].

Overall, no single serum marker is sensitive or specific enough to diagnose intestinal ischemia, and only the association of two or more factors has proved helpful in predicting the progression of incarcerated hernia toward bowel necrosis [69, 103].

Imaging studies are useful in doubtful diagnosis and in patients with complicated inguinal hernia, particularly if bowel ischemia is suspected [14, 19, 75, 104]. Without intra-abdominal complications, groin ultrasound (US) should be the initial imaging modality to evaluate a suspected incarcerated inguinal hernia [105, 106]. Sonographic signs of incarceration include free fluid in hernia sac and within the dilated bowel loop, intestine thickened wall (> 2,5 cm), and "back-and-forth" peristalsis sign [20, 107, 108]. Moreover, sonographic reduction of Doppler color flow within the bowel loops, the absence of peristalsis, and free air in the intestinal wall are signs of strangulation [104, 109].

Multidetector computed tomography (MDCT) is considered the modality of choice in incarcerated inguinal hernia since it supplies the surgeon with decisive information to clear a doubtful diagnosis, to detect signs of peritonitis, and to evaluate bowel necrosis and its severity [18, 110–113]. Analysis of the overall diagnostic performance of MDCT for detecting ischemic bowel has shown contrasting results, with a sensitivity reaching almost 100% and, by contrast, specificity reported in some studies as low as 61% [114, 115]. The low specificity rate is probably because some CT signs found in ischemic bowel are also observed in other conditions, especially in inflammatory bowel diseases and peritonitis in which no vascular compromise is involved [16]. CT diagnosis of bowel ischemia is based on the presence of two or more of the following signs: bowel wall thickening, a high attenuation of the bowel wall on unenhanced CT, mesenteric edema, fluid in the hernia sac, asymmetric bowel wall enhancement on IV contrast-enhanced CT, and pneumatosis in advanced stage [103, 116, 117]. In conclusion, in patients with incarcerated inguinal hernia, MDCT allows identifying patients at high risk of bowel necrosis, regardless of surgical risk, and requiring an emergent surgical repair [110, 118–120].

6. Treatment

Inguinal hernia is a common problem occurring in about 15% of adult men [121], and inguinal hernioplasty is probably the most common operation performed by a general surgeon [122].

The definitive therapy for inguinal hernia is surgery; generally, patients are referred for surgical treatment after diagnosis [23, 123]. The main reason for this strategy is the fear of hernia incarceration, which requires emergency operations [124–128]. In addition, elective surgical hernia repair is a safe and effective treatment for rare and minor complications, as well as in elderly patients [129, 130].

By contrast, several studies have shown that emergent inguinal hernia repair has a high morbidity and mortality rate, estimated at around 30 and 13,4%, respectively [84, 87, 131, 132].

Therefore, in contemporary practice, the majority of patients, regardless of age and symptoms and who are healthy enough, are referred to surgery [23, 133, 134].

Lichtenstein mesh tension-free technique is the procedure of choice [2, 135–138] due to its safety and efficacy with a low recurrence rate ranging from 0.002 to 0.48% [87].

However, many elderly people have several comorbidities and present a high surgical risk. A watchful-waiting approach is warranted for this group of patients, particularly if they are asymptomatic or minimally symptomatic [134, 139, 140].

Proponents of this strategy argue that the risk of incarceration is low, occurring in only 2–4% of patients followed up as long as 11.5 years and that only 7% of operations are performed emergently [24, 141, 142]. Furthermore, there is no difference in pain relief between patients operated on and those treated with a watchful strategy [143].

However, despite these positive results, it should be remembered that around two-thirds of patients treated with a watchful-waiting approach cross over to surgery within 10 years mainly because of pain or incarceration of hernia [144–146].

Things change when a hernia becomes incarcerated since this complication is life-threatening and needs prompt treatment [147–149].

In high-surgical risk patients without signs of strangulation, a manual non-invasive reduction of incarcerated hernia, performed under analgesia/sedation (Taxis maneuver), is considered a safe and reliable treatment [4, 72, 150]. The procedure can also be performed under US guidelines increasing the safety and efficacy of the technique [151]. The success of this approach is reported in 70% of cases, and it is also considered the treatment of choice in pediatric patients [149]. The advantage of the manual reduction procedure is to avoid emergency operations in critically ill patients with an increased risk of morbidity and mortality [72, 150]. In addition, definitive surgical repair can be scheduled early after a successful Taxis maneuver ("two-stage procedure"), providing better anatomical conditions for operation [47, 152].

Unfortunately, a manual reduction procedure may carry the risk of reducing necrotic bowel into the abdomen, the event that leads to diffuse peritonitis which needs an emergent surgical treatment [153, 154]. However, cases are rare, and since bowel strangulation occurs with a very narrow hernia orifice, the risk of reducing a necrotic bowel is very low [149].

In current practice, the role of manual reduction is still under debate, and, anyway, the procedure should be considered a temporary treatment due to the high incidence of re-incarceration [154]. Furthermore, the technique is not even mentioned in a recent update of different society's guidelines for the emergency repair of abdominal wall hernias [4, 71, 155].

Incarcerated inguinal hernia associated with intestinal obstruction and/or suspected bowel ischemia represents a mandatory indication for emergent surgery [23, 71, 147]. Unfortunately, complications after urgent repair, particularly in elderly patients, are common, and the reported morbidity and mortality are high, ranging from 19 to 30% and from 1.4 to 13.4%, respectively [131, 156, 157].

Several factors have been investigated in order to predict surgical risk and outcome in this group of patients [84, 85, 158]. Age over 70 years is considered a negative prognostic factor, and it is estimated that postoperative mortality increases 1% with every year of age [8, 159, 160]. However, old age "per se" seems not to be responsible for poor outcomes, but only if it is associated with comorbidities [133, 161] or with a "frailty" status [162]. Cardiovascular disease, diabetes mellitus, COPD, and obesity are also associated with increased postoperative complications [6, 163, 164]. Furthermore, patients with ASA (America Society of Anesthesiologist) III-IV class show mortality 2,5 times higher than those with ASA I-II class [100, 134, 160]. Smoking seems to hinder the oxygenation of the surgical field, impairing the wound-healing process [56, 165, 166].

However, among risk factors, probably the most important is the necrosis of incarcerated bowel, which demands intestine resection [6, 83, 84, 157]. It is estimated that bowel resection increases mortality by 3 to 4 times [28], although this result is disputed by other studies, which show that intestinal resection is a predictor of morbidity but not of mortality [7, 85, 167].

Intestinal ischemia includes different grades of severity, ranging from reversible stage to transmural necrosis with possible wall perforation [168]. This "acute bowel injury," also in an early phase of its development, leads to bacterial translocation, absorption of bacterial endotoxin, systemic inflammatory response syndrome (SIRS), and may progress to multiorgan dysfunction syndrome (MOS) [71, 169, 170]. Therefore, early diagnosis of ischemic bowel and prompt surgical treatment assume great clinical value in these patients [151, 171].

Incarcerated inguinal hernia may be treated with different surgical approaches, and the choice of the technique depends on several factors including anesthetic considerations, surgeon's expertise, suspect of bowel necrosis, and contamination of the surgical field [147, 148]. The most common technique, especially in elderly patients, is the open anterior mesh tension-free repair. In this regard, the Lichtenstein procedure has gained great acceptance and has become the technique of choice in emergency settings and high-risk patients [172–175]. The mesh guarantees excellent repair results, but its use in complicated hernia is controversial due to the increased risk of wound infection [176–179]. However, several studies have shown that mesh can be safely implanted in complicated hernia without increased risk of wound infection, even in the case of bowel resection [156, 180, 181]. The choice of mesh is crucial for the success of the operation [182, 183]. Polypropylene is the ideal material to be used in contaminated fields since its macroporous structure allows contact among bacteria and the patient's immune system cells, allowing the recovery from infection [184, 185].

In conclusion, the mesh can be safely used in clean and clean-contaminated surgical fields (CDC Class I-II), whereas its use in cases of bowel perforation and in grossly contaminated-dirty surgical fields (CDC Class III-IV) is not recommended [23, 71, 186].

When mesh is contraindicated, a primary tissue repair is required. Several techniques can be employed such as Bassini, Shouldice, and Mc Vay procedures [187–189].

The Shouldice technique is considered the most effective procedure, particularly in specialized centers [22, 190]. However, all "pure tissue repair" techniques are burdened with high postoperative morbidity and can show a recurrence rate as high as 34%, especially when employed in an emergency setting [87, 191].

Therefore, to obviate the poor results of the suture tissue repair technique and perform a mesh tension-free repair also in a contaminated field and, at the same time, trying to avoid the risk of wound infection, the use of absorbable mesh has been proposed [192, 193].

The laparoscopic approach has recently become popular, and it is considered a reliable procedure for the repair of bilateral inguinal hernia and recurrent hernia, and also for unilateral inguinal hernia [194–198]. Furthermore, a series of studies have confirmed that the laparoscopic approach can be safely performed in old-age patients with an ASA I-II class without increasing the incidence of complications and mortality [25, 199, 200]. However, some concerns still exist regarding emergent laparoscopic repair of incarcerated inguinal hernia, and little evidence exists about the technique's efficacy [4, 201]. In addition, it is reported that the laparoscopic procedure has some limitations. A minimally invasive approach requires general anesthesia, is time-consuming, has a long learning curve, is not cost-effective, and entails specific complications such as bladder, vascular, and visceral injuries, which are unusual in an open approach and sometimes result in the death of the patient [202–205]. Only 10% of all inguinal hernia repairs are estimated to be performed *via* laparoscopic approach in the United States [202, 203].

However, several studies have shown that minimally invasive technique presents several advantages over open repair, even for the treatment of incarcerated inguinal hernia [206–209]. For example, laparoscopy allows a careful reduction of herniated bowel, an accurate assessment of its viability, reduces the postoperative pain, and allows faster recovery, and, finally, the procedure shows a lesser or similar recurrence rate compared to the open approach [210–212].

Among laparoscopic techniques, either transabdominal pre-peritoneal repair (TAPP) or totally extraperitoneal approach (TEP) is a feasible and reliable method [213, 214], although an increased risk of recurrence is reported for TEP repair [203].

An interesting use of the laparoscopic technique is the hernia sac laparoscopy, also known as hernioscopy [215]. This method, defined as a mixed laparoscopic-open surgical approach, can be employed to assess the viability of the intestine in case of spontaneous reduction of the sac content during an open emergent inguinal repair before the assessment of the viability of the intestine [216, 217]. This event, which occurs in about 1% of patients during anesthetic induction, poses the risk of leaving the necrotic bowel inside the abdomen with the consequent development of peritonitis [218]. In this circumstance, hernioscopy is a reliable and accurate method to assess the viability of the retracted intestine, and allows to avoid unnecessary laparotomy in high-risk patients [219, 220].

The choice of anesthetic methods is an important issue in inguinal hernia repair, especially in elderly patients and in complicated hernias [221–223]. Virtually, all anesthetic techniques such as general, regional (epidural and spinal), and local anesthesia can be used [224–226]. However, epidemiological data show that nearly 80% of inguinal hernia repairs are performed under general anesthesia, although the evidence to support this choice is low [21, 227]. Furthermore, these data contrast those originating from specialized centers where local anesthesia is used in more than 95% of patients [228, 229].

The choice of anesthetic technique depends on several factors including patient or surgeon preference, technique feasibility in a given patient, and intra- and postoperative pain control [230]. However, general anesthesia is usually preferred in emergency inguinal repair since the technique provides the surgeon with optimal operating conditions in terms of immobility and muscular relaxation [231]. Furthermore, general anesthesia remains the method of choice in anxious or uncooperative patients, in morbid obesity, and in cases where intestine ischemia is suspected, and bowel resection could be performed [5, 71, 222].

Regional anesthesia offers some advantages compared with general technique. For example, control of postoperative pain favors the regional approach; nausea and vomiting are less frequent, just like deep vein thrombosis and pulmonary edema [232–234]. However, regional anesthesia is burdened with common complications such as postdural puncture headache, hypotension, and urinary retention [233]. Furthermore, meta-analysis does not show definitive data concerning the advantage of regional over general anesthesia [235].

Local anesthesia has become a popular technique for inguinal hernia repair, and it is strongly recommended in elderly patients and in those with comorbidities [236–238]. Moreover, European Hernia Society Guidelines (EHS) suggest that this technique should be used in patients with ASA III or IV class. Local anesthesia has advantages over general and regional anesthesia such as less postoperative pain, shorter hospital stay, early mobilization, and avoiding urinary retention and cognitive dysfunction [231, 237, 239]. Despite these advantages, the role of local anesthesia for inguinal hernia repair is still under debate, especially in emergency settings [225, 240, 241]. Incarcerated hernia has a complicated local anatomy, tissues are swollen, the patient often complains of pain, and muscle relaxation is not satisfactory [242]. Furthermore, local anesthesia is considered a risk factor for recurrence [240]. For these reasons, the technique is rarely used in emergencies, although some studies have shown the feasibility and safety of local anesthesia for treating incarcerated inguinal hernia in high-risk patients [236, 237, 241].

7. Conclusion

Incarcerated inguinal hernia represents a serious clinical problem. Moreover, its incidence is high in elderly people with several comorbidities and presents a high surgical risk. An early diagnosis is of paramount importance in order to establish a prompt and tailored patient treatment. Surgical open tension-free repair is still the treatment of choice, especially in high-risk patients, and should be performed under general/regional anesthesia if bowel necrosis is suspected. The laparoscopic approach has grown in popularity and is currently considered a valid option to open surgery for incarcerated inguinal hernias in old-age patients.

Author details

Fabrizio Ferranti
Division of General Surgery, San Paolo Hospital, ASL Roma, Rome, Italy

*Address all correspondence to: fabrizio.ferranti@fastwebnet.it

References

[1] Primatesta P, Goldrace MJ. Inguinal hernia repair: Incidence of elective and emergency surgery, readmission and mortality. International Journal of Epidemiology. 1996;**25**(4):835-839. DOI: 10.1093/ije/25.4.835

[2] Kingsnorth A, LeBlanc K. Hernias: Inguinal and incisional. Lancet. 2003;**362**(9395):1561-1571. DOI: 10.1016/S0140-6736(03)14746-0

[3] Compagna R, Rossi R, Fappiano F, Bianco T, Accurso A, et al. Emergency groin hernia repair: Implications in elderly. BMC Surgery. 2001;**13**(Suppl. 2):S29. DOI: 10.1186/1471-2482-13-S2-S29

[4] Simons MP, Aufenacker T, Bay-Nielsen M, Bouillot JL, Campanelli G, et al. European hernia society guidelines on the treatment of inguinal hernia in adult patients. Hernia. 2009;**13**(4):343-403. DOI: 10.1007/s10029-009-0529-7

[5] Hair A, Duffy K, Mclean J, Taylor SH, et al. Groin hernia repair in Scotland. The British Journal of Surgery. 2000;**87**(12):1722-1726. DOI: 10.1046/j.1365-2168.2000.01598.x

[6] Dai W, Chen Z, Zuo J, Tan J, Tan M. Risks factors of postoperative complications after emergency repair of incarcerated groin hernia for adult patients: A retrospective cohort study. Hernia. 2019;**23**(2):267-276. DOI: 10.1007/s10029-018-1854-5

[7] Kurt N, Oncel M, Ozkan Z, Bingul S. Risk and outcome of bowel resection in patients with incarcerated groin hernias: Retrospective study. World Journal of Surgery. 2003;**27**(6):741-743. DOI: 10.1007/s00268-003-6826-x

[8] Ge BJ, Huang Q, Liu LM, Bian HP, Fan YZ. Risk factors for bowel resection and outcome in patients with incarcerated groin hernias. Hernia. 2010;**14**(3):259-264. DOI: 10.1007/s10029-009-0602-2

[9] Chiow AKH. Inguinal hernias: A current review of an old problem. Proceedings of Singapore Healthcare. 2010;**19**(3):202-211. DOI: 10.1177/201010581001900306

[10] Koizumi M, Sata N, Kaneda Y, Endo K, Sasanuma H, et al. Optimal timeline for emergency surgery in patients with strangulated groin hernias. Hernia. 2014;**18**(6):845-848. DOI: 10.1007/s10029-014-1219-7

[11] Proctor VK, O'Connor OM, Burns FA, Green S, Sayers AE, et al. Management of acutely symptomatic hernia (MASH) study. The British Journal of Surgery. 2022;**109**(8):754-762. DOI: 10.1093/bjs/znac107

[12] Ahmad N, Sadaqat AK, Abid KJ. Management of strangulated inguinal hernia in adults. Pakistan Journal of Medical and Health Sciences. 2014;**8**(1):34-37

[13] Helgstrand F, Rosenberg J, Kehlet H, Bisgaard T. Outcomes after emergency versus elective ventral hernia repair: A prospective nationwide study. World Journal of Surgery. 2013;**37**(10):2273-2279. DOI: 10.1007/s00268-013-2123-5

[14] van den Berg JC, de Valois JC, Go PM, Rosenbusch G. Detection of groin hernia with physical examination, ultrasound, and MRI compared with laparoscopic findings. Investigative Radiology. 1999;**34**(12):739-743

[15] Hariprasad S, Srinivas T. Clinical study on complicated presentations

of groin hernias. International Journal of Research in Medical Sciences. 2017;**5**(8):3303-3308. DOI: 10.18203/2320-6012.ijrms20173159

[16] Frager D, Baer JW, Medwid SW, Rothpearl A, Bossart P. Detection of intestinal ischemia in patients with acute small-bowel obstruction due to adhesions or hernia: Efficacy of CT. AJR. American Journal of Roentgenology. 1996;**166**(1):67-71. DOI: 10.2214/ajr.166.1.8571907

[17] Geffroy Y, Boulay-Coletta I, Julles MC, Nakache S, Taourel P, et al. Increased unenhanced bowel-wall attenuation at multidetector CT is highly specific of ischemia complicating small-bowel obstruction. Radiology. 2013;**270**(1):159-167. DOI: 10.1148/radiol.13122654

[18] Cherian PT, Parnell AP. The diagnosis and classification of inguinal and femoral hernia on multisection spriral CT. Clinical Radiology. 2008;**63**(2):184-192. DOI: 10.1016/j.crad.2007.07.018

[19] Suzuki S, Furui S, Okinaga K, Sakamoto T, Murata J, et al. Differentiation of femoral versus inguinal hernia: CT findings. AJR. American Journal of Roentgenology. 2007;**189**(2):W78-W83. DOI: 10.2214/AJR.07.2085

[20] Gottlieb M, Peksa GD, Pandurangadu AV, Nakitende D, Takhar S, Seethala RR. Utilization of ultrasound for the evaluation of small bowel obstruction: A systematic review and meta-analysis. The American Journal of Emergency Medicine. 2018;**36**(2):234-242. DOI: 10.1016/j.ajem.2017.07.085

[21] Bay-Nielsen M, Kehlet H, Strand L, Malmstrom J, Andersen FH, Wara P, et al. Quality assessment of herniorraphies in Denmark: A prospective nationwide study. Lancet. 2001;**358**(9288):1124-1128. DOI: 10.1016/S0140-6736(01)06251-1

[22] Amato B, Moja L, Panico S. Shouldice technique versus other open techniques for inguinal hernia repair. Cochrane Database of Systematic Reviews. 18 Apr 2012;**2012**(4):CD001543. DOI: 10.1002/14651858.CD001543.pub4

[23] HerniaSurge Group. International guidelines for groin hernia management. Hernia. 2018;**22**(1):1-165. DOI: 10.1007/s10029-017-1668-x

[24] Fitzgibbons RJ Jr, Ramanan B, Arya S, Turner SA, Li X, et al. Long-term results of a randomized controlled trial of nonoperative strategy (watchful waiting) for men with minimally symptomatic inguinal hernias. Annals of Surgery. 2013;**258**(3):508-515. DOI: 10.1097/SLA.0b013e3182a19725

[25] He Z, Hao X, Li J, Zhang Y, Feng B, et al. Laparoscopic inguinal hernia repair in elderly patients. Single center experience in 12 years. Annals of Laparoscopic and Endoscopic Surgery. 2017;**2**(5):88. DOI: 10.21037/ales.2017.04.04

[26] Yeh DD, Alam HB. Hernia emergencies. Surgical Clinics of North America. 2014;**94**(1):97-130. DOI: 10.1016/j.suc.2013.10.009

[27] Rutkow IM. Demographic and socioeconomics aspects of hernia repair in the United States in 2003. The Surgical Clinics of North America. 2003;**83**(5):1045-1051. DOI: 10.1016/S0039-6109(03)00132-4

[28] Kulah B, Kulacoglu IH, Orruc MT, et al. Presentation and outcome of incarcerated external hernias in adults. American Journal of Surgery. 2001;**18**(2):101-104. DOI: 10.1016/s0002-9610(00)00563-8

[29] Le Blanc KA. Current considerations in laparoscopic incisional and ventral herniorraphy. JSLS. 2000;**4**(2):121-139

[30] Dabbas N, Adams K, Pearson K, Royle G. Frequency of abdominal wall hernias: Is classical teaching out of date? JRSM Short Reports. 2011;**2**(1):5. DOI: 10.1258/shorts.2010.010071

[31] Gallegos NC, Dawson J, Jarvis M, Hobsley M. Risk of strangulation in groin hernias. The British Journal of Surgery. 1991;**78**(10):1171-1173. DOI: 10.1002/bjs.1800781007

[32] Neutra R, Velez A, Ferrada R, Galan R. Risk of incarceration of inguinal hernia in Cali, Colombia. Journal of Chronic Diseases. 1981;**34**(11):561-564. DOI: 10.1016/0021-9681(81)90018-7

[33] Abrahamson J. Etiology and pathophysiology of primary and recurrent groin hernia formation. The Surgical Clinics of North America. 1998;**78**(6):953-972. DOI: 10.1016/S0039-6109(05)70364-9

[34] Romain B, Chemaly R, Meyer N, Brigand C, Steinmetz JP, et al. Prognostic factors of postoperative morbidity and mortality in strangulated groin hernia. Hernia. 2012;**16**(4):405-410. DOI: 10.1007/s10029-012-0937-y

[35] Brasso K, Nielsen KL, Christiansen J. Long-term results of surgery for incarcerated groin hernia. Acta Chirurgica Scandinavica. 1989;**155**(11-12):583-585

[36] Gurer A, Ozdogan M, Ozlem N, Yildirim A, Kulacoglu H, et al. Uncommon content in groin hernia sac. Hernia. 2006;**10**(2):152-155. DOI: 10.1007/s10029-005-0036-4

[37] Kouraklis G, Glinavou A, Andromanakos N, Karatzas G. Perforation of a solitary diverticulum of sigmoid colon in an incarcerated scrotal hernia. Digestive Diseases and Sciences. 2004;**49**(5):883-884. DOI: 10.1023/b:ddas.0000030104.86885.a2

[38] Abbasov A, Yanar TH. Incarcerated appendix epiploica in a right inguinal hernia sac. Ulusal Travma ve Acil Cerrahi Dergisi. 2022;**28**(12):1744-1746. DOI: 10.14744/tjtes.2021.35724

[39] Schizas D, Katsaros I, Tsapralis D, Moris D, Michalinos A, et al. Littre's hernia: A systematic review of the literature. Hernia. 2019;**23**(1):125-130. DOI: 10.1007/s10029-018-1867-0

[40] Tajti J, Pieler J, Abrahàm S, Simonka Z, Paszt A, et al. Incarcerated gallbladder in inguinal hernia: A case report and literature review. BMC Gastroenterology. 2020;**20**:45. DOI: 10.1186/s12876-020-01569-5

[41] Thomas WE, Vowles KD, Williamson RC. Appendicitis in external herniae. Annals of the Royal College of Surgeons of England. 1982;**64**(2):121-122

[42] D'Alia C, Lo Schiavo MG, Tonante A, Taranto F, Gagliano E, et al. Amyand's hernia: Case report and review of the literature. Hernia. 2003;**7**(2):89-91. DOI: 10.1007/s10029-002-0098-5

[43] Burchart J, Pommergaard HC, Bisgaard T, Rosenberg J. Patient-related risk factors for recurrence after inguinal hernia repair:A systematic review and meta-analysis of observational studies. Surgical Innovation. 2015;**22**(3):303-317. DOI: 10.1177/1553350614552731

[44] Ruhl CE, Evhart JE. Risk factors for inguinal hernia among adults in the US population. American Journal of Epidemiology. 2007;**165**(10):1154-1161. DOI: 10.1093/aje/kwm011

[45] Rosemar A, Angeras U, Rosengren A. Body mass index and

groin hernia: A 34-year follow-up study in Swedish men. Annals of Surgery. 2008;**247**(6):1064-1068. DOI: 10.1097/SLA.0b013e31816b4399

[46] Koskimaki J, Hakama M, Hutala H, Tammela TL. Association of non urologic diseases with lower urinary tract symptoms. Scandinavian Journal of Urology and Nephrology. 2001;**35**(5):377-381. DOI: 10.1080/003655901753224431

[47] Kapur P, Caty MG, Glick PL. Pediatric hernias and hydroceles. Pediatric Clinics of North America. 1998;**45**(4):773-789. DOI: 10.1016/s0031-3955(05)70044-4

[48] van Veen RN, van Wessem KJ, Halm JA, Simons MP, Plaisier PW, et al. Patent processus vaginalis in the adult as a risk factor for the occurrence of indirect inguinal hernia. Surgical Endoscopy. 2007;**21**(2):202-205. DOI: 10.1007/s00464-006-0012-9

[49] Van Wessm KJ, Simons MP, Plaisier PW, Lange JF. The etiology of indirect inguinal hernias: Congenital and/or acquired? Hernia. 2003;**7**(2):76-79. DOI: 10.1007/s10029-002-0108-7

[50] Kl W, Poola AS, Gould JL, Sharp SW, St. Peter SD, et al. The risk of developing a symptomatic inguinal hernia in children with an asymptomatic patent processus vaginalis. Journal of Pediatric Surgery. 2017;**52**(1):60-64. DOI: 10.1016/j.jpedsurg.2016.10.018

[51] Liem MS, van der Graaf Y, Beemer FA, van Vroonhoven TJ. Increased risk for inguinal hernia in patients with Ehlers-Danlos syndrome. Surgery. 1997;**122**(1):114-115. DOI: 10.1016/s0039-6060(97)90273-7

[52] Oberg S, Andresen K, Rosenberg J. Etiology of inguinal hernias: A comprehensive review. Frontiers in Surgery. 2017;**4**:52. DOI: 10.3389/fsurg.2017.00052

[53] Rafetto JD, Cheung Y, Fisher JB, Cantelmo NL, Watkins MT, et al. Incision and abdominal wall hernias in patients with aneurysm or occlusive aortic disease. Journal of Vascular Surgery. 2003;**37**(6):1150-1154. DOI: 10.1016/s0741-5214(03)00147-2

[54] Peeters E, De Hertogh G, Junge K, Klinge U, Miserez M. Skin as a marker for collagen type I/III ratio in abdominal wall fascia. Hernia. 2014;**18**(4):519-525. DOI: 10.1007/s10029-013-1128-1

[55] Henriksen NA, Mortensen JH, Sorensen LT, Bay-Jensen AC, Agren MS, et al. The collagen turnover profile is altered in patients with inguinal and incisional hernia. Surgery. 2015;**157**(2):312-321. DOI: 10.1016/j.surg.2014.09.006

[56] Sorensen LT, Jorgensen S, Petersen LJ, Hemmingsen U, Bulow J, et al. Acute effects of nicotine and smoking on blood flow, tissue oxygen, and aerobe metabolism of the skin and subcutis. The Journal of Surgical Research. 2009;**152**(2):224-230. DOI: 10.1016/j.jss.2008.02.066

[57] Vad MV, Frost P, Rosenberg J, Andersen JH, Svendsen SW. Inguinal hernia repair among men in relation to occupational mechanical exposures and lifestyle factors: A longitudinal study. Occupational and Environmental Medicine. 2017;**74**(11):769-775. DOI: 10.1136/oemed-2016-104160

[58] Cobb WS, Burns JM, Kercher KW, Matthews BD, James Norton H, et al. Normal intra abdominal pressure in healthy adults. The Journal of Surgical Research. 2005;**120**(2):231-235. DOI: 10.1016/j.jss.2005.06.015

[59] Svendsen SW, Frost P, Vad MV, Andersen JH. Risk and prognosis

of inguinal hernia in relation to occupational mechanical exposures-a systematic review of the epidemiologic evidence. Scandinavian Journal of Work, Environment & Health. 2013;**39**(1):5-26. DOI: 10.5271/sjweh.3305

[60] Vad MV, Frost P, Bay-Nielsen M, Svendsen SW. Impact of occupational mechanical exposures on risk of lateral and medial inguinal hernia requiring surgical repair. Occupational and Environmental Medicine. 2012;**69**(11):802-809. DOI: 10.1136/oemed-2012-100787

[61] Stedman TL. Stedman's Medical Dictionary. 28th ed. Philadelphia, PA: Lippincott Williams and Wilkins; 2005

[62] Sartelli M, Coccolini F, van Ramshorst GH, Campanelli G, Mandalà V, et al. WSES guidelines for emergency repair of complicated abdominal wall hernias. World Journal of Emergency Surgery: WJES. 2013;**8**:50. DOI: 10.1186/1749-7922-8-50

[63] Nyhus LM. Classification of inguinal hernias: Milestones. Hernia. 2004;**8**(2):87-88. DOI: 10.1007/s10029-003-0173-6

[64] Zollinger RM. An updated traditional classification of inguinal hernias. Hernia. 2004;**8**(4):318-322. DOI: 10.1007/s10029-004-0245-2

[65] Rutkow IR, Robbins AW. Classification systems and groin hernias. The Surgical Clinics of North America. 1998;**78**(6):1117-1127,vii. DOI: 10.1016/S0039-6109(05)70373-X

[66] Gilbert AI. An anatomic and functional classification for the diagnosis and treatment of inguinal hernia. American Journal of Surgery. 1989;**157**(3):331-333. DOI: 10.1016/0002-9610(89)90564-3

[67] Simmons BP. Guidelines for prevention of surgical wound infections. American Journal of Infection Control. 1983;**11**(4):133-143. DOI: 10.1016/0196-6553(83)90030-5

[68] Schumpelick V, Treutner KH, Arlt G. Classification of inguinal hernias. Chirurg. 1994;**65**(10):331-333

[69] Sarr MG, Bulkley GB, Zuidema GD. Preoperative recognition of intestinal strangulation obstruction. Prospective evaluation of diagnostic capability. American Journal of Surgery. 1983;**145**(1):176-182. DOI: 10.1016/0002-9610(83)90186-1

[70] Miserez M, Alexandre JH, Campanelli G, Corcione F, Cuccurullo D, et al. The European hernia society groin hernia classification: Simple and easy to remember. Hernia. 2007;**11**(2):113-116. DOI: 10.1007/s10029-007-0198-3

[71] Birindelli A, Sartelli M, Di Saverio S, Coccolini F, Ansaloni L, et al. Update of the WSES guidelines for emergency repair of complicated abdominal wall hernias. Hernia. 2017;**2017**(12):37. DOI: 10.1186/s13017-017-0149-y

[72] East B, Pawlak M, de Beaux AC. A manual reduction of hernia under analgesia/sedation (Taxis) in the acute inguinal hernia: A useful technique in COVID-19 times to reduce the need for emergency surgery-a literature review. Hernia. 2020;**24**(5):937-941. DOI: 10.1007/s10029-020-02227-1

[73] Shattla A, Chamberlain B, Webb W. Current status of diagnosis and management of strangulation obstruction of the small bowel. American Journal of Surgery. 1978;**132**(3):299-302. DOI: 10.1016/0002-9610(76)90379-2

[74] Kang SK, Burnett CA, Freund E, Sestito J. Hernia: Is it a

work-related condition? American Journal of Industrial Medicine. 1999;**36**(6):638-644. DOI: 10.1002/(sici)1097-0274(199912)36:6<638::aid-ajim6>3.0.co;2-w

[75] Pathak S, Poston GJ. It is highly unlikely that the development of an abdominal wall hernia can be attributable to a single strenuous event. Annals of the Royal College of Surgeons of England. 2006;**88**(2):168-171. DOI: 10.1308/003588406X95093

[76] Jenkins JT, O'Dwyer PJ. Inguinal hernias. BMJ. 2008;**336**(7638):269-272. DOI: 10.1136/bmj.39450.428275.AD

[77] Kappikeri VS, Sangamesh JM. A clinical study of complicated inguinal hernias. Rajv Gandhi University of Health Science Journal of Medical Sciences. 2018;**8**(2):60-70. DOI: 10.26463/rjms.8_2_4

[78] Oishi SN, Oage CP, Schwesinger WH. Complicated presentations of groin hernias. American Journal of Surgery. 1991;**162**(6):568-571. DOI: 10.1016/0002-9610(91)90110-y

[79] Gough IR. Strangulation adhesive small-bowel obstruction with normal radiographs. The British Journal of Surgery. 1978;**65**(6):431-434. DOI: 10.1002/bjs.1800650618

[80] Otamari T, Sjodahl R, Ihse I. Intestinal obstruction with strangulation of the small bowel. Acta Chirurgica Scandinavica. 1987;**153**(4):307-310

[81] Bekoe S. Prospective analysis of management of incarcerated and strangulated inguinal hernia. American Journal of Surgery. 1973;**126**(5):665-668. DOI: 10.1016/s0002-9610(73)80018-2

[82] Aguirre DA, Santosa AC, Casola G, Sirlin CB. Abdominal wall hernias: Imaging features, complications, and diagnostic pitfalls at multi-detector row CT. Radiographics. 2005;**25**(6):1501-1520. DOI: 10.1148/rg.256055018

[83] Dal F, Topal U, Sozuer EM, Akyuz M, Talih T, et al. Evaluation of the factors related to strangulation and, mortality in patients with incarcerated abdominal wall hernias. Iranian Red Crescent Medical Journal. 2022;**24**(2):e1800. DOI: 10.32592/ircmj.2021.23.5.366

[84] Gul M, Aliosmanoglu KM, Onder A, Taskesen F, et al. Factors affecting morbidity and mortality in patients who underwent emergency operation for incarcerated abdominal wall hernia. International Surgery. 2012;**97**(4):305-309. DOI: 10.9738/CC114.1

[85] Kulah B, Duzgun AP, Moran M, Kulacoglu IH, Ozmen MM, et al. Emergency hernia repairs in elderly patients. American Journal of Surgery. 2001;**182**(5):455-459. DOI: 10.1016/s0002-9610(01)00765-6

[86] Abi-Haidar Y, Sanchez V, Itani KMF. Risk factors and outcomes of acute versus elective groin hernia surgery. Journal of the American College of Surgeons. 2011;**213**(3):363-369. DOI: 10.1016/j.jamcollsurg.2011.05.008

[87] Alvarez Pèrez JA, Baldonedo RF, Bear IG, Solis JAS, Alvarez P, et al. Incarcerated groin hernias in adults: Presentation and outcome. Hernia. 2004;**8**(2):121-126. DOI: 10.1007/s10029-003-0186-1

[88] Askew G, Williams GT, Brown SC. Delay in presentation and misdiagnosis of strangulated hernia: Prospective study. Journal of the Royal College of Surgeons of Edinburgh. 1992;**37**(1):37-38

[89] Markogiannakis H, Memos N, Messaris E, Dardamanis D, Larentzakis A, et al. Predictive value of procalcitonin for bowel ischemia and

necrosis in bowel obstruction. Surgery. 2011;**149**(3):394-403. DOI: 10.1016/j.surg.2010.08.007

[90] O'Leary MP, Neville AL, Keeley JA, Kim DY, de Virgilio C, et al. Predictors of ischemic bowel in patients with small bowel obstruction. The American Surgeon. 2016;**82**(10):992-994

[91] Icoz G, Makay O, Sozbilen M, et al. Is D-dimer a predictor of strangulated intestinal hernia ? World Journal of Surgery. 2006;**30**(12):2165-2169. DOI: 10.1007/s00268-006-0138-x

[92] Ten Broek RPG, Krielen P, Di Saverio S, Coccolini F, Biffi WL, et al. Bologna guidelines for diagnosis and management of adhesive small bowel obstruction (ASBO): 2017 update of the evidence based guidelines from the world society of emergency surgery ASBO working group. World Journal of Emergency Surgery : WJES. 2018;**13**:24. DOI: 10.1186/s13017-018-0185-2

[93] Zielenski MD, Eiken PW, Bannon MP, Heller SF, Lohse CM, et al. Small bowel obstruction-who needs an operation? A multivariate prediction model. World Journal of Surgery. 2010;**34**(5):910-919. DOI: 10.1007/s00268-010-0479-3

[94] Lange H, Jackel R. Usefulness of plasma lactate concentration in the diagnosis of acute abdominal disease. The European Journal of Surgery. 1994;**160**(6-7):381-384

[95] Tanaka K, Hanyu N, Iida T, et al. Lactate levels in the detection of preoperative bowel strangulation. The American Surgeon. 2012;**78**(1):86-88

[96] Graeber G, O'Neil J, Wolf R, Wukich D, Caffery P, Harman J. Elevated levels of peritoneal serum creatine phosphokinase with strangulated small bowel obstruction. Archives of Surgery. 1983;**118**(7):837-840. DOI: 10.1001/archsurg.1983.01390070045009

[97] Moller L, Kristensen TS. Plasma fibrinogen and ischemic hearth disease risk factors. Arteriosclerosis and Thrombosis. 1991;**11**(2):344-350. DOI: 10.1161/01.atv.11.2.344

[98] Kahramanca S, Kaya O, Ozgehan G, Guzel H, Azili C, et al. Are fibrinogen and complete blood count parameters predictive in incarcerated abdominal hernia repair? International Surgery. 2014;**99**(6):723-728. DOI: 10.9738/INTSURG-D-13-00107.1

[99] Napoli MD, Singh P. Is plasma fibrinogen useful in evaluating ischemic stroke? Why, how, and when. Stroke. 2009;**40**(5):1549-1552. DOI: 10.1161/STROKEAHA.108.537084

[100] Lin YP, Lee J, Chao HC, Kong MS, Lai MW, et al. Risk factors for intestinal gangrene in children with small-bowel volvulus. Journal of Pediatric Gastroenterology and Nutrition. 2011;**53**(4):417-422. DOI: 10.1097/MPG.0b013e3182201a7c

[101] Keeley JA, Kaji A, Kim DY, Putman B, Neville A. Predictors of ischemic bowel in patients with incarcerated hernias. Hernia. 2019;**23**(2):277-280. DOI: 10.1007/s10029-019-01884-1

[102] Riedel S, Melendez JH, An AT, Rosenbaum JE, Zenilman JM. Procalcitonin as a marker for the detection of bacteremia and sepsis in the emergency department. American Journal of Clinical Pathology. 2011;**135**(2):182-189. DOI: 10.1309/AJCP1MFYINQLECV2

[103] Jancelewicz T, Vu LT, Shawo AE, Yeh B, Gasper WJ, et al. Predicting strangulated small bowel obstruction: An old problem revisited. Journal of

Gastrointestinal Surgery. 2009;**13**(1): 93-99. DOI: 10.1007/s11605-008-0610-z

[104] Ogata M, Mateer JR, Condon RE. Prospective evaluation of abdominal sonography for the diagnosis of bowel obstruction. Annals of Surgery. 1996;**223**(3):237-241. DOI: 10.1097/00000658-199603000-00002

[105] American College of Radiology, ACR Appropriateness Criteria Hernia, Expert Panel on Gastrointestinal Imaging, Garcia EM, Pietryga JA, Kim DH, et al. Journal of the American College of Radiology. 2022;**19**(11S):S329-S340. DOI: 10.1016/j.jacr.2022.09.016

[106] Bradley M, Morgan J, Pentlow B, Roe A. The positive predictive value of diagnostic ultrasound for occult hernias. Annals of the Royal College of Surgeons of England. 2006;**88**(2):165-167. DOI: 10.1308/003588406X95110

[107] Lee RK, Griffith JF, Ng WH. High accuracy of ultrasound in diagnosing the presence and type of groin hernia. Journal of Clinical Ultrasound. 2015;**43**(9):538-547. DOI: 10.1002/jcu.22271

[108] Hefny AF, Corr P, Abu-Zidan FM. The role of ultrasound in the management of intestinal obstruction. Journal of Emergencies, Trauma, and Shock. 2012;**5**(1):84-86. DOI: 10.4103/0974-2700.93109

[109] Jamadar DA, Jacobson JA, Morag Y, Girish G, Dong Q, el al. Characteristic locations of inguinal region and anterior abdominal hernias: Sonographic appearances and identification of clinical pitfalls. AJR. American Journal of Roentgenology. 2007;**188**(5):1356-1364. DOI: 10.2214/AJR.06.0638

[110] Silva AC, Pimenta M, Guimaraes LS. Small bowel obstruction: What to look for. Radiographics. 2009;**29**(2):423-439. DOI: 10.1148/rg.292085514

[111] Balthazar EJ, Liebeskind ME, Macari M. Intestinal ischemia in patients in whom small-bowel obstruction is suspected: Evaluation of accuracy, limitations, and clinical implications of CT in diagnosis. Radiology. 1997;**205**(2):519-522. DOI: 10.1148/radiology.205.2.9356638

[112] Mullan CP, Siewert B, Eisenberg RL. Small bowel obstruction. AJR. American Journal of Roentgenology. 2012;**198**(2):W105-W117. DOI: 10.2214/AJR.10.4998

[113] Piga E, Zetner D, Andresen K, Rosenberg J. Imaging modalities for inguinal hernia diagnosis: A systematic review. Hernia. 2020;**24**(5):917-926. DOI: 10.1007/s10029-020-02189-4

[114] Mallo RD, Salem L, Lalani T, Flum DR. Computed tomography diagnosis of complete obstruction in small obstruction: A systematic review. Journal of Gastrointestinal Surgery. 2005;**9**(5):690-694. DOI: 10.1016/j.gassur.2004.10.006

[115] Millet I, Taourel P, Ruyer A, Molinari N. Value of CT findings to predict surgical ischemia in small bowel obstruction: A systematic review and meta-analysis. European Radiology. 2015;**25**(6):1823-1835. DOI: 10.1007/s00330-014-3440-2

[116] Zins M, Millet I, Taourel P. Adhesive small bowel obstruction: Predictive radiology to improve patient management. Radiology. 2020;**296**(3):480-491. DOI: 10.1148/radiol.2020192234

[117] Murphy KP, O'Connor OJ, Maher MM. Adult abdominal hernias. AJR. American Journal of Roentgenology. 2014;**202**(6):W506-W5011. DOI: 10.2214/AJR.13.12071

[118] Paulson EK, Thompson WM. Review of small-bowel obstruction: The diagnosis and when to worry. Radiology. 2015;**275**(2):332-342. DOI: 10.1148/radiol.15131519

[119] Scrima A, Lubner MG, King S, Pankratz J, Kennedy J, et al. Value of MDCT and clinical an laboratory data for predicting the need for surgical intervention in suspected bowel obstruction. AJR. American Journal of Roentgenology. 2017;**208**(4):785-793. DOI: 10.2214/AJR.16.16946

[120] Shadbolt CL, Heinze SB, Dietrich RB. Imaging of groin masses: Inguinal anatomy and pathologic conditions revisited. Radiographics. 2001;**21**:S261-S271. DOI: 10.1148/radiographics.21.suppl_1.g01oc17s261

[121] Purkayastha S, Chow A, Athanasiou T, Tekkis P, Darzi A. Inguinal hernia. BMJ Clinical Evidence. 2008;**16**:0412

[122] Matthews RD, Neumayer L. Inguinal hernia in the 21st century: An evidence-based review. Current Problems in Surgery. 2008;**45**(4):261-312. DOI: 10.1067/j.cpsurg.2008.01.002

[123] Kulacoglu H. Current options in inguinal hernia repair in adult patients. Hippokratia. 2011;**15**(3):223-231

[124] Malik AM, Khan A, Talpur KA, Laghari AA. Factors influencing morbidity and mortality in elderly population undergoing inguinal hernia surgery. The Journal of the Pakistan Medical Association. 2010;**60**(1):45-47

[125] Turrentine FE, Wang H, Simpson VB, Jones RS. Surgical risk factors, morbidity, and mortality in elderly patients. Journal of the American College of Surgeons. 2006;**203**(6):865-877. DOI: 10.1016/j.jamcollsurg.2006.08.026

[126] Orchard MR, Wright JA, Kelly A, McCabe DJ, Hewes. The impact of healthcare rationing on elective and emergency hernia repair. Hernia. 2016;**20**(3):405-409. DOI: 10.1007/s10029-015-1441-y

[127] Davies M, Davies C, Morris-Stiff G, Shute K. Emergency presentation of abdominal hernias: Outcome and reasons for delay in treatment- a prospective study. Annals of the Royal College of Surgeons of England. 2007;**89**(1):47-50. DOI: 10.1308/003588407X160855

[128] Nilsson H, Stylianidis G, Haapamaki M, Nilsson E, Nordin P. Mortality after groin hernia surgery. Annals of Surgery. 2007;**245**(4):656-660. DOI: 10.1097/01.sla.0000251364.32698.4b

[129] Gianetta E, Cian FD, Cunea S, Friedman D, Vitale B, et al. Hernia repair in elderly patients. The British Journal of Surgery. 2005;**84**(7):983-985. DOI: 10.1002/bjs.1800840721

[130] Allen PIM, Zager N, Goldman M. Elective repair of groin hernias in the elderly. The British Journal of Surgery. 1987;**74**(11):987. DOI: 10.1002/bjs.1800741109

[131] Dunne JR, Malone DL, Tracy GK, Napolitano LM. Abdominal wall hernias: Risk factors for infection and resource utilization. The Journal of Surgical Research. 2003;**111**(1):78-84. DOI: 10.1016/s0022-4804(03)00077-5

[132] McEntee G, O'Carroll A, Mooney B, Egan T, Delaney P. Timing of strangulations in adults hernias. The British Journal of Surgery. 1989;**76**(7):725-726. DOI: 10.1002/bjs.1800760724

[133] Malek S, Torella F, Edwards P. Emergency repair of groin herniae:

Outcome and implication of elective surgery waiting times. International Journal of Clinical Practice. 2004;**58**(2):207-209. DOI: 10.1111/j.1368-5031.2004.0097.x

[134] Ceresoli M, Carissimi F, Nigro A, Fransvea P, Lepre L, et al. Emergency hernia repair in the elderly: Multivariate analysis of morbidity and mortality from an Italian registry. Hernia. 2022;**26**(1):165-175. DOI: 10.1007/s10029-020-02269-5

[135] Amid PK, Shulman AG, Lichtenstein IL. Open "tension free" repair of inguinal hernias: The Lichtenstein technique. The European Journal of Surgery. 1996;**162**(6):447-553

[136] Amid PK. Lichtenstein tension-free hernioplasty: Its inception, evolution, and principles. Hernia. 2004;**8**(1):1-7. DOI: 10.1007/s10029

[137] Bisgaard T, Bay-Nielsen M, Christensen IJ, Kehlet H. Risk of recurrence 5 years or more after primary Lichtenstein mesh and sutured inguinal hernia repair. The British Journal of Surgery. 2007;**94**(8):1038-1040. DOI: 10.1002/bjs.5756

[138] Scott NW, McCormack K, Graham P, Go PM, Ross SJ, et al. Open mesh versus non-mesh for repair of femoral and inguinal hernia. Cochrane Database of Systematic Reviews. 2002;**4**:CD002197. DOI: 10.1002/14651858.CD002197

[139] O'Dwyer PJ, Chung L. Watchful waiting was as safe as surgical repair for minimally symptomatic inguinal hernias. Evidence-Based Medicine. 2006;**11**(3):73. DOI: 10.1136/ebm.11.3.73

[140] Fitzgibbons RJ, Giobbie-Hurder A, Gibbs JO, Dunlop DD, Reda DJ, et al. Watchful waiting vs.repair of inguinal hernia in minimally symptomatic men: A randomized clinical trial. JAMA. 2006;**295**(3):285-292. DOI: 10.1001/jama.295.3.285

[141] van den Heuvel B, Dwars BJ, Klassen DR, Bonjer HJ. Is surgical repair of asymptomatic groin hernia appropriate? A review. Hernia. 2011;**15**(3):251-259. DOI: 10.1007/s10029-011-0796-y

[142] O'Dwyer PJ, Norrie J, Alani A, Walker A, Duffy F, Horgan P. Observation or operation for patients with an asymptomatic inguinal hernia. Annals of Surgery. 2006;**244**(2):167-173. DOI: 10.1097/01.sla.0000217637.69699.ef

[143] INCA Trialists Collaboration. Operation compared with watchful waiting in elderly male inguinal hernia patients: A review and data analysis. Journal of the American College of Surgeons. 2011;**212**(2):251-259. DOI: 10.1016/j.jamcollsurg.2010.09.030

[144] Reistrup H, Fonnes S, Rosenberg J. Watchful waiting vs repair for asymptomatic or minimally asymptomatic inguinal hernia in men: A systematic review. Hernia. 2021;**25**(5):1121-1128. DOI: 10.1007/s10029-020-02295-3

[145] Miserez M, Peeters E, Aufenacker T, Bouillot JL, Campanelli G, et al. Update with level 1 studies of the European hernia society guidelines on the treatment of inguinal hernia in adult patients. Hernia. 2014;**18**(2):151-163. DOI: 10.1007/s10029-014-1236-6

[146] Gong W, Li J. Operation versus watchful waiting in asymptomatic or minimally symptomatic inguinal hernias: The meta-analysis results of randomized controlled trials. International Journal of Surgery. 2018;**52**:120-125. DOI: 10.1016/j.ijsu.2018.02.030

[147] Weber G. Principles of the management of adult inguinal hernia: Recommendations by the European hernia society. Magyar Sebészet. 2010;**63**(5):287-296. DOI: 10.1556/MaSeb.63.2010.5.1

[148] Rai S, Chandra SS, Smile SR. A study of the risk of strangulation and obstruction in groin hernias. The Australian and New Zealand Journal of Surgery. 1998;**68**(9):650-654. DOI: 10.1111/j.1445-2197.1998.tb04837.x

[149] Harissis JV, Doutsis E, Fatouros M. Incarcerated hernia: To reduce or not reduce? Hernia. 2009;**13**(3):263-266. DOI: 10.1007/s10029-008-0467-9

[150] Pawlak M, Niebuhr H, Bury K. Dynamic inguinal ultrasound: A diagnostic tool for hernia surgeons. Hernia. 2015;**19**(6):1033-1034. DOI: 10.1177/145749691009900307

[151] Chen SC, Lee CC, Liu YP, Yen ZS, Wuang HP, et al. Ultrasound may decrease the emergency surgery rate of incarcerated inguinal hernia. Scandinavian Journal of Gastroenterology. 2005;**40**(6):721-724. DOI: 10.1080/00365520510015485

[152] Isil RG, Yazici P, Demir U, Kaya C, Bostanci O, et al. Approach to inguinal hernia in high-risk geriatric patients: Should it be elective or emergent? Ulusal Travma ve Acil Cerrahi Dergisi. 2017;**23**(2):122-127. DOI: 10.5505/tjtes.2016.36932

[153] Smith G, Wrigth JE. Reduction of gangrenous small bowel by taxis on an inguinal hernia. Pediatric Surgery International. 1996;**11**(8):582-583. DOI: 10.1007/BF00626074

[154] Nehme AE. Groin hernias in elderly patients: Management and prognosis. American Journal of Surgery. 1983;**146**(2):257-260. DOI: 10.1016/0002-9610(83)90386-0

[155] De Simone B, Birindelli A, Ansaloni L, Sartelli M, Coccolini F, et al. Emergency repair of complicated abdominal wall hernias: WSES guidelines. Hernia. 2020;**24**(2):359-368. DOI: 10.1007/s10029-019-02021-8

[156] Venara A, Hubner M, Le Naoures P, Hamel GF, Hamy A. Surgery for incarcerated hernia: Short-term outcome with or without mesh. Langenbeck's Archives of Surgery. 2014;**399**(5):571-577. DOI: 10.1007/s00423-014-1202-x

[157] Bessa SS, Katri KM, Abdel Salam WN, Abdel-Baki NA. Early results from the use of Lichtenstein repair in the management of strangulated groin hernia. Hernia. 2007;**11**(3):239-242. DOI: 10.1007/s10029-007-0207-6

[158] Derici H, Unlap HR, Bozdag AD, Nazil O, Tansung T, Kamer E. Factors affecting morbidity and mortality in incarcerated abdominal wall hernias. Hernia. 2007;**11**(4):341-346. DOI: 10.1007/s10029-007-0226-3

[159] Martinez-Serrano MA, Pereira JA, Sancho JJ, Lòpez-Cano M, Bombuy E, et al. Study Group of Abdominal Hernia Surgery of the Catalan Society of Surgery. Risk of death after emergency repair of abdominal wall hernias: Still waiting for improvement. Langenbeck's Archives of Surgery. 2010;**395**(5):551-556. DOI: 10.1007/s00423-009-0515-7

[160] Isil RG, Yazici P, Demir U, Kaya C, Bostanci O, et al. Outcomes of geriatric patients who underwent incarcerated inguinal hernia repair. The Medical Bullettin of Sisli Etfal Hospital. 2016;**50**(2):103-109

[161] Pavlidius TE, Symeonidis NG, Rafailidis SE, Psarras K, Ballas KD, et al. Tension-free by mesh-plug technique for inguinal hernia repair in elderly patients. Scandinavian

Journal of Surgery. 2010;**99**(3):137-141. DOI: 10.1177/145749691009900307

[162] Morley JE, Vellas B, van Kan GA, Anker SD, Bauer JM. Frailty consensus: A call to action. Journal of the American Directors Association. 2013;**14**(6):392-397. DOI: 10.1016/j.jamda.2013.03.022

[163] Hellspong G, Gunnarson U, Dahlstrand U, Sandblom G. Diabetes as a risk factor in patients undergoing groin hernia surgery. Langenbeck's Archives of Surgery. 2017;**402**(2):219-225. DOI: 10.1007/s00423-016-1519-8

[164] Atila K, Guler S, Inal A. Prosthetic repair of acutely incarcerated groin hernias: A prospective clinical observational cohort study. Langenbeck's Archives of Surgery. 2010;**395**(5):563-568. DOI: 10.1007/s00423-008-0414-3

[165] Kaoutzanis C, Leichtle SW, Mouwad NJ, Welch KB, Lampman RM, et al. Risk factors for postoperative wound infections and prolonged hospitalization after ventral/incisional hernia repair. Hernia. 2015;**19**(1):113-123. DOI: 10.1007/s10029-013-1155-y

[166] Suljagic V, Jevtic M, Djorjevic B, Jovelic A. Surgical site infections in a tertiary health care center; prospective cohort study. Surgery Today. 2010;**40**(8):763-771. DOI: 10.1007/s00595-009-4124-4

[167] Abete P, Cherubini A, Di Bari M, Vigorito C, Viviani G, et al. Does comprehensive geriatric assessment improve the estimate of surgical risk in elderly patients? An Italian multicenter observational study. American Journal of Surgery. 2016;**211**(1):76-83. DOI: 10.1016/j.amjsurg.2015.04.016

[168] Sagar PM, MacFie J, Sedman P, May J, Mancey-Jones B, et al. Intestinal obstruction promotes gut translocation of bacteria. Diseases of the Colon and Rectum. 1995;**38**(6):640-644. DOI: 10.1007/BF02054126

[169] Beltran MA, Cruces KS. Are the outcomes of emergency Lichtenstein hernioplasty similar to the outcomes of elective Lichtenstein hernioplasty? International Journal of Surgery. 2007;**5**(3):198-204. DOI: 10.1016/j.ijsu.2006.04.006

[170] Cheng J, Wei Z, Liu X, Li X, Yuan Z, et al. The role of intestinal mucosa injury induced by intra-abdominal hypertension in the development of abdominal compartment syndrome and multiple organ dysfunction syndrome. Critical Care. 2013;**17**(6):R283. DOI: 10.1186/cc13146

[171] Chen P, Huang L, Yang W, He D, Liu X, et al. Risk factors for bowel resection among patients with incarcerated groin hernias: A meta-analysis. The American Journal of Emergency Medicine. 2020;**38**(2):376-383. DOI: 10.1016/j.ajem.2019.09.023

[172] Elsebae MM, Nasr M, Said M. Tension-free repair versus Bassini technique for strangulated inguinal hernia: a controlled randomized study. International Journal of Surgery. 2008;**6**(4):302-305. DOI: 10.1016/j.ijsu.2008.04.006

[173] Hentati H, Dougaz W, Dziri C. Mesh repair versus non mesh repair for strangulated inguinal hernia: Systematic with meta-analysis. World Journal of Surgery. 2014;**38**(11):2784-2790. DOI: 10.1007/s00268-014-2710-0

[174] Kockerling F, Heine T, Adolf D, Zarras K, Weyhe D, et al. Trends in emergent groin hernia repair-An analysis from the herniamed registry. Frontiers in Surgery. 2021;**8**:655755.3. DOI: 10.3389/fsurg.2021.655755

[175] Lichtenstein IL, Shulman AG, Amid PK, Montllor MM. The tension-free hernioplasty. American Journal of Surgery. 1989;**157**(2):188-193. DOI: 10.1016/0002-9610(89)90526-6

[176] Nieuwenhiuzen J, van Ramshorst GH, ten Brinke JG, de Wit T, van der Harst E, et al. The use of mesh in acute hernia: Frequency and outcome in 99 cases. Hernia. 2011;**15**(3):297-300. DOI: 10.1007/s10029-010-0779-4

[177] Taylor SG, O'Dwyer PJ. Chronic groin sepsis following tension-free inguinal hernioplasty. The British Journal of Surgery. 1999;**86**(4):562-565. DOI: 10.1046/j.1365-2168.1999.01072.x

[178] Falagas ME, Kasiakou SK. Mesh-related infections after hernia repair surgery. Clinical Microbiology and Infection. 2005;**11**(1):3-8. DOI: 10.1111/j.1469-0691.2004.01014.x

[179] Klinge U, Klosterhalfen B. Modified classification of surgical meshes for hernia repair based on the analyses of 1,000 explanted meshes. Hernia. 2012;**16**(3):251-258. DOI: 10.1007/s10029-012-0913-6

[180] Ueda J, Nomura T, Sasaki J, Shigrhara K, Yamahatsu K, et al. Prosthetic repair of an incarcerated groin hernia with small intestinal resection. Surgery Today. 2012;**42**(4):359-362. DOI: 10.1007/s00595-011-0019-2

[181] Wysocki A, Pozniczek KJ, Bolt L. Use of polypropylene prostheses for strangulated inguinal and incisional hernias. Hernia. 2001;**5**(2):106-106. DOI: 10.1007/s100290100013

[182] Robinson TN, Clarke JH, Schoen J, Walsh MD. Major mesh-related complications following hernia repair: Events reported to the Food and Drug Administration. Surgical Endoscopy. 2005;**19**(12):1556-1660. DOI: 10.1007/s00464-005-0120-y

[183] Coda A, Lamberti R, Martorana S. Classification of prosthetics used in hernia repair based upon weight and biomaterial. Hernia. 2012;**16**(1):9-20. DOI: 10.1007/s10029-011-0868-z

[184] D'Ambrosio R, Capasso L, Sgueglia S, Iarrobino G, Buonoincontro S, et al. The meshes of polypropylene in emergency surgery for strangulated hernias and incisional hernias. Annali Italiani di Chirurgia. 2004;**75**(5):569-573

[185] Franciosi C, Romano F, Caprotti R, De Fina S, Colombo G, et al. Hernia repair with prolene mesh according to the Lichtenstein technique. Results of 692 cases. Minerva Chirurgica. 2000;**55**(9):593-597

[186] Carbonel AM, Criss CN, Cobb WS, Novitsky YW, Rosen MJ. Outcomes of synthetic mesh in contaminated ventral hernia repairs. Journal of the American College of Surgeons. 2013;**217**(6):991-998. DOI: 10.1016/j.jamcollsurg.2013.07.382

[187] Tse W, Johns W, maher J, Rivers J, Miller T. Bassini inguinal repair: Obsolete or still a viable surgical option. A single center cohort study. International Journal of Surgery Open. 2021;**36**:100415. DOI: 10.1016/j.ijso.2021.100415

[188] Rutledge RH. Cooper's ligament repair: A 25 year experience with a single technique for all groin hernias in adults. Surgery. 1998;**103**(1):1-10

[189] Shouldice EB. The Shouldice repair for groin hernias. The Surgical Clinics of North America. 2003;**83**(5):1163-1187,vii. DOI: 10.1016/S0039-6109(03)00121-X

[190] Simons MP, Kleijnen J, van Geldere D, Hoitsma HF, Obertop H. Role

of the Shouldice technique in inguinal hernia repair: A systematic review of controlled trials and meta-analysis. The British Journal of Surgery. 1996;**83**(6):734-738. DOI: 10.1002/bjs.1800830606

[191] Beets GL, Oosterhhuis KJ, Go PM, Baeten CG, Kootstra G. Long term follow up (12-15 years) of a randomized controlled trial comparing Bassini-Stetten, Shouldice, and high ligation with narrowing of the internal ring for primary inguinal hernia repair. Journal of the American College of Surgeons. 1997;**185**(4):352-357

[192] Guzzo JL, Bochicchio GV, Henry S, Keller E, Scalea TM. Incarcerated inguinal hernia in the presence of Fournier's gangrene: A novel approach to a complex problem. The American Surgeon. 2007;**73**(1):93-95

[193] Puccio F, Solazzo M, Marciano P. Comparison of three different mesh materials in tension-free inguinal repair: Prolene versus Vypro versus surgisis. International Surgery. 2005;**90**(3 Suppl):S21-S23

[194] Payiziwula J, Zhao PJ, Aierke A, Yao G, Apaer S, et al. Laparoscopy versus open incarcerated inguinal hernia repair in octogenarians; single-center experience with world review. Surgical Laparoscopy, Endoscopy & Percutaneous Techniques. 2019;**29**(2):138-140. DOI: 10.1097/SLE.0000000000000629

[195] Pallati PK, Gupta PK, Bichala S, Gupta H, Fang X, et al. Short-term outcomes of inguinal hernia repair in octogenarians and nonagenarians. Hernia. 2013;**17**(6):723-727. DOI: 10.1007/s10029-012-1040-0

[196] Velasco JM, Vallina VL, Esposito DJ, Theodore S. Laparoscopic herniorrhaphy in the geriatric population. The American Surgeon. 1988;**64**(7):633-637

[197] Bittner R, Sauerland S, Schmedt CG. Comparison of endoscopic techniques vs Shouldice and other non open mesh techniques for inguinal hernia repair: A meta-analysis of randomized controlled trials. Surgical Endoscopy. 2005;**19**(5):605-615. DOI: 10.1007/s00464-004-9049-9

[198] Mahon D, Decadt B, Rhodes M. Prospective randomized trial of laparoscopic (transabdominal preperitoneal) vs open (mesh) repair for bilateral and recurrent inguinal hernia. Surgical Endoscopy. 2003;**17**(9):1386-1390. DOI: 10.1007/s00464-002-9223-x

[199] Zu X, Liu Z, Shen J, Liu J, Tang R. Comparison of open and laparoscopic inguinal-hernia repair in octogenarians. Asian Journal of Surgery. 2023;**46**(2):738-741. DOI: 10.1016/j.asjsur.2022.06.149

[200] Dallas KB, Froylich D, Choi JJ, Rosa JH, Lo C, et al. Laparoscopic versus open inguinal hernia repair in octogenarians: A follow-up study. Geriatrics and Gerontology International. 2013;**13**(2):329-333. DOI: 10.1111/j.1447-0594.2012.00902.x

[201] Motson EW. Why does NICE not recommend laparoscopic herniorraphy? BMJ. 2002;**324**(7345):1092-1094. DOI: 10.1136/bmj.324.7345.1092

[202] Memon MA, Cooper NJ, Memon B, Memon MI, Abrams KR. Meta-analysis of randomized controlled trials comparing open and laparoscopic inguinal repair. The British Journal of Surgery. 2003;**90**(12):1479-1482. DOI: 10.1002/bjs.4301

[203] Neumayer L, Giobbie-Hurder A, Jonasson O, Fitzgibbons R Jr, Dunlop D, et al. Open mesh versus laparoscopic mesh repair of inguinal hernia. The New England Journal of Medicine. 2004;**350**(18):1819-1827. DOI: 10.1056/NEJMoa040093

[204] O'Reilly EA, Burke JP, O'Connel PR. A meta-analysis of surgical morbidity and recurrence after laparoscopic and open repair of primary unilateral inguinal hernia. Annals of Surgery. 2012;**255**(5):846-853. DOI: 10.1097/SLA.0b013e31824e96cf

[205] Hynes DM, Stroupe KT, Luo P, Giobbe-Hurder A, Reda D, et al. Cost effectiveness of laparoscopic versus open mesh hernia operation: Results of a Department of Veterans Affairs randomized clinical trial. Journal of the American College of Surgeons. 2006;**203**(4):447-457. DOI: 10.1016/j.jamcollsurg.2006.05.019

[206] Coco D, Leanza S. Open versus laparoscopic incarcerated or strangulated inguinal hernia repair- a review. IJMBS. 2020;**4**(12):103-109. DOI: 10.32553/ijmbs.v4i12.1551

[207] Wake BL, McCormack K, Fraser C, Vale PJ, Grant AM. Transabdominal pre- peritoneal (TAPP) versus totally extraperitoneal (TEP) laparoscopic techniques for inguinal hernia repair. Cochrane Database of Systematic Reviews. 2005;**2005**(1):CD004703.pub2. DOI: 10.1002/14651858.CD004703.pub2

[208] Legnani GL, Rasini M, Pastori S, Sarli D. Laparoscopic trans-peritoneal hernioplasty (TAPP) for the acute management of strangulated inguino-crural hernias: A report of nine cases. Hernia. 2008;**12**(2):185-188. DOI: 10.1007/s10029-007-0305-5

[209] Liu J, Shen Y, Nie Y, Zhao X, Wang F, et al. If laparoscopic technique can be used for treatment of acutely incarcerated/strangulated inguinal hernia? World Journal of Emergency Surgery : WJES. 2021;**16**(1):5. DOI: 10.1186/s13017-021-00348-1

[210] Choi YY, Kim Z, Hur Y. Laparoscopic total extraperitoneal repair for incarcerated inguinal hernia. Journal of the Korean Surgical Society. 2011;**80**(6):426-430. DOI: 10.4174/jkss.2011.80.6.426

[211] Landau O, Kyzer S. Emergent laparoscopic repair of incarcerated incisional and ventral hernia. Surgical Endoscopy. 2004;**18**(9):1374-1376. DOI: 10.1007/s00464-003-9116-7

[212] Yang GPC. Laparoscopy in emergency hernia repair. Annals of Laparoscopic and Endoscopic Surgery. 2017;**2**:107. DOI: 10.21037/ales.2017.05.05

[213] Deeba S, Purkayastha S, Athanasiou T, Darzi A, Zacharakis E. Laparoscopic approach to incarcerated and strangulated inguinal hernias. JSLS. 2009;**13**(3):327-331

[214] Kurumiya Y, Mizuno K, Sekogouchi E, Sugawara G. Comparative study of open approach and laparoscopic surgery for emergent groin hernias. International Surgery Journal. 2019;**6**(4):1047-1050. DOI: 10.18203/2349-2902.isj20191249

[215] Binderow SR, Klapper AS, Bufalini B. Hernioscopy: Laparoscopy via an inguinal hernia sac. Journal of Laparoendoscopic Surgery. 1992;**2**(5):229-233. DOI: 10.1089/lps.1992.2.229

[216] Sajid MS, Ladwa N, Colucci G, Miles WF, Baig MK, et al. Diagnostic laparoscopy through deep inguinal ring: A literature-based review on the forgotten approach to visualize the abdominal cavity during emergency and elective groin hernia repair. Surgical Laparoscopy, Endoscopy & Percutaneous Techniques. 2013;**23**(3):251-254. DOI: 10.1097/SLE.0b013e31828dacc5

[217] Agresta F, Ansaloni L, Baiocchi GL, Bergamini C, Campanile FC, et al.

Laparoscopic approach to acute abdomen from the consensus development conference of the Società Italiana di Chirurgia Endoscopica e nuove tecnologie (SICE), Associazione Chirurghi Ospedalieri Italiani (ACOI), Società Italiana di Chirurgia (SIC), Società Italiana di Chirurgia d'Urgenza e del trauma (SICUT), Società Italiana dell'Ospedalità Privata (SICOP), and the European Association for Endoscopic Surgery (EAES). Surgical Endoscopy. 2012;**26**(8):2134-2164. DOI: 10.1007/s00464-012-2331-3

[218] Morris-Stiff G, Hassn A. Hernioscopy: A useful technique for the evaluation of incarcerated hernias that retract under anaesthesia. Hernia. 2008;**12**(2):133-135. DOI: 10.1007/s10029-007-0296-2

[219] Sgourakis G, Radkte A, Sotiropoulos GC, Dedemadi G, Fouzas I, Karaliotas C. Assessment of strangulated content of spontaneously redudec inguinal hernia via hernia sac laparoscopy: Preliminary results of a prospective randomized study. Surgical Laparoscopy, Endoscopy & Percutaneous Techniques. 2009;**19**(2):133-137. DOI: 10.1097/SLE.0b013e31819d8b8b

[220] Al-Naami MY, Al-Shawi JS. The use of laparoscopy to assess viability of slipped content in incarcerated hernia inguinal hernia: A case report. Surgical Laparoscopy, Endoscopy & Percutaneous Techniques. 2003;**13**(4):292-294. DOI:10.1097/00129689-200308000-00016

[221] Balentine CJ, Meier J, Berger M, Reisch J, Cullum M, et al. Using local Anesthesia for inguinal hernia repair reduces complications in older patients. The Journal of Surgical Research. 2021;**258**:64-72. DOI: 10.1016/j.jss.2020

[222] Bakota B, Kopljar M, Baranovic S, Miletic M, Marinovis M, et al. Should we abandon regional anesthesia in open inguinal hernia repair in adults? European Journal of Medical Research. 2015;**20**(1):76. DOI: 10.1186/s40001-015-0170-0

[223] Fredman B, Zohar E, Philipov A, Olsfanger D, Shalev M, et al. The induction, maintenance, and recovery characteristics of spinal versus general anesthesia in elderly patients. Journal of Clinical Anesthesia. 1998;**10**(8):623-630. DOI: 10.1016/s0952-8180(98)00099-3

[224] Kulacoglu H, Alptekin A. Current options in local anesthesia for groin hernia repairs. Acta Chirurgica Iugoslavica. 2011;**58**(3):25-35. DOI: 10.2298/aci1103025k

[225] Teasdale C, AM MC, Williams NB, et al. A randomized controlled trial to compare local with general anaesthesia for short-stay inguinal hernia repair. Annals of the Royal College of Surgeons of England. 1982;**64**(4):238-242

[226] Reece-Smith AM, Maggio AQ, Tang TY, Walsh SR. Local anaesthetic vs general anaesthetic for inguinal hernia repair: Systematic review and meta-analysis. International Journal of Clinical Practice. 2009;**63**(12):1739-1742. DOI: 10.1111/j.1742-1241.2009.02131.x

[227] Bhattacharya P, Mandal MC, Mukhopadhyay S, Das S, Pal PP, et al. Unilateral paravertebral block: An alternative to conventional spinal anaesthesia for inguinal hernia repair. Acta Anaesthesiologica Scandinavica. 2010;**54**(2):246-251. DOI: 10.1111/j.1399-6576.2009.02128.x

[228] Nordin P, Zetterstrom H, Carsson P, Nilsson E. Cost-effectiveness analysis of local, regional, and general anaesthesia for inguinal hernia repair using data from a randomized clinical trial. The British Journal of Surgery. 2011;**94**(4):500-555. DOI: 10.1002/bjs.5543

[229] Amid PK, Shulman AG, Lichtenstein IL. Local anesthesia for inguinal hernia repair step-by-step procedure. Annals of Surgery. 1994;**220**(6):735-737. DOI: 10.1097/00000658-199412000-00004

[230] Kehlet H, White PF. Optimizing anesthesia for inguinal herniorrhaphy: General, regional, or local anesthesia? Anesthesia and Analgesia. 2001;**93**(6):1367-1369. DOI: 10.1097/00000539-200112000-00001

[231] Sanjay P, Woodward A. Inguinal hernia repair: Local or general anaesthesia? Annals of the Royal College of Surgeons. 2007;**89**(5):497-503. DOI: 10.1308/003588407X202056

[232] Ozgun H, Kurt MN, Kurt I, Cevikel MH. Comparison of local, spinal, and general anaesthesia for inguinal herniorrhaphy. The European Journal of Surgery. 2002;**168**(8-9):455-459. DOI: 10.1080/110241502321116442

[233] Burney RE, Prabhu MA, Greenfield ML, Shanks A, O'Reilly. Comparison of spinal vs general anesthesia via laryngeal mask airway in inguinal hernia repair. Archives of Surgery. 2004;**139**(2):183-187. DOI: 10.1001/archsurg.139.2.183

[234] Rodgers A, Walker N, Schug S, McKee A, Kehlet H, et al. Reduction of postoperative mortality and morbidity with epidural or spinal anaesthesia: Results from overview of randomized trials. BMJ. 2000;**321**(7275):1493. DOI: 10.1136/bmj.321.7275.1493

[235] Neuman MD, Silber JH, Elkassabany NM, Ludwig JM, Fleisher LA. Comparative effectiveness of regional versus general anesthesia for hip fracture surgery in adults. Anesthesiology. 2012;**117**(1):72-92. DOI: 10.1097/ALN.0b013e3182545e7c

[236] Chen T, Zhang Y, Wang H, Ni Q, Yang L, et al. Emergency inguinal hernia repair under local anesthesia: A 5-year experience in a teaching hospital. BMC Anesthesiology. 2016;**16**:17. DOI: 10.1186/s12871-016-0185-2

[237] Amato B, Compagna R, Della Corte GA, Martino G, Bianco T, et al. Feasibility of inguinal hernioplasty under local anaesthesia in elderly patients. BMC Surgery. 2012;**12**(Suppl 1):S2. DOI: 10.1186/1471-2482-12-S1-S2

[238] Callessen T, Bech K, Kehlet H. One thousand consecutive inguinal hernia repairs under unmonitored local anesthesia. Anesthesia and Analgesia. 2001;**93**(6):1373-1376. DOI: 10.1097/00000539-200112000-00004

[239] Kehelet H, Aasvang E. Groin hernia repair: Anesthesia. World Journal of Surgery. 2005;**29**(8):1058-1061. DOI: 10.1007/s00268-005-7969-8

[240] Kehelet H, Bay-Nielsen M. Local anaesthesia as a risk factor for recurrence after groin hernia repair. Hernia. 2008;**12**(5):507-509. DOI: 10.1007/s10029-008-0371-3

[241] Nordin P, Zetterstrom H, Gunnarsson U, Nilsson E. Local, regional, or general anaesthesia in groin hernia repair: Multicenter randomized trial. Lancet. 2003;**362**(9378):853-858. DOI: 10.1016/S0140-6736(03)14339-5

[242] Kurman A, Fisher H, Dell-Kuster S, et al. Effect of intraoperative infiltration with local anesthesia on the development of chronic pain after postoperative after inguinal hernia repair: A randomized triple-blinded, placebo controlled trial. Surgery. 2015;**157**(1):144-154. DOI: 10.1016/j.surg.2014.07.008

Chapter 9

Open Hernia Repair

Kumar Hari Rajah and M. Somanathan

Abstract

Inguinal hernias are a common clinical condition that is present to the surgical clinic and open inguinal hernias repairs are one of the most common operations that are performed by general surgeons. Open inguinal hernia repairs have evolved from tension repairs like the Bassini and darning repair to the shouldice repair. As these procedures were under tension and hence the recurrence rates were high. The Lichtenstein repair was a tension free repair that uses mesh, revolutionized hernia repair as the procedure was simple and the recurrence rates were low whether the procedure was performed by a junior or senior surgeon. The Lichtenstein repair is now the most popular repair for inguinal hernias. Variants to this include the plug and patch repair and the prolene hernia system, which uses various types of tension free mesh repairs. This chapter investigates the various open hernia techniques with emphasis on the tension free repairs which involve the use of mesh (Lichtenstein) and not the use of mesh (Desarda). The older tension repairs like the Shouldice and Bassini repairs are also reviewed.

Keywords: open hernia repair, Lichtenstein repair, Desarda repair, Shouldice repair, Bassini repair

1. Introduction

Inguinal hernias are protrusions that occur through the inguinal canal, and they are classified as direct and indirect inguinal hernias. They are far more common in males than females. They can also be classified as reducible or irreducible inguinal hernias [1].

The treatment of inguinal hernias has always been surgical repair and they can be divided into open and laparoscopic repair. The open inguinal hernia repairs are further classified into (1) Tension free repair and (2) Tissue-suture repair [2].

The tension free repair operations are Lichtenstein's tension free repair, the prolene hernia system repair and the plug, patch technique and the desarda technique. The tissue suture repair includes the Bassini's repair, The Mcvay's repair and the Shouldice repair [3].

The Lichtenstien tension free repair is the most common open hernia operation that is performed as it is associated with low recurrence rate, and it is reproducible by all non-specialist surgeons [4].

In choosing the technique of hernia repair will depend on the patient characteristics and the experience of the surgeon as well as understanding the evidence that is available to achieve the best outcome for the patient [5].

1.1 Lichtenstein tension free repair

This technique was introduced by lichtenstein in 1984 and it is the most popular open hernia technique because it does not require a long learning curve and it has a low recurrence and complication rate [6].

The Lichtenstein procedure involves the placement of a prolene mesh over the posterior wall of the inguinal canal and anchoring it to the inguinal ligament with non-absorbable sutures and slit is made to accommodate the cord and the upper edge of the mesh is anchored with non-absorbable sutures. Sakorafas et al. conducted a retrospective study on 540 patients who underwent the Lichtenstein procedure for hernia repair and there were no complications like wound infection and the recurrence rate was 0.2% [7].

The advantage of this procedure is that it can be performed under local anesthesia and hence it is cost effective. The placement of the mesh over the posterior wall of the inguinal canal and adjustments to the size of the mesh and suture technique has been associated with the reduced rates of post operative complications. Just et al. in their prospective study in 1592 patients who underwent the Lichtenstein repair confirmed this [8].

The prospective study by Yamamoto et al. which performed this repair on 314 patients and the results showed no mortality and decreased wound infection rate and they concluded that the lichtenstein repair can be safely performed by trainee surgeons with minimal complications [9].

Praviz et al. performed the lichtenstein hernia repair on 3480 patients with inguinal hernia and they were performed under local anesthesia. The postoperative wound infection rate was low, and the postoperative analgesia and recurrence was low and the stay in hospital and cost were low [10].

The Hernia surge group guidelines also concluded that the Lichtenstein tension free hernia repair is the preferred method of open hernia repair due to its low complications and recurrence rate [11].

Metzger et al. conducted a retrospective study on 440 patients who underwent inguinal hernia repair of which the Lichtenstein repair was the predominant repair, and the results showed this repair can be conducted as a daycare procedure as it is associated with reduced cost and post operative complications [12].

Alabi et al. conducted a systemic review on mesh fixation techniques in inguinal hernia. Twenty systemic reviews were included in the study and the conclusion was that glue fixation and non-suture fixation was associated with better outcomes with regards to recurrence and chronic pain when compared to suture fixation of mesh. Further randomized control trials with large sample sizes may be needed to further evaluate this [13].

Ladwa et al. also conducted a systemic review and meta-analysis comparing suture mesh fixation to glue mesh fixation. Seven trials including 1259 patients of which 628 underwent suture mesh repair and 653 underwent glue mesh fixation. The results showed there were no differences with regards to recurrence rates and chronic pain, but further randomized trials may be needed to further evaluate the effectiveness of glue mesh fixation [14].

The Lichtenstein repair was also compared with the plug mesh repair by Wilasrusmee et al. who performed at study on 94 patients with inguinal hernias of which 25 underwent the plug mesh repair, 26 underwent the Lichtenstein repair and 36 underwent the Bassani repair. There were no complication or recurrence rates in the plug mesh and Lichtenstein repair groups. This concluded that both the plug mesh and Lichtenstein repair were effective in the management of inguinal hernias [15].

Singh et al. also compared the Lichtenstein repair with the plug and patch mesh repair on 200 patients who underwent primary hernia repair. There were no differences in the duration of surgery, post operative infection rates and chronic pain, hence it concluded that both procedures were effective in the treatment of primary inguinal hernias [16].

The prolene hernia system uses a special mesh with a three-dimensional theoretical effect of strengthening and maintaining the anterior and posterior wall of the inguinal canal without tension. It consists of an underlay patch and overlay patch with an intervening connector. This procedure was associated with a shorter hospital stay and reduced post operative pain and is a viable alternative to the Lichtenstein procedure [17].

The use of the prolene hernia system in a regional hospital as demonstrated by Berende et al. in their retrospective study on 193 patients who underwent this type of hernia repair. The patients were followed up and the wound infection rates and recurrence rates were low demonstrating its use in non-hernia specific centers [18].

The Lichtenstein, prolene hernia system and the ultrapro hernia system were compared by a prospective randomized trial by Magnusson et al. in the management of primary inguinal hernias. Three hundred nine patients were involved in the study and the conclusion was that recurrence rates and chronic pain rates were the same in all the groups hence the Lichtenstein repair should be the first choice in the management of primary inguinal hernias [19].

The Plug and Patch technique which was popularized by Rudkow and Robbins involves a cone shaped plug made of polypropylene that is inserted into the inguinal canal in an indirect hernia and followed by placement of a mesh patch that is sewn over the spermatic cord and laid on top of the posterior wall. This repair was prospectively studied by Bringman et al. and it was associated with a recurrence rate that is equivalent to the Lichtenstein repair [20].

The conclusion from these studies is that the Lichtenstein hernia repair is a safe and effective treatment option for inguinal hernia (**Figure 1**).

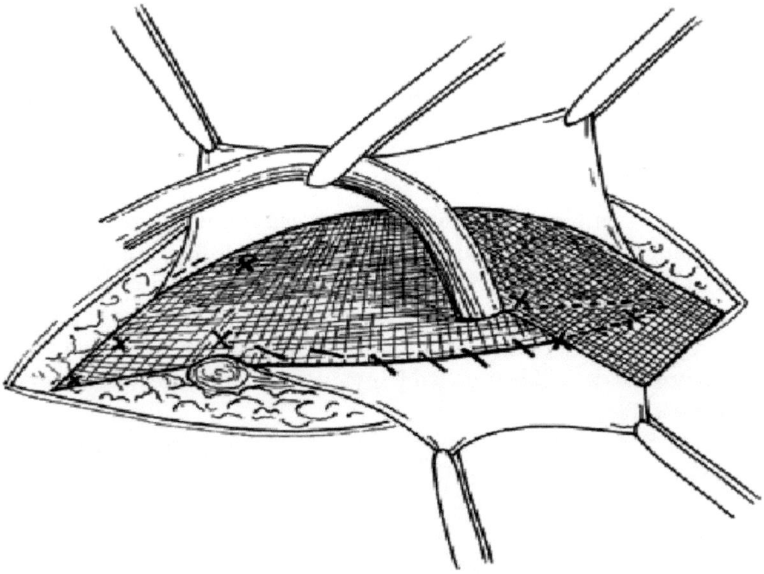

Figure 1.
The Lichtenstein repairs.

1.2 Desarda hernia repair

This procedure was introduced by Dr. M.P. Desarda in 2001 and he performed a hernia repair by strengthening the posterior wall by incising the external oblique aponeurosis and the undetached strip is sutured to the inguinal ligament to form a new posterior wall. This procedure does not use any foreign material like mesh and hence it has a decreased risk of wound infection and chronic pain. Desarda et al. performed a prospective study on 860 patients with inguinal hernias and all the patients underwent this type of hernia repair. The patients were followed up and there were no reported wound infection rates, and no recurrence were observed [21].

Desarda performed a further prospective study on 229 patients with this hernia repair and they were followed up and there were no reported recurrence or chronic groin pain with this hernia repair [22].

Gurgenidze et al. also performed a prospective study on 118 patients who underwent a desarda hernia repair for inguinal hernia. The patients were followed up and the wound infection rates were low and there was no recurrence. This showed that the Desarda hernia repair was good in the management of inguinal hernias [23].

Khairy et al. performed the desarda hernia repair on 100 patients with inguinal hernias. All the procedures were done under spinal anesthesia and there were no post operative complications like wound infection and seroma formation. There was also no recorded recurrence on follow up of these patients. This study showed the advantage of using the desarda hernia repair technique in the management of inguinal hernias [24].

Bashir et al. performed the desarda hernia technique on 50 patients with inguinal hernias. This was a prospective study, and the patients were followed up and there were no wound infection rates and there were also no recurrence rates. The conclusion from this study was that the desarda hernia repair was a safe and effective hernia repair technique [25].

Ge Hua et al. conducted a systemic review to compare the surgical outcomes of both the desarda repair and the Lichtenstein repair. Eight articles which included 4 randomized control trials and 4 nonrandomized control trials were included in the study. A total of 1014 patients of which 500 underwent the desarda repair and 514 underwent the Lichtenstein repair. The conclusion of this systemic review was that there was no difference in the surgical outcomes post operative wound infection, chronic pain, and recurrence rates. The limitation of this study was the small sample size and limited randomized control trials [26].

Pereira et al. also conducted a systematic review and meta-analysis on the desarda technique versus the Lichtenstein repair in the treatment of primary inguinal hernias, comparing both outcomes. Five randomized control trials including 536 patients were included in the study, 310 underwent the desarda repair and 226 underwent the Lichtenstein repair. The conclusion from this study showed that both procedures were comparable in terms of post operative infection rates and recurrence rates, but larger randomized control trials will be needed to evaluate the long-term outcomes of the desarda technique [27].

The conclusion from these studies is that the desarda technique is a good technique but further trials may be needed for further evaluation (**Figure 2**).

1.3 The shouldice repair

This repair was performed at the shouldice hospital, and it involves the division of the fascia transversalis and reconstruction of the posterior wall of the inguinal canal

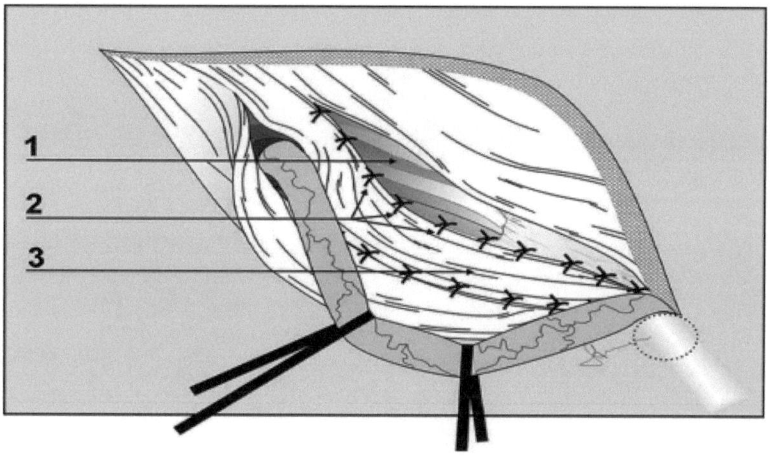

Figure 2.
Desarda hernia repair.

done with continuous stainless-steel sutures. Two continuous suture lines are used starting from the pubic crest and extending up to the transversalis fascia, transverses abdominus and internal oblique muscle. These sutures start from the pubic crest and advance towards the internal ring and the same sutures are reversed back towards the pubic crest including the shelving edge of the inguinal ligament. The second suture line begins laterally including the internal oblique and transversus muscle, extending medially, and including the inner line of the external oblique muscle and extending towards the pubic tubercle and then reverses back to the internal ring while picking up the inner aspect of the external oblique aponeurosis [28].

Amato et al. conducted a review to evaluate the efficacy of the shouldice repair against other open techniques of open repair. Sixteen trials were reviewed with 2566 shouldice repairs were done against 1121 mesh repairs and 1608 non mesh repairs. The conclusion of this review was that the shouldice repair was the best non mesh hernia repair, but recurrence rates were much lower in the mesh hernia repair group. Hence if mesh is not available, the shouldice repair is the best alternative for hernia repair [29].

Bracale et al. conducted a systemic review and network meta-analysis comparing the shouldice and desarda hernia repair in the treatment of primary hernia repairs. Fourteen randomized control trials involving 2791 patients and the conclusion of this study was that the recurrence rates were similar but the total operative time was reduced in the desarda group, hence the shouldice repair is still considered the best non-mesh hernia repair but the desarda repair is slowly emerging as an alternative non-mesh hernia repair [30].

Hay et al. conducted a multicentric trial on 1578 patients who underwent the shouldice repair for primary inguinal hernias. The patients were followed up to 5 years and the mean recurrence rate was 5% and the post operative infection rates were negligible. This showed that the shouldice repair is considered the best non mesh inguinal hernia repair (**Figure 3**) [31].

1.4 Other hernia repairs

The Bassini hernia repair has long been regarded as the first inguinal hernia repair, it involves suturing the transversalis fascia and conjoint tendon to the

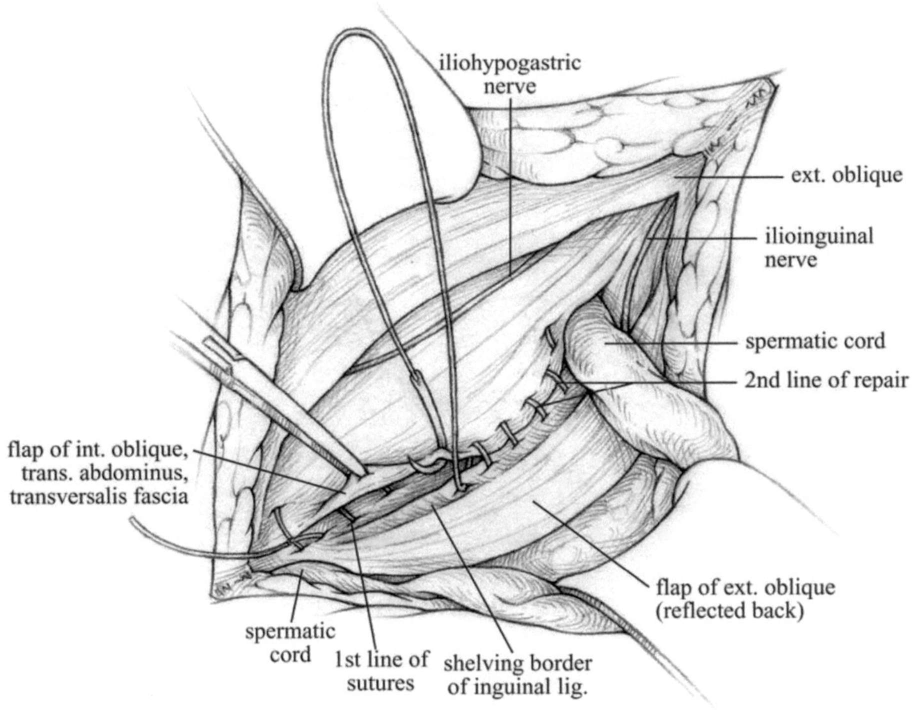

Figure 3.
The shouldice repair.

inguinal ligament behind the spermatic cord and is frequently associated with a tanner slide (vertical relaxing incisions over the anterior rectus sheath). This procedure was the most popular procedure before the introduction of tension free repair with mesh. Its main indication now is for primary inguinal hernia repair in patients who do not want to use mesh. Wayne et al. in their study on the use of the bassini repair in the treatment of inguinal hernias showed a recurrence rate of 3.7% to 4.8%, but they are much higher than the Lichtenstein repair. Another downside of this procedure is the need to avoid excessive tension over the inguinal region by not lifting heavy objects [32, 33].

The darning technique is another operation that is performed for primary inguinal hernias, and it involves the approximation of the conjoint tendon to the inguinal ligament with monofilament nylon from the pubic tubercle to the internal ring and back to the pubicle tubercle with forcibly bringing the tissues together. This procedure is relative tension free tissue repair with studies done by Olalekan et al. which showed a recurrence rate of 1.5% [34].

The advantage of the darning technique is the cost and early recovery, but the recurrence rate is still higher when compared with the Lichtenstein repair as demonstrated by the prospective clinical trial that was conducted by boonnithi et al. [35].

The Lotheissen/McVay repair is a tissue repair which is complex and rarely performed nowadays. The repair involves the splitting of the transversalis fascia and dissecting the cooper ligament. The hernia is repaired by suturing the transversalis fascia, transverses abdominus and internal oblique to the pectineal ligament (**Figure 4**) [36].

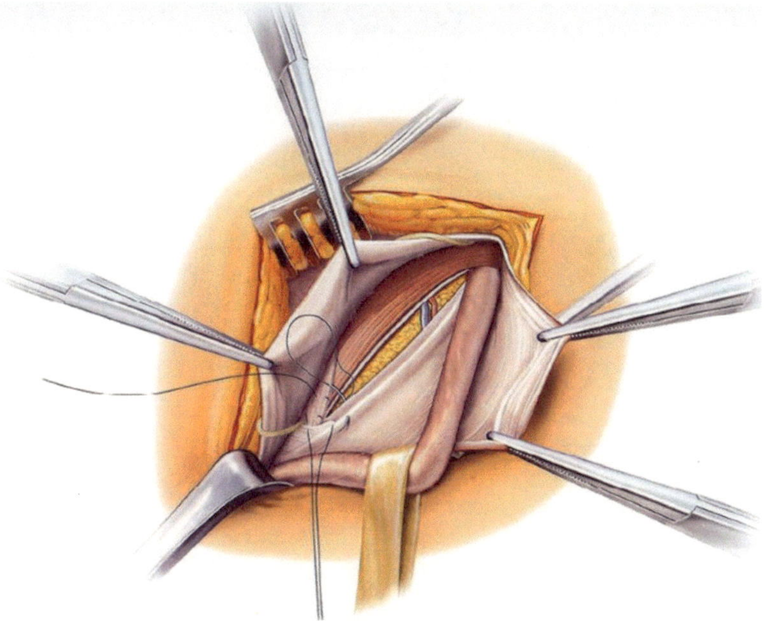

Figure 4.
The Bassini inguinal hernia repair.

2. Conclusion

Open inguinal hernia repair has evolved over time from pure tissue-based repair to mesh repair. The introduction of the tension free Lichtenstein repair with its low recurrence rate and low cost of operation has revolutionized the management of inguinal hernia repair and has become the most common open inguinal hernia repair. The Lichtenstein repair is easy to learn for junior surgeons and can be applied in various settings. It has replaced all tissue-based repair. The shouldice repair is the open tissue based inguinal hernia repair that is associated with the lowest recurrence rate and is indicated in patients where insertion of mesh is contraindicated. The Desarda repair is slowly emerging as an alternative for tension free inguinal hernia repair, but more studies are required to evaluate its recurrence rate. The Lichtenstein repair continues to be the most popular open inguinal hernia operation that is being performed worldwide as it can be performed under local anesthesia and hence be able to reduce the cost of the procedure. It is for this reason that open inguinal hernia repairs will continue to be a common surgical procedure that is being performed by general surgeons.

Conflict of interest

"The authors declare no conflict of interest."

Author details

Kumar Hari Rajah* and M. Somanathan
Taylor's University School of Medicine and Health Science, Selangor, Malaysia

*Address all correspondence to: kharirajah@yahoo.com.my

References

[1] Wib O, Ge N. Inguinal hernia. A review. Journal of Surgery and Operative Care. 2016;**1**(2):1-10

[2] Kulacoglu H. Current options in inguinal hernia repair in adult patients. Hippokratia. 2011;**15**(3):223-231

[3] Ismaila BO, Alayande BT, Ojo EO, Sule AZ. Inguinal hernia repair in Nigeria: A survey of surgical trainees. Hernia. 2019;**23**(3):625-629. DOI: 10.1007/s10029-019-01885-0. Epub 2019 Jan 17

[4] Jenkins JT, O'Dwyer PJ. Inguinal hernias. BMJ. 2008;**336**:269-272

[5] Kah, Heng Chiow A, Keong Chong C, Tan SM. Inguinal hernias: A current review of an old problem. Proceedings of Singapore Healthcare. 2010;**19**:202-211

[6] Campanelli G, Canziani M, Frattini F, Cavalli M, Agrusti S. Inguinal hernia: State of the art. International Journal of Surgery. 2008;**6**(Suppl. 1):526-528

[7] Sakorafas GH, Halikias I, Nissotakis C, Kotsifopoulos N, Stavrou A, Antonopoulos C, et al. Open tension free repair of inguinal hernias; the Lichtenstein technique [Internet]. 2001. Available from: http://www.biomedcentral.com/1471-2482/1/3

[8] Just E, Botet X, Martínez S, Escolà D, Moreno I, Duque E. Reduction of the complication rate in Liechtenstein hernia repair. International Journal of Surgery. 2010;**8**(6):462-465

[9] Yamamoto S, Maeda T, Uchida Y, Yabe SI, Nakano M, Sakano S, et al. Open tension-free mesh repair for adult inguinal hernia: Eight years of experience in a community hospital. Asian Journal of Surgery. 2002;**25**(2):121-125

[10] Amid PK. Lichtenstein tension-free hernioplasty: Its inception, evolution, and principles. Hernia. 2004;**8**(1):1-7. DOI: 10.1007/s10029-003-0160-y. Epub 2003 Sep 20

[11] Tran H. Endorsement of the HerniaSurge guidelines by the Australasian hernia society. In: Hernia. Vol. 22. France: Springer-Verlag; 2018. p. 177

[12] Metzger J, Lutz N, Laidlaw I. Guidelines for inguinal hernia repair in everyday practice. Annals of the Royal College of Surgeons of England. 2001;**83**:209-212

[13] Alabi A, Haladu N, Scott NW, Imamura M, Ahmed I, Ramsay G, et al. Mesh fixation techniques for inguinal hernia repair: An overview of systematic reviews of randomised controlled trials. Hernia. Springer-Verlag Italia s.r.l. Aug 2022;**26**(4):973-987

[14] Ladwa N, Sajid MS, Sains P, Baig MK. Suture mesh fixation versus glue mesh fixation in open inguinal hernia repair: A systematic review and meta-analysis. International Journal of Surgery. 2013;**11**:128-135

[15] Horharin P, Wilasrusmee C, Cherudchayaporn K, Pinyaku N, Phanpradi O, Phromsopha N. Comparative study of tailor-made mesh plug herniorrhaphy versus lichtenstein herniorrhaphy versus bassini operation: A prospective clinical trial. Asian Journal of Surgery. 2006;**29**(2):74-78

[16] Singh R, Gupta A, Shah A, Singh A. A study about inguinal hernia mesh repairs: Plug and patch versus lichtenstein mesh repair technique. International Surgery Journal. Nov 2016;**3**(4):1967-1974

[17] Gilbert AI, Graham MF, Voigt WJ. A bilayer patch device for inguinal hernia repair. Hernia. 1999;**3**(3):161-166

[18] Berende CAS, Ruurda JP, Hazenberg CEVB, Olsman JG, Geffen HJAA. Inguinal hernia treatment with the Prolene hernia system in a Dutch regional training hospital. Hernia. 2007;**11**(4):303-306

[19] Magnusson J, Nygren J, Thorell A. Lichtenstein, Prolene hernia system, and UltraPro hernia system for primary inguinal hernia repair: One-year outcome of a prospective randomized controlled trial. Hernia. 2012;**16**(3):277-285

[20] Bringman S, Ramel S, Nyberg B, Anderberg B. Introduction of Herniorraphy with Mesh Plug and Patch [Internet]. 2000. Available from: https://academic.oup.com/ejs/article/166/4/310/6040444

[21] Desarda MP. Physiological repair of inguinal hernia: A new technique (study of 860 patients). Hernia. 2006;**10**(2):143-146. DOI: 10.1007/s10029-005-0039-1. Epub 2005 Dec 9

[22] Desarda MP. No-mesh inguinal hernia repair with continuous absorbable sutures: A dream or reality? (a study of 229 patients). Saudi Journal of Gastroenterology. 2008;**14**(3):122-127. DOI: 10.4103/1319-3767.41730

[23] Gurgenidze M, Datuashvili G. Desarda technique for inguinal hernia repair. Georgian Medical News. Jul-Aug 2018;**280-281**:7-10

[24] Khairy M, Madbouly AEW, Sharaf M. Evaluation of Desarda technique in inguinal Herniorrhaphy. Al-Azhar International Medical Journal. 2020;**1**(2):193-197

[25] Bashir S, Afzal MO, Rafi Y. Desarda Technique for Inguinal Hernia Repair, a multicenter experience. 2016;**9**:311-313

[26] Ge H, Liang C, Xu Y, Ren S, Wu J. Desarda versus Lichtenstein technique for the treatment of primary inguinal hernia: A systematic review. International Journal of Surgery. Elsevier Ltd. 2018;**50**:22-27

[27] Pereira C, Varghese B. Desarda non-mesh technique versus Lichtenstein technique for the treatment of primary inguinal hernias: A systematic review and meta-analysis. Pereira Cureus. 18 Nov 2022;**14**(11)

[28] Bendavid R. The Shouldice technique: A canon in hernia repair. Canadian Journal of Surgery. 1997;**40**(3):199-205 207

[29] Amato B, Moja L, Panico S, Persico G, Rispoli C, Rocco N, et al. Shouldice technique versus other open techniques for inguinal hernia repair. Cochrane Database of Systemic Reviews. 18 Apr 2012;**2012**(4):CD001543

[30] Bracale U, Melillo P, Piaggio D, Pecchia L, Cuccurullo D, Milone M, et al. Is Shouldice the best NON-MESH inguinal hernia repair technique? A systematic review and network metanalysis of randomized controlled trials comparing Shouldice and Desarda. International Journal of Surgery. 2019;**62**:12-21

[31] Hay JM, Boudet MJ, Fingerhut A, Pourcher J, Hennet H, Habib E, et al. S L E N Shouldice inguinal hernia repair in the male adult: The gold standard? A multicenter controlled trial in 1578 patients. Annals of Surgery. Dec 1995;**222**(6):719-727

[32] Naveen N, Srinath R. A comparative study between modified bassini's repair

and lichtenstein mesh repair of inguinal hernias in rural population. Journal of Clinical and Diagnostic Research. 2014;**8**(2):88-91

[33] Tse W, Johns W, Maher J, Rivers J, Miller T. Bassini inguinal hernia repair: Obsolete or still a viable surgical option? A single center cohort study. International Journal of Surgery Open. 2021:36

[34] Oo O, Oa A, Aa E, Ce A, Ak O, Om A. A 5-year review of darning technique of inguinal hernia repair. Nigerian Journal of Surgery. 2015;**21**(1):52

[35] Boonnithi N, Kongkham K. A prospective clinical trial comparing darn vs Bassini vs Lichtenstein inguinal Herniorrhaphy. The Thai Journal of Surgery. 2010;**31**:125-129

[36] Junge K. Lotheissen/McVay Repair [Internet]. 2019. Available from: https://www.ebsco.com/terms-of-use

Chapter 10

Individualized Treatment of Inguinal Hernia in Children

George Sakellaris, Konstantinos Zachos, Maria Athanasopoulou, Antonios Panagidis, Vasileios Alexopoulos, Ioannis Spyridakis, Anastasia Vareli and Xenophon Sinopidis

Abstract

The inguinal hernia is the commonest type of hernia in children. Either scheduled or as an emergency, hernia surgery is performed daily in every pediatric surgical institution worldwide, regardless of age or gender. In this chapter, we discuss the embryology of the inguinal canal and its pathophysiological association with hernia formation. We also present the most frequent clinical and diagnostic issues of the pediatric hernia. The management of strangulated hernia, differential diagnosis, and the particular uncommon hernia types are presented as well. We finally present the evolution of hernia surgery from the classical operative methods to the modern laparoscopic techniques.

Keywords: pediatric inguinal hernia, pediatric hernia surgery, laparoscopic hernia surgery uncommon inguinal pediatric hernias, strangulated inguinal hernia, open inguinal pediatric hernia surgery, pediatric hernia complications

1. Introduction

Inguinal hernia is the most common congenital disorder in daily pediatric surgical practice. It may be managed in a tactical manner or appear as an organ and life-threatening event that requires urgent treatment in cases of testis, ovary, or intestinal entrapment (incarceration and strangulation of hernia). In this chapter, the particular characteristics, the diagnosis, and the current management of inguinal hernia in children are described in detail.

2. Incidence

A hernia is defined as a protrusion of an organ or tissue, through an abnormal opening. Congenital inguinal hernia is one of the most frequent congenital conditions, most commonly encountered from birth until the age of 6 years [1]. It may be divided into two types, the indirect (prevailing in childhood, 99% of cases) and the direct which is rare in children. The accurate incidence of indirect inguinal hernia is unknown as an effect of factors, such as prematurity, associated disease, and medical accessibility. However, indirect inguinal hernia is observed approximately in 1–5% of the term males, who outnumber females with a predominancy of 80% [2]. It is mostly encountered on the right side (60%). A total of 10% of the cases are bilateral [1–3].

There is a higher incidence of indirect inguinal hernia in preterm infants as well as in conditions of increased intra-abdominal pressure. Abnormal abdominal content as with ascites or during peritoneal dialysis, as well as abnormal abdominal wall disorders, such as exomphalos, gastroschisis, and bladder exstrophy, may increase the incidence of indirect inguinal hernia. Prematurity also seems to increase the incidence (2–30%) and the frequency of incarceration (1–6% during the first 6 months of life). Therefore, correction is strongly advised before hospital discharge [4]. Cystic fibrosis, congenital collagen conditions such as Ehlers-Danlos syndrome, mucopolysaccharidoses (Hunter-Hurler syndrome), and congenital hip dislocation are frequently associated with higher incidence of hernia rates. Cystic fibrosis has higher inguinal hernia incidence, up to eight times the general population and mucopolysaccharidoses are associated with a recurrence rate of 50%. Recurrence may be a primary symptom of the disease in these patients [4, 5]. Direct inguinal hernia is rare in children, mainly diagnosed during surgery, and may be a result of inguinal floor trauma after surgical reconstruction of indirect hernia or as a result of higher intra-abdominal pressure.

3. Bilateral inguinal hernia

The incidence of bilateral inguinal hernia is not clearly defined. This occurs because the consideration of the patent processus vaginalis as a potential for causing actual hernia is still under debate. However, there are predisposing factors, such as gender, age, and the side of the precedent hernia, which seem to favor bilateral presentation and the necessity of simultaneous treatment of both sides [5]. Female gender, left-sided hernia, and prematurity seem to favor postoperative contralateral hernia appearance. Collagen disorders, cystic fibrosis, and ventricular-peritoneal shunts are followed by higher bilateral rates and present higher risk of anesthesia complications.

Bilateral management is recommended in preterm infants due to high incarceration risk, and in infants and young children with the prementioned disorders, in patients with a history of incarcerated hernia, and in patients under increased anesthetic risk. The final medical decision is patient-personalized in cooperation with the parent and in accordance with the current data.

4. Embryology and pathophysiology

To fully understand the inguinal hernia embryology and pathophysiology, some evidence of the inguinal canal formation and the testicular descent should be recalled.

4.1 Formation of the inguinal canal

The dynamic development of the inguinal canal is closely connected to differentiation of the gonads and their migration into the scrotum. The inguinal canal is established in both sexes even though testicular descent occurs in the male, while in the female the ovary remains inside the pelvis as the Fallopian tube acts as a barrier. In the female, the gubernaculum becomes the round ligament [6].

4.2 Testicular descent

The intra-abdominal differentiation of the male gonad is followed by its descent through the inguinal canal, guided by the gubernaculum. The gubernaculum originates in two triangular mesenchymal condensations, the inguinal plica dorsal to the Wolffian duct and the inguinal crista opposite the plica [6, 7]. The growth and differentiation of the gubernaculum is induced by insulin-like factor 3 (INSL3), which is secreted by Leydig cells [8, 9]. The pelvic portion of the gubernaculum is created by merging the mesonephric and inguinal portions. The inguinal portion continues to extend as far as the superficial inguinal ring, which is formed by the external oblique muscle. Condensation of the mesenchyme progresses caudally to form the scrotal part of the ligament. Notably, the gubernaculum is not connected to the gonads at any time during embryogenesis. At the end of this period, the vaginal process appears as a protrusion and evagination of the peritoneum that surrounds the pelvic and inguinal portion of the gubernaculum.

It is controversial as to whether the gubernaculum acts as a guide through the inguinal canal or actively pulls the testis into the scrotum. In contrast to males, in females it is remodeled into the round ligament in female fetuses. Herein, the vaginal process reaches only the initial section of the inguinal canal and the ovaries do not reach the abdominal wall [7].

At the 32–35th gestational week, the gubernaculum descends from the region of the internal inguinal ring, accompanied by a parietal peritoneal diverticulum, the future vaginal process (processus vaginalis), to its final destination in the scrotum, through the anterior wall muscles [6]. More specifically, it is accompanied by the transversalis fascia, and the internal and external oblique abdominal muscles, which form the final testicular layers in the scrotum. During further development, the vaginal process elongates and eventually envelops the gubernaculum.

The vaginal process normally obliterates around the 35th week of gestation and becomes the tunica and processus vaginalis. Failure of this obliteration leads to a persistent vaginal process that may result in an inguinal hernia or a hydrocele depending on what the content is, either an intraperitoneal organ or a peritoneal fluid. In both cases, the final management target is occlusion of the processus vaginalis [6].

The testicular vessels and vas deferens are retroperitoneal structures that exit the internal ring behind the gubernaculum and the vaginal process. As a result, *the future processus vaginalis lies anteriorly and slightly medially to the spermatic cord structures*. When the processus remains patent, a potential hernia results, and may become an actual hernia when an intra-abdominal content exits the cavity into it. The sac of hernia can be extremely thin or thick according to the age of the patient, the symptoms, or the incarceration occurrence [6, 7].

5. Clinical presentation

Indirect inguinal hernia may present as an inguinal protruding mass toward the scrotum in boys or descending toward the labia in girls. It is easily observed in conditions of enhanced intra-abdominal pressure and may spontaneously reduce after gentle lateral pressure.

It is not unusual for a bulge to be felt by the patient during clinical examination. The silken cord sign may be revealed by careful palpation, as thickening and slipperiness of the cord structures during examination of the inguinal channel [10]. In general, a careful history in combination with a careful examination set the diagnosis [11].

When there is no sign during examination and only a pediatric note is available, a good history-referring to a recurrent inguinal bulge, which is spontaneously reduced or gradually becoming difficult in reducing, is adequate to proceed with surgery. An ultrasound may seem useful. A firm, tender mass occupying the inguinal canal and possibly extending to the scrotum may be the first sign of an inguinal hernia (possible acute obstructed hernia) and requires urgent management [11].

Direct inguinal hernia is rare, noticed as a protruding inguinal mass close to the epigastric vessels, either spontaneously or after provoked higher intra-abdominal pressure. A history of previously surgically corrected ipsilateral inguinal hernia may be noted.

6. Diagnosis

The clinical features, combined with a careful history and an inguinal ultrasound occasionally, set the diagnosis. Inguinal hernia should be differentiated from a hydrocele. Differential diagnosis includes the potential acute scrotum etiology in cases of a painful inguinal mass not previously noticed. All the potential inguinal mass situations include torsion of the testis or the testicular appendages (Sinopidis [12]), infection, and trauma. A careful history, a thorough physical examination, and a regional ultrasound may differentiate all these situations from a hernia.

The hydroceles are asymptomatic inguinal, scrotal, or inguinoscrotal, nonsensitive masses that can be intermittently seen. An empty scrotum in the morning, which progressively enlarges throughout the day, is typical of a communicating hydrocele. It can be slowly reduced by sustained pressure during examination. The transillumination sign can be diagnostically helpful. Hydroceles are corrected with surgery only in children older than 12–18 months, when the process vaginalis is unlikely to close. The idiopathic scrotal edema appears as edema of the scrotum in total accompanied with external irritability and regional erythema. There is no processus vaginalis or testis interference. Finally, a tumor may occur, although a rarity [11].

7. Uncommon hernia types

Content of hernia sac usually includes omentum, small and large intestines, lateral ankle of bladder, and ovary in female [Scott]. Rarely, content may include the appendix (Amyand's hernia), Meckel's diverticulum (Littré's hernia), or only a part of the small intestine (Richter's hernia).

7.1 Amyand's hernia

Amyand's hernia is a hernia that contains the vermiform appendix. It is extremely rare, with an incidence of 0.5–1%. It mainly occurs in the right inguinal region, but it may be found as well in the left inguinal area, due to mobile cecum, malrotation, or situs inversus [13]. The presence of a noninflamed appendix in the inguinal hernia is three times more common in children than in adults, due to the persistent patency of the processus vaginalis in infancy and childhood [13]. The pathophysiology of acute appendicitis in the inguinal canal is under controversy. It is not certain whether a relationship exists between incarceration and inflammation, or whether it is incidental [14]. Amyand's hernia is usually diagnosed during surgical exploration of the groin, though ultrasound can prove helpful in children [14, 15]. Neonatal appendicitis is extremely rare (0.1% of appendicitis cases in infancy, which constitutes 2% of pediatric appendicitis). Premature neonates account for 50% of these cases, and in one third of these, the inflamed appendix lies within a hernia. Enterocutaneous fistula secondary to appendicitis in an Amyand's hernia is also extremely rare [14].

7.2 Littré's hernia

Meckel's diverticulum (MD) occurs as a result of incomplete obliteration of the omphalomesenteric duct during fetal development. It is typically found at the antimesenteric border of the ileum, usually located from 30 to 90 cm from the ileocecal valve, presenting occasionally ectopic gastric or pancreatic mucosa, and remains asymptomatic in 91–96%. When symptomatic, it appears frequently as hemorrhage, perforation, inflammation, and obstruction [16]. Involvement of a MD in a hernia is known as Littré's hernia (LH) [17]. In LH, a protrusion of the MD through a remaining patent processus vaginalis is observed in less than 1% of MD cases, usually on the right side and it is difficult to diagnose before surgery. It is more frequent in boys, but overall rare in children [18]. LH has been divided into two distinct subtypes. A true one, which is more common, contains Meckel's diverticulum. A mixed type contains a segment of small bowel in addition to MD and is less commonly reported [18]. The clinical preoperative diagnosis remains difficult, even in cases of strangulated inguinal hernias, whereas obstruction can occur if the base of the diverticulum is broad enough to cause narrowing of the intestinal lumen [19].

7.3 Richter's hernia

Richter's hernia is formed when the antimesenteric border of intestine protrudes into the hernial sac, but it never involves all the intestine. Such a protrusion through the inguinal canal is a rare clinical entity and evolves 12–36% of all presentations. The femoral ring (36–88%), postincision hernias (4–25%), spigelian hernias, and the umbilicus (extremely rare) are other possible locations [20, 21] The hernial sac usually contains a segment of the distal ileum, however any part of the gastrointestinal tract may be involved. Pediatric evidence is scarce, and our knowledge is mainly based on the adult population [20]. Clinical presentation is often misleading. An abnormal internal ring predisposes to strangulation and blood supply compromise, leading to ischemia and intestinal necrosis. Compared with patients with other hernias, patients with Richter's hernias have greater preoperative delay, rate of bowel resection, length of hospital stay, and postoperative morbidity and mortality rates [21].

8. Complications

Inguinal hernias can be strangulated and incarcerated. Premature children are susceptible to hernia incarceration (up to 60% during the first 6 months of life) [11]. The intestine as well as the ovaries or the fallopian tube can be incarcerated. The patient presents irritability and complains of groin pain. When the bowel is strangulated, cramping abdominal pain, vomiting nonbilious at first but rapidly progressing to bilious one, signs of ileus can be found. The physical examination reveals a firm, painful nonreducible mass in the inguinal area or even extending to the scrotum. Blood may be revealed in rectal examination in cases of intestinal necrosis. A history of known hernia in the affected area might be noted. Incarceration might sometimes be the first clinical presentation of an inguinal hernia. Incarcerated hernias with no signs of strangulation can be reduced nonoperatively in 80% of cases, followed by surgery in elective time. However, failure of reduction after three manual attempts or a hernia that remains unreduced after 2 h, including after attempt of gentle manual reduction, requires urgent surgical reduction and repair as further delay may jeopardize the sac contents, as well as the testis in the male [11].

9. Surgical management

Surgical repair is the definitive treatment of an inguinal hernia. Although such an operation is one of the most common methods in pediatric surgery, many issues arise, concerning the kind of anesthesia, the technique used in either elective or urgent fashion, the timing of the repair, especially for the preterm infants, and the contralateral exploration during surgery for unilateral inguinal hernia.

10. Anesthesia

General anesthesia is a golden standard option in pediatric surgery. In expert hands, there is a very low risk of complications, with postoperative apnea being the most common. Moreover, the use of antidotes makes this technique more suitable for short duration procedures [22]. However, general anesthetics and sedatives have been accused of having possible, harmful effects on the developing brain of a child [23]. General anesthesia, especially in preterm infants, can cause apnea and bradycardia postoperatively, meaning a reduced blood flow to the brain [24]. Such a decrease in oxygen supply could negatively affect the development of the central nervous system [25]. Although not the most appropriate for small duration procedures, regional central anesthesia is gaining ground. It is more cost effective than general anesthesia [26], creates minimal cardiorespiratory disturbances [22, 27], prevents the complications of high-risk patients with difficult intubation, is better tolerated in patients with respiratory diseases [28], and decreases neuroendocrine stress as a response to surgery [29].

One of the major issues of spinal anesthesia is the high failure rate that can reach 20% of the cases [30]. On the contrary, there is no mention of failure for general anesthesia. No fatal incidents have been reported during regional central anesthesia. The complications of this technique are usually minor. The most usual are post-dural puncture headache (2–4%), back pain (5–10%), and transient neurological symptoms (3–4%) [31].

11. Timing of operation

One of the most debated issues, concerning inguinal hernia repair in children, is the timing of operation, especially in preterm infants. It is common knowledge among pediatric surgeons that in full-term infants and children of any age, without other comorbidities, an inguinal hernia should be repaired soon after diagnosis [32].

However, in preterm infants. The optimal timing to perform surgical repair (before or after hospital or neonatal intensive care (NICU) discharge) remains controversial, due to the difficulty of balancing the risk of incarceration against the risk of intraoperative and postoperative complications [33, 34]. One of the first attempts to overcome this problem was the choice of many pediatric surgeons in the late 1990s and early 2000s, to opt for an operation when the child was at least 2 kg of weight, trying in such manner to minimize as possible the risk of strangulation concurrently with the risk of intraoperative and postoperative complications, although a lot has changed since then.

Some researchers argue that the risk of incarceration in infants is increased at least twofold, if the surgical repair gets delayed 14 days after diagnosis, reaching 60% of the cases, especially in preterm infants [35, 36]. On the other hand, many studies have demonstrated no significant difference in incarceration rates between patients undergoing hernia repair before (18.1%) and after (11.3%) discharge [37–41]. Of note, weight (either at birth or at incarceration), prematurity, sex, and side did not significantly correlate with the incidence of incarceration [42]. Many surgeons have also reported that early surgery for inguinal hernia in preterm infants increases five times the risk for postoperative apnea and ventilator dependence, with a maximum percentage of 4.7 in case of infants with postconceptional age less than 45 weeks [41, 43]. More specifically, respiratory problems were reported in 5.1 and 3.3% of the patients with early and late repair, respectively [37–40, 44]. Moreover, many surgeons have observed a 1–9% possibility of recurrence, if preterm babies were operated before discharge, due to the small anatomic area during surgery and the friable hernia sac [42, 45, 46]. Between preterm patients with early repair of inguinal hernia and those with late repair, the recurrence rate was 5.7% against 1.8% [37–40].

The European Pediatric Surgeons' Association Evidence and Guideline Committee concluded that no significant differences were found for incarceration between early and late surgical intervention in preterm infants with inguinal hernia. However, the late repair of a hernia after discharge from the hospital or NICU in a preterm infant will have better outcomes in terms of respiratory complications and hernia recurrence [41]. To sum up, a hernia in healthy full-term children should be electively repaired soon after diagnosis. On the other hand, the perfect timing for the repair of a hernia in a preterm infant is not 100% clear and every single case should be considered according to the specific needs of the patient.

12. Contralateral exploration

The exploration and repair of a contralateral patent processus vaginalis is still a matter of debate. It has been reported that gender, age, and birth weight have no influence on the development of a contralateral metachronous hernia [47, 48]. Many surgeons prefer to explore and repair the contralateral side, especially if the patient has birth weight less than 1500 gr, if it is a female, and if the operation is scheduled for a left-sided hernia [42]. It can be understood that during laparoscopic surgery, the inspection of the contralateral side is very easy to perform, but in case of open surgery, the exploration of the other side implies an increased risk of vas deferens and vessels' injury.

According to literature, the likelihood of a patent processus vaginalis in the opposite side ranges from 20 to 70% [36, 41, 49–51]. However, the overall presentation of a metachronous hernia in an initially asymptomatic contralateral processus vaginalis does not exceed 11.6% [41, 47, 48, 51–54]. Although the fact that such a percentage increases if the patient is preterm or less than 1 year of age, female, with a left-sided initial hernia, it must be underlined that the routine repair of a contralateral explored, asymptomatic patent processus vaginalis during laparoscopy or the choice to proceed to the opposite side during open surgery may result in overtreatment [42, 50, 53].

As regards laparoscopic procedures where the contralateral side is easily explored for a patent processus vaginalis, 20 procedures must be performed to avoid one metachronous inguinal hernia [51, 54]. For these reasons, European guidelines affirm that exploration and repair of the opposite site during surgery for unilateral inguinal hernia in children may prevent the development of a metachronous one, but such practice should not become the routine method because of the extensive heterogeneity among the currently available evidence [41].

13. Surgical technique through inguinal incision

The most common approach for repair of an inguinal hernia in children is through an inguinal incision. With the patient in supine position, a small cut is made through the dermis in the middle of the line that connects the anterior superior iliac spine and the pubic tubercle. The incision continues down to the subcutaneous fat, Camber's and Scarpa's fascia. Ladd and Gross, the fathers of pediatric surgery, preferred to open the external oblique muscle and perform reconstruction of the inguinal canal (Ferguson procedure), while others avoid entering the inguinal canal (Mitchell-Banks repair) [55].

The internal and external rings in the neonate are almost overlapping anatomically. As the patient grows, some distance is observed between the two, which in the adults results in 4 cm. The external oblique muscle is opened with a longitudinal incision to its fibers. The sac is identified beneath the transversalis fascia and the cremasteric muscle, which is dissected taking care not to traumatize the ileofemoral and ileoinguinal nerves. The hernia sac is grasped, and the cord structures are dissected gently, without injuring the vas deferens and the spermatic vessels in males, while in females such risk does not exist.

The sac is clamped, ligated, and divided. The distal part may be left without ulterior manipulation, due to the risk of injury of the testicle. The proximal part is dissected until the level of the internal ring twisted on itself and double ligated with monofilament absorbable suture and ligated. Routine inspection of the testis is not needed, but if so, particular care should be taken to place the testis in its right position inside the hemiscrotum. The surgical wound is closed in layers according to the right anatomical order. The skin is closed with subcutaneous suture for a better esthetic result. A dressing protects the wound from stools and urine.

In females, 40% of the inguinal hernias are sliding hernias. For this reason, the proximal part of the sac is opened, explored, and any structures are reduced inside the abdominal cavity. If the ovary or the fallopian tube makes part of the wall of the inguinal sac, the closure of the sac is performed by placing an external purse-string stitch above the level of protruding structure and then invert the sac in the internal ring, which is closed with sutures (Bevan repair) [56].

14. Laparoscopic procedure

The first to report a laparoscopic hernia repair was El-Gohary, but he only operated in females [57]. The *transabdominal purse-string stitch technique* was presented for the first time by Montupet and Esposito in 1999, which was, also, the first successful laparoscopic inguinal hernia repair in boys [58]. It is one of the most used among pediatric surgeons, although multiple laparoscopic techniques have been proposed. Scier described his *intracorporeal repair with z-stitches of the processus vaginalis* in females only and 12 years later, he described a similar procedure in males, but used several interrupted stitches than the z-suture to close the sac [59].

Many other techniques for transabdominal repair have been presented with small novelties, such as injection of normal saline (2 ml) into the extraperitoneal space to elevate the peritoneum away from the vas deferens and the testicular vessels, division and suture of the patent processus vaginalis at the level of the internal inguinal ring, use of the peritoneum to cover the processus vaginalis, and circumferential division of the peritoneum at the deep ring by purse-string closure of the proximal peritoneum [60–63].

Prasad et al. in 2003 presented for the first time the *extraperitoneal repair* [64]. Since then, a variety of devices and slight modifications have been described to improve the extracorporeal technique [65–73].

Some researchers have combined the open and laparoscopic techniques for a better overall result [74]. The *transabdominal laparoscopic hernia repair* is performed with the patient in the supine position. A foley catheter is always placed, to avoid injury to the bladder. After the placement of a 5 mm trocar transumbilically, pneumoperitoneum is achieved with a pressure of 8–12 mmHg, according to the size of the patient. Two 3 mm small incisions in the right and left lower quadrants are made and two 3 mm trocars are placed. Usually, the surgeon is positioned in the contralateral side of the hernia and the monitor in the ipsilateral side. Obviously, any hernia contents are reduced before beginning repair of the hernia. In males, the cord structures are identified and carefully excluded from the purse-string stitch that will close the sac, while in females many include the round ligament in the purse-string stitch. After completion of the operation, the gas used is removed from the peritoneal cavity. The 3 mm wounds do not require stitches and can be closed with steri-strips or skin glue. The wound of the umbilicus is closed with absorbable stitches in layers according to the right anatomical order. The contralateral side can be easily evaluated, and bilateral repair can be performed if necessary.

In the *extracorporeal procedure*, the only port used is the one in the umbilicus. The level of the internal ring is identified with palpation and compression. A small incision is made anterolateral to the ring itself. A curved awl that bears a suture is passed around the lateral half of the internal ring. After half of the sac is surrounded by the suture, the awl pierces the peritoneum, and the suture is grasped. The empty awl is withdrawn and reinserted into the wound. It passes around the medial half of the internal ring and once more enters the peritoneum at the same point the suture is left, previously, in the abdominal cavity. Care must be taken to exclude the vas deferens and vessels. The suture is passed through the awl and the awl is pulled out of the abdomen completing the purse string. The knot is tied extracorporeally and buried in the subcutaneous tissue.

A special note must be made for the extraperitoneal repair described by Patkowski et al. (percutaneous internal ring suturing, PIRS) and used as minimal invasive procedure by many surgeons in the modern era [68]. An 18-gauge injection needle, with a nonabsorbable 2–0 monofilament thread inside the barrel of the needle, is introduced into the abdominal cavity under laparoscopic guidance, leaving the ends of the thread outside the patient's body. By moving the tip of the needle, the thread passes under the peritoneum, over the half of the internal ring including a part of the ligament and adjacent tissue. The thread is pushed through the barrel of the needle and a loop is created. The needle is pulled out and one of the ends of the thread is introduced once again inside the peritoneal cavity in the same manner as that described before. Care is taken to puncture with the needle the same point on the skin. This time the thread surrounds the other half of the internal inguinal ring including once more part of the ligament. To avoid injury to the vas deferens and vessels, a small space is left above these structures. The end of the thread goes through the barrel of the needle into the loop and the needle is withdrawn. The thread loop is pulled out of the abdominal cavity, with the thread end caught by the loop. In this way, the thread is placed around the internal ring under the peritoneum, and both ends exit from the same point on the skin. A knot is made to close the inguinal ring and placed under the skin.

Single-port laparoscopy procedures, intracorporeal and extracorporeal, have been described. Such techniques seem to be a feasible and safe alternative to repairing inguinal hernia in the pediatric population [75, 76].

15. Open versus laparoscopic hernia surgery

When comparing the open procedure with the laparoscopic methods, we evaluate the operative time, the recurrence rates, metachronous hernia rates, the lengths of hospitalization, and the complications. Perioperative complications include injury of the vas deferens and spermatic vessels in males and ovaries in females, bleeding, and bowel trauma. Postoperative complications are testicular atrophy, iatrogenic ascent testis, hematoma, edema, hydrocele, and wound infection.

Unilateral repair of inguinal hernia in children has no difference in operative time between open and laparoscopic techniques, although most of the researchers agree that in females, both procedures last less [77–82]. Some of them have presented shorter operative time with the laparoscopic repair for unilateral hernia, especially with the PIRS procedure, but insist that the learning curve and, thus, the experience of the surgeon is of great importance [41, 82–84]. Recurrence rates are similar in both techniques, ranging from 0 to 6.3% for open surgery and from 0 to 5.7% for the laparoscopic procedures [77, 79–82, 85]. Some researchers argue that the risk of recurrence after laparoscopic surgery is much higher, even reaching 26.7% of the cases [86]. Such a high percentage of recurrence is justified by many, because of the surgeon's inexperience and comorbidities of the patients, especially pulmonary diseases [87, 88]. Moreover, most of the studies present an average follow-up of 2–3 years of the patients who have undergone surgery, while some studies claim that a follow-up of at least 5 years is necessary to put on display the majority of the recurrences [89].

As regards the rates of metachronous contralateral hernia, the results are controversial. On the one hand, there are researchers who claim that no difference is demonstrated between open and laparoscopic procedures [79, 82, 90, 91]. On the other hand, there are studies that present a percentage of 5.9% of metachronous hernia in the open repair and near to zero in the laparoscopic procedures. This is, easily, understood, because of the easy inspection of the contralateral side in a laparoscopic surgery, although, as mentioned, a treatment of every patent processus vaginalis can result in overtreatment [91–95]. The length of hospitalization (4–6 h), postoperative pain, and, consequently, the time for a full recovery do not show significant differences between the two techniques [77, 79–82, 90].

Perioperative complications like bleeding (5.7%) testicular injury or trauma of the vas deferens or the vessels (0.13–1.6%) and ovarian lesion seem to have the same rates between open and laparoscopic procedures [77, 81, 85, 89, 91]. With regard to postoperative complications, most of them conclude that there are no significant disparities between open and laparoscopic procedures, although testicular compromise can range from 2.6 to 13%, especially in case of strangulated hernias [77, 79, 80, 89–91]. Nonetheless, some claim that open and laparoscopic repairs present slightly different rates for some postoperative complications. For example, *testicular atrophy can range from 0 to 13% of the cases in open repair, while in laparoscopic procedures this percentage is almost zero*. The same applies to injury of the spermatic vessels, which in open procedures reaches a percentage of 1.6%. The risk of iatrogenic ascent testis was more pronounced in laparoscopic surgery (3.2%), whereas in open surgery it was 1.2–2.7%. Hydrocele formation was seen in 2.9 and 5.7% of the cases in open and laparoscopic procedures, respectively [81, 91, 96, 97]. Finally, most studies concur that the cosmetic results of the laparoscopic procedures are superior if compared with those of the open surgery [70, 71, 79–81, 85, 92, 98].

16. Management of strangulated hernia

If the surgeon is certain that there is no compromise of an internal organ, a reduction maneuver can be attempted. The patient is laid in a supine position. The sac with the incarcerated bowel lies in front and anteriorly of the external inguinal ring in such a fashion that the ridge of the ring is covered by the sac and its content. Standing next to the patient, the surgeon must perform a maneuver of gentle continuous pressure of the herniated bulge with one hand, while with the other hand, firm pressure to the margins of the external ring is applied, to prevent overlapping the ridge, and obtain reduction into the inguinal canal.

The success of the procedure can be understood by the relief of the patient and from a sensation of sudden liberation in the fingers that apply pressure to the bottom of the hernia, usually accompanied with a characteristic sound. This maneuver can last for several minutes and can be facilitated by light sedation or intramuscular administration of pethidine. It is recommended to conduct the follow-up of the patient for 24 to 48 h, to observe the stools, since reduction of gangrenous intestine has been reported [99]. The definitive repair of the hernia should be delayed for at least 48 h, due to edema of the tissues.

In case of peritonitis or signs of shock, due to serious bowel compromise or if the manual reduction fails, broad-spectrum antibiotics are administered, a nasogastric tube and a foley catheter are placed, and the patient is promptly brought to the operation room. We should mention that in females, the strangulated organ can be a part of the intestine or the bladder, but, also, an ovary, a fallopian tube, or the mesosalpinx. General anesthesia is, sometimes, sufficient for the reduction of the hernia, nonetheless the operation should proceed.

The operation with a standard inguinal incision is used by most surgeons. Others prefer an incision in the longitudinal axes of the inguinal canal, which will make the surgery easier in case of a compromise bowel that needs to be excised. The external inguinal ring is cut. If the hernia contents are present, the hernia sac is opened, and the bowel is inspected. If not compromised, the content is reduced, and the procedure continues in the standard fashion. If the internal ring is still constringing the sac or if the bowel is not viable, the inferior epigastric vessels are ligated and part of the floor of the inguinal canal is opened to enlarge the external ring. Any necrotic bowel must be excised, and an end-to-end anastomosis is performed through the inguinal incision. During closure, the floor of the inguinal canal must be repaired.

If the content of the hernia is reduced before it can be inspected, the surgeon should search for indirect signs of intestinal necrosis, such as foul smell or blood-stained fluid. In dubious cases, a camera can be placed through a port in the umbilicus and if compromised intestine is found, the incision of the umbilicus is enlarged, and the bowel is brought out for repair.

Laparoscopy is gaining ground for the repair of a strangulated hernia and according to some researchers, it presents certain advantages from a technical point of view [99]. It is straightforward that with laparoscopy the incarcerated organ can be easily inspected. It is not necessary to wait a few days for the tissue edema to abate and there is no manipulation of the structures of the cord. Depending on the experience of the surgeon, some prefer to reduce and inspect the bowel through laparoscopy and proceed with herniorrhaphy through the standard inguinal incision [100].

17. Conclusions

Inguinal hernia is the most common surgical disease in children. Although a daily issue in pediatric surgical routine, there are still debates on certain characteristics regarding management decisions and surgical technique. Both open and laparoscopic surgical procedures present their advantages and their risks. However, if we remember the declaration of the Hippocratic oath for the good of the patients according to our ability and judgment, we shall avoid overtreatment and any unnecessary impact on patients and their families. Furthermore, we must have in mind that the future is in minimal invasive surgery. If used with prudence and with a proper learning curve, as technology gets better and more specific, there will be only profit for the health of pediatric patients.

Author details

George Sakellaris[1*], Konstantinos Zachos[2], Maria Athanasopoulou[2], Antonios Panagidis[2], Vasileios Alexopoulos[2], Ioannis Spyridakis[3], Anastasia Vareli[2] and Xenophon Sinopidis[4]

1 Department of Pediatric Surgery, University General Hospital of Crete, Herakleion, Greece

2 Department of Pediatric Surgery, Patras Children's Hospital, Patras, Greece

3 Department of Pediatric Surgery, Aristotle University of Thessaloniki School of Medicine, Thessaloniki, Greece

4 Department of Pediatric Surgery, University of Patras School of Medicine, Patras, Greece

*Address all correspondence to: georgesakellaris97@gmail.com

References

[1] Yeap E, Pacilli M, Nataraja RM. Inguinal hernias in children. The Australian Journal of General Practice. 2020;**49**:38-43. DOI: 10.31128/AJGP-08-19-5037

[2] Palmer LS. Hernias and hydroceles. Pediatrics in Review. 2013;**34**:457-464. DOI: 10.1542/pir.34-10-457

[3] Alshahwani N, Briatico D, Lee W, Farrokhyar FJ. Review and quality assessment of systematic reviews and meta-analyses on the management of pediatric inguinal hernias: A descriptive study. The Journal of Surgical Research. 2022;**278**:404-417. DOI: 10.1016/j.jss.2022.04.008

[4] Chan YY, Durbin-Johnson B, Kurzrock EA. Pediatric inguinal and scrotal surgery-practice patterns in U.S. academic centers. Journal of Pediatric Surgery. 2016;**51**:1786-1790. DOI: 10.1016/j.jpedsurg.2016.07.019

[5] Akinkuotu AC, Roberson M, Strassle PD, Phillips MR, McLean SE, Hayes-Jordan A. Factors associated with inguinal hernia repair in premature infants during neonatal admission. Journal of Pediatric Surgery. 2022;**57**:369-374. DOI: 10.1016/j.jpedsurg.2021.08.014

[6] Taghavi K, Geneta VP, Mirjalili SA. The pediatric inguinal canal: Systematic review of the embryology and surface anatomy. Clinical Anatomy. 2016;**29**:204-210. DOI: 10.1002/ca.22633

[7] Pechriggl E, Blumer M, Tubbs RS, Olewnik Ł, Konschake M, Fortélny R, et al. Embryology of the abdominal wall and associated malformations-a review. Frontiers in Surgery. 2022;**9**:891896. DOI: 10.3389/fsurg.2022.891896

[8] Panagidis A, Kostopoulou E, Rojas Gil AP, Sinopidis X, Kourea H, Skiadopoulos S, et al. Correlation between insulin-like peptide 3 and appendix testis length in congenital cryptorchidism. Journal of Paediatrics and Child Health. 2020;**56**:1283-1289. DOI: 10.1111/jpc.14924

[9] Sinopidis X, Mourelatou R, Kostopoulou E, Karvela A, Rojas-Gil AP, Tsekoura E, et al. Novel combined insulin-like 3 variations of a single nucleotide in cryptorchidism. Journal of Pediatric Endocrinology & Metabolism. 2019;**32**:987-994. DOI: 10.1515/jpem-2018-0547

[10] Aneiros Castro B, Cano Novillo I, García VA. The accuracy of silk glove sign compared with inguinal bulge in the diagnosis of indirect inguinal hernia in children. Journal of Laparoendoscopic & Advanced Surgical Techniques. 2019;**29**:1349-1351. DOI: 10.1089/lap.2019.0126

[11] Scott V, Davenport M, Fisher RM. Inguinal hernias and hydroceles. In: Sinha CK, Davenport M, editors. Handbook of Pediatric Surgery. London: Springer-Verlag; 2010. pp. 229-233. DOI: 10.1007/978-1-84882-132-3_33

[12] Sinopidis X, Panagidis A, Kourea E, Kostopoulou E, Rojas-Gil AP, Skiadopoulos S, et al. New insights into the expression of androgen and estrogen receptors of the appendix testis in congenital cryptorchidism. Journal of Pediatric Endocrinology & Metabolism. 2020;**33**:503-508. DOI: 10.1515/jpem-2019-0392

[13] Michalinos A, Moris D, Vernadakis S. Amyand's hernia: A review. American Journal of Surgery. 2014;**207**:989-995. DOI: 10.1016/j.amjsurg.2013.07.043

[14] Panagidis A, Sinopidis X, Zachos K, Alexopoulos V, Vareli A, Varvarigou A, et al. Neonatal perforated Amyand's hernia presenting as an enterocutaneous scrotal fistula. Asian Journal of Surgery. 2015;**38**:177-179. DOI: 10.1016/j.asjsur.2014.03.001

[15] Sun SL, Chen KL, Gauci C. Appendiceal abscess within a giant Amyand's hernia: A case report. Cureus. 2023;**15**:e36947. DOI: 10.7759/cureus.36947

[16] Sinopidis X, Fouzas S, Kambouri K, Panagidis A, Alexopoulos V, Karatza A, et al. Predictive model of heterotopy in Meckel's diverticulum in children. ANZ. 2019;**89**:E241-E245. DOI: 10.1111/ans.15226

[17] Qin D, Liu G, Wang Z. Littre's hernia in a paediatric patient. African Journal of Paediatric Surgery. 2014;**11**:351-353. DOI: 10.4103/0189-6725.143168

[18] Bakal Ü, Tartar T, Saraç M, Kazez A. Littre hernia in children: A clinical aspect. The Turkish Journal of Gastroenterology. 2019;**30**:101-104. DOI: 10.5152/tjg.2018.18228

[19] Odongo CN, Godier-Furnemont A, Moro J, Oyania F. A case report of an asymptomatic necrotic Meckel's diverticulum in an inguinal hernia during elective surgery in a resource limited setting: Littre's hernia. International Journal of Surgery Case Reports. 2023;**105**:108011. DOI: 10.1016/j.ijscr.2023.108011

[20] Kadirov S, Sayfan J, Friedman S, Orda RJ. Richter's hernia-a surgical pitfall. The American College of Surgeons. 1996;**182**:60-62

[21] Moleiro Bilbao A, Hernández-Siverio GN. Richter's hernia in the newborn as cause of testicular infarction. Cirugía Pediátrica. 2009;**22**:226-228

[22] Gupta A, Saha U. Spinal anesthesia in children: A review. Journal of Anaesthesiology Clinical Pharmacology. 2014;**30**:10-18. DOI: 10.4103/0970-9185.125687

[23] Andropoulos DB, Greene MF. Anesthesia and developing brains-implications of the FDA warning. The New England Journal of Medicine. 2017;**376**:905-907. DOI: 10.1056/NEJMp1700196

[24] McCannME,WithingtonDE,ArnupSJ, Davidson AJ, Disma N, Frawley G, et al. GAS consortium. Differences in blood pressure in infants after general anesthesia compared to awake regional anesthesia (GAS study-a prospective randomized trial). Anesthesia and Analgesia. 2017;**125**:837-845. DOI: 10.1213/ANE.0000000000001870

[25] Davidson AJ, Disma N, de Graaff JC, et al. Neurodevelopmental outcome at 2 years of age after general anaesthesia and awake-regional anaesthesia in infancy (GAS): An international multicentre, randomised controlled trial. Lancet. 2016;**387**:239-250. DOI: 10.1016/S0140-6736(15)00608-X

[26] Imbelloni LE, Vieira EM, Sperni F, Guizellini RH, Tolentino AP. Spinal anesthesia in children with isobaric local anaesthetics: Report on 307 patients under 13 years of age. Pediatric Anaesthesia. 2006;**16**:43-48. DOI: 10.1111/j.1460-9592.2005.01680.x

[27] Davidson AJ, Morton NS, Arnup SJ, de Graaff JC, Disma N, Withington DE, et al. General anesthesia compared to spinal anesthesia (GAS) consortium. Apnea after awake regional and general anesthesia in infants: The general anesthesia compared to

spinal anesthesia study–comparing apnea and neurodevelopmental outcomes, a randomized controlled trial. Anesthesiology. 2015;**123**:38-54. DOI: 10.1097/ALN.0000000000000709

[28] López T, Sánchez FJ, Garzón JC, Muriel C. Spinal anesthesia in pediatric patients. Minerva Anestesiologica. 2012;**78**:78-87. DOI: 10.1111/j.1460-9592.2011.03769.x

[29] Wolf AR, Doyle E, Thomas E. Modifying infants stress responses to major surgery: Spinal vs extradural vs opioid analgesia. Paediatric Anaesthesia. 1998;**8**:305-311. DOI: 10.1046/j.1460-9592.1998.00239.x

[30] Frawley G, Bell G, Disma N, Withington DE, de Graaff JC, Morton NS, et al. Predictors of failure of awake regional anesthesia for neonatal hernia repair: Data from the general anesthesia compared to spinal anesthesia study-comparing apnea and neurodevelopmental outcomes. Anesthesiology. 2015;**123**:55-65. DOI: 10.1097/ALN.0000000000000708

[31] Kokki H. Spinal blocks. Paediatric Anaesthesia. 2012;**22**:56-64. DOI: 10.1111/j.1460-9592.2011.03693.x

[32] Levitt MA, Ferraracio D, Arbesman MC, Brisseau GG, Glick PL. Variability of inguinal hernia surgical technique: A survey of north American pediatric surgeons. Journal of Pediatric Surgery. 2002;**37**:745-751. DOI: 10.1053/jpsu.2002.32269

[33] Choo SC, Chen Y, McHoney M. Delayed versus early repair of inguinal hernia in preterm infants: A systematic review and meta-analysis. Journal of Pediatric Surgery. 2022;**57**:527-533. DOI: 10.1016/j.jpedsurg.2022.07.001

[34] Baird R, Gholoum S, Laberge JM, Puligandla P. Prematurity, not age at operation or incarceration, impacts complication rates of inguinal hernia repair. Journal of Pediatric Surgery. 2011;**46**:908-911. DOI: 10.1016/j.jpedsurg.2011.02.059

[35] Zamakhshary M, To T, Guan J, Langer JC. Risk of incarceration of inguinal hernia among infants and young children awaiting elective surgery. CMAJ. 2008;**179**:1001-1005. DOI: 10.1503/cmaj.070923

[36] Wang KS, Committee on Fetus and Newborn, American Academy of Pediatrics; Section on Surgery, American Academy of Pediatrics. Assessment and management of inguinal hernia in infants. Pediatrics. 2012;**130**:768-773. DOI: 10.1542/peds.2012-2008

[37] Crankson SJ, Al Tawil K, Al Namshan M, Al Namshan M, Baylon BJ, Gieballa M, et al. Management of inguinal hernia in premature infants: 10-year experience. Journal of Indian Association of Pediatric Surgeons. 2015;**20**:21-24. DOI: 10.4103/0971-9261.145440

[38] Khan FA, Zeidan N, Larson SD, Taylor JA, Islam S. Inguinal hernias in premature neonates: Exploring optimal timing for repair. Pediatric Surgery International. 2018;**34**:1157-1161. DOI: 10.1007/s00383-018-4356-8

[39] Pandey R, Dako J, Venus S, Kumar D, Mhanna M. Early versus late inguinal hernia repair in extremely low-birthweight infants. The Journal of Maternal-Fetal & Neonatal Medicine. 2017;**30**:2457-2460. DOI: 10.1080/14767058.2016.1253059

[40] Takahashi A, Toki F, Yamamoto H, Otake S, Oki Y, Kuwano H. Outcomes of herniotomy in premature infants: Recent 10-year experience. Pediatrics International. 2012;**54**:491-495. DOI: 10.1111/j.1442-200X.2012.03607.x

[41] Morini F, Dreuning KMA, Janssen Lok MJH, Wester T, Derikx JPM, Friedmacher F, et al. Surgical management of pediatric inguinal hernia: A systematic review and guideline from the European pediatric surgeons' association evidence and guideline committee. European Journal of Pediatric Surgery. 2022;**32**:219-232. DOI: 10.1055/s-0040-1721420

[42] Pini Prato A, Rossi V, Mosconi M, Disma N, Mameli L, Montobbio G, et al. Inguinal hernia in neonates and ex-preterm: Complications, timing and need for routine contralateral exploration. Pediatric Surgery International. 2015;**31**:131-136. DOI: 10.1007/s00383-014-3638-z

[43] Ozdemir T, Arıkan A. Postoperative apnea after inguinal hernia repair in formerly premature infants: Impacts of gestational age, postconceptional age and comorbidities. Pediatric Surgery International. 2013;**29**:801-804. DOI: 10.1007/s00383-013-3330-8

[44] Lee SL, Gleason JM, Sydorak RM. A critical review of premature infants with inguinal hernias: Optimal timing of repair, incarceration risk, and postoperative apnea. Journal of Pediatric Surgery. 2011;**46**:217-220. DOI: 10.1016/j.jpedsurg.2010.09.094

[45] Fette AM, Hollwarth ME. Special aspects of neonatal inguinal hernia and herniotomy. Hernia. 2001;**5**:92-96. DOI: 10.1007/s100290100011

[46] Masoudian P, Sullivan KJ, Mohamed H, Ahmed N. Optimal timing for inguinal hernia repair in premature infants: A systematic review and meta-analysis. Journal of Pediatric Surgery. 2019;**54**:1539-1545. DOI: 10.1016/j.jpedsurg.2018.11.002

[47] Hoshino M, Sugito K, Kawashima H, Goto S, Kaneda H, Furuya T, et al. Prediction of contralateral inguinal hernias in children: A prospective study of 357 unilateral inguinal hernias. Hernia. 2014;**18**:333-337. DOI: 10.1007/s10029-013-1099-2

[48] Wenk K, Sick B, Sasse T, Moehrlen U, Meuli M, Vuille-dit-Bille RN. Incidence of metachronous contralateral inguinal hernias in children following unilateral repair-a meta-analysis of prospective studies. Journal of Pediatric Surgery. 2015;**50**:2147-2154. DOI: 10.1016/j.jpedsurg.2015.08.056

[49] Weaver KL, Poola AS, Gould JL, Sharp SW, St Peter SD, Holcomb GW III. The risk of developing a symptomatic inguinal hernia in children with an asymptomatic patent processus vaginalis. Journal of Pediatric Surgery. 2017;**52**:60-64. DOI: 10.1016/j.jpedsurg.2016.10.018

[50] Kokorowski P, Wang HHS, Routh JC, Hubert KC, Nelson CP. Evaluation of the contralateral inguinal ring in clinically unilateral inguinal hernia: A systematic review and meta-analysis. Hernia. 2014;**18**:311-324. DOI: 10.1007/s10029-013-1146-z

[51] Muensterer OJ, Gianicolo G. Contralateral processus closure to prevent metachronous inguinal hernia: A systematic review. International Journal of Surgery. 2019;**68**:11-19. DOI: 10.1016/j.ijsu.2019.06.001

[52] Casaccia G, Arnoldi R, Pini PA. Timing and management of inguinal hernia in the premature baby. European Journal of Pediatric Surgery. 2017;**27**:472-477. DOI: 10.1055/s-0037-1608802

[53] Maillet OP, Garnier S, Dadure C, Bringuier S, Podevin G, Arnaud A, et al. Inguinal hernia in premature boys: Should we systematically explore the contralateral side? Journal of

Pediatric Surgery. 2014;**49**:1419-1423. DOI: 10.1016/j.jpedsurg.2014.01.055

[54] Zhao J, Chen Y, Lin J, Jin J, Yang H, Wang F, et al. Potential value of routine contralateral patent processes vaginalis repair in children with unilateral inguinal hernia. The British Journal of Surgery. 2017;**104**:148-151. DOI: 10.1002/bjs.10302

[55] Sachs M, Damm M, Encke A. Historical evolution of inguinal hernia repair. World Journal of Surgery. 1997;**21**:218-223. DOI: 10.1007/s002689900220

[56] Bevan A. Sliding hernias of the ascending colon and caecum, the descending colon, sigmoid and the bladder. Annals of Surgery. 1930;**92**:754. DOI: 10.1097/00000658-193010000-00026

[57] El-Gohary MA. Laparoscopic ligation of inguinal hernia in girls. Pediatric Endosurgery & Innovative Techniques. 1997;**1**:185-188. DOI: 10.1089/pei.1997.1.185

[58] Montupet P, Esposito C. Laparoscopic treatment of congenital inguinal hernia in children. Journal of Pediatric Surgery. 1999;**34**:420-423. DOI: 10.1016/s0022-3468(99)90490-6

[59] Schier F. Laparoscopic herniorrhaphy in girls. Journal of Pediatric Surgery. 1998;**33**:1495-1497. DOI: 10.1016/s0022-3468(98)90483-3

[60] Chan KL, Tam PKH. A safe laparoscopic technique for the repair of inguinal hernias in boys. Journal of the American College of Surgeons. 2003;**196**:987-989. DOI: 10.1016/S1072-7515(03)00121-2

[61] Becmeur F, Philippe P, Lemandt-Schultz A, Moog R, Grandadam S, Lieber A, et al. A continuous series of 96 laparoscopic inguinal hernia repairs in children by a new technique. Surgical Endoscopy. 2004;**18**:1738-1741. DOI: 10.1007/s00464-004-9008-5

[62] Yip KF, Tam PKH, Li MKW. Laparoscopic flip-flap hernioplasty: An innovative technique for pediatric hernia surgery. Surgical Endoscopy. 2004;**18**:1126-1129. DOI: 10.1007/s00464-003-9155-0

[63] Wheeler AA, Matz ST, Schmidt S, Pimpalwar A. Laparoscopic inguinal hernia repair in children with transperitoneal division of the hernia sac and proximal purse string closure of peritoneum: Our modified new approach. European Journal of Pediatric Surgery. 2011;**21**:381-385. DOI: 10.1055/s-0031-1291181

[64] Prasad R, Lovvorn HN, Wadie GM, Lobe TE. Early experience with needlescopic inguinal herniorrhaphy in children. Journal of Pediatric Surgery. 2003;**38**:1055-1058. DOI: 10.1016/s0022-3468(03)00191-x

[65] Harrison MR, Lee H, Albanese CT, Farmer DL. Subcutaneous endoscopically assisted ligation (SEAL) of the internal ring for repair of inguinal hernias in children: A novel technique. Journal of Pediatric Surgery. 2005;**40**:1177-1180. DOI: 10.1016/j.jpedsurg.2005.03.075

[66] Takehara H, Yakabe S, Kameoka K. Laparoscopic percutaneous extraperitoneal closure for inguinal hernia in children: Clinical outcome of 972 repairs done in 3 pediatric surgical institutions. Journal of Pediatric Surgery. 2006;**41**:1999-2003. DOI: 10.1016/j.jpedsurg.2006.08.032

[67] Oue T, Kubota A, Okuyama H, Kawahara H. Laparoscopic percutaneous extraperitoneal closure (LPEC) method

for the exploration and treatment of inguinal hernia in girls. Pediatric Surgery International. 2005;**21**:964-968. DOI: 10.1007/s00383-005-1556-9

[68] Patkowski D, Czernik J, Chrzan R, Jaworski W, Apoznan W. Percutaneous internal ring suturing: A simple minimally invasive technique for inguinal hernia repair in children. Journal of Laparoendoscopic & Advanced Surgical Techniques. 2006;**16**:513-517. DOI: 10.1089/lap.2006.16.513

[69] Bharathi SR, Arora M, Baskaran V. How we "SEAL" internal ring in pediatric inguinal hernias. Surgical Laparoscopy, Endoscopy & Percutaneous Techniques. 2008;**18**:192-194. DOI: 10.1097/SLE.0b013e31816a0645

[70] Endo M, Ukiyama E. Laparoscopic closure of patent Processus Vaginalis in girls with inguinal hernia using a specially devised suture needle. Pediatric Endosurgery & Innovative Techniques. 2001;**5**:187-191. DOI: 10.1089/10926410152403147

[71] Endo M, Watanabe T, Nakano M, Yoshida F, Ukiyama E. Laparoscopic completely extraperitoneal repair of inguinal hernia in children: A single-institute experience with 1,257 repairs compared with cut-down herniorrhaphy. Surgical Endoscopy. 2009;**23**:1706-1712. DOI: 10.1007/s00464-008-0300-7

[72] Muensterer OJ, Georgeson KE. Inguinal hernia repair by single-incision pediatric endosurgery (SIPES) using the hydrodissection-lasso technique. Surgical Endoscopy. 2011;**25**:3438-3439. DOI: 10.1007/s00464-011-1713-2

[73] Li S, Li M, Wong KKY, Liu L, Tam PKH. Laparoscopically assisted simple suturing obliteration (LASSO) of the internal ring using an epidural needle: A handy single-port laparoscopic herniorrhaphy in children. Journal of Pediatric Surgery. 2014;**49**:1818-1820. DOI: 10.1016/j.jpedsurg.2014.09.027

[74] Yeung CK, Lee KH. Inguinal herniotomy: Laparoscopic-assisted extraperitoneal technique. In: Bax KMA, Georgeson KE, Rothenberg SS, Valla JS, Yeung CK, editors. Endoscopic Surgery in Infants and Children. Berlin, Heidelberg: Springer-Verlag; 2008. pp. 591-596

[75] Yilmaz E, Afsarlar CE, Senel E, Cavusoglou YH, Karaman I, Karaman A, et al. A novel technique for laparoscopic inguinal hernia repair in children: Single-port laparoscopic percutaneous extraperitoneal closure assisted by an optical forceps. Pediatric Surgery International. 2015;**31**:639-646. DOI: 10.1007/s00383-015-3722-z

[76] Ahmed A, Elgaffar H. Laparoscopic single instrument closure of inguinal hernia in female children: A novel technique. Journal of Pediatric Surgery. 2015;**50**:1613-1616. DOI: 10.1016/j.jpedsurg.2015.05.003

[77] Kantor N, Travis N, Wayne C, Nasr A. Laparoscopic versus open inguinal hernia repair in children: Which is the true gold-standard? A systematic review and meta-analysis. Pediatric Surgery International. 2019;**35**:1013-1026. DOI: 10.1007/s00383-019-04521-1

[78] Shehata SMK, El Attar AA, Attia MA, Hassan AM. Laparoscopic herniotomy in children: Prospective assessment of tertiary center experience in a developing country. Hernia. 2013;**17**:229-234. DOI: 10.1007/s10029-012-1031-1

[79] Chan KL, Hui WC, Tam PKH. Prospective randomized single center, single-blind comparison of laparoscopic vs open repair of pediatric inguinal hernia. Surgical Endoscopy.

2005;**19**:927-932. DOI: 10.1007/s00464-004-8224-3

[80] Gause CD, Casamassima MGS, Yang J, Hsiung G, Rhee D, Salazar JH, et al. Laparoscopic versus open inguinal hernia repair in children ≤ 3: A randomized controlled trial. Pediatric Surgery International. 2017;**33**:367-376

[81] Shalaby R, Ibrahem R, Shahin M, Yehya A, Abdalrazek M, Alsayaad I, et al. Laparoscopic hernia repair versus open herniotomy in children ≤ 3: A controlled randomized study. Minimully Invasive Surgery. 2012;**2012**:484135. DOI: 10.1155/2012/484135

[82] Dreuning K, Maat S, Twisk J, van Heurn E, Derikx J. Laparoscopic versus open pediatric inguinal hernia repair: State-of-the-art comparison and future perspectives from a meta-analysis. Surgical Endoscopy. 2019;**33**:3177-3191. DOI: 10.1007/s00464-019-06960-2

[83] Wolak PK, Strzelecka A, Piotrowska A, Dąbrowska K, Wolak PP, Piotrowska I, et al. The operative time for unilateral inguinal hernia repair in children performed with percutaneous internal ring suturing (PIRS) or open approach method. Journal of Clinical Medicine. 2021;**10**:1293. DOI: 10.3390/jcm10061293

[84] Thomas DT, Göcmen KB, Tulgar S, Boga I. Percutaneous internal ring suturing is a safe and effective method for the minimal invasive treatment of pediatric inguinal hernia: Experience with 250 cases. Journal of Pediatric Surgery. 2016;**51**:1330-1335. DOI: 10.1016/j.jpedsurg.2015.11.024

[85] Celebi S, Uysal AI, Inal FY, Yildiz A. A single-blinded, randomized comparison of laparoscopic versus open bilateral hernia repair in boys. Journal of Laparoendoscopic & Advanced Surgical Techniques. Part A. 2014;**24**:117-121. DOI: 10.1089/lap.2013.0397

[86] Hassan ME, Mustafawi AR. Laparoscopic flip-flap technique versus conventional inguinal hernia repair in children. JSLS. 2007;**11**:90-93

[87] Abd-Alrazek M, Alsherbiny H, Mahfouz M, Alsamahy O, Shalaby R, Shams A, et al. Laparoscopic pediatric inguinal hernia repair: A controlled randomized study. Journal of Pediatric Surgery. 2017;**52**:1539-1544. DOI: 10.1016/j.jpedsurg.2017.07.003

[88] Antao B, Samuel M, Curry J, Kiely E, Drake D. Open inguinal herniotomy in infants. Pediatric Endosurgery & Innovative Techniques. 2004;**8**:302309. DOI: 10.1089/pei.2004.8.302

[89] Grosfeld JL, Minnick K, Shedd F, West KW, Rescorla FJ, Vane DW. Inguinal hernia in children: Factors affecting recurrence in 62 cases. Journal of Pediatric Surgery. 1991;**26**:283-287. DOI: 10.1016/0022-3468(91)90503-L

[90] Koivusalo AI, Korpela R, Wirtavuori K, Piiparinen S, Rintala RJ, Pakarinen MPA. A single-blinded, randomized comparison of laparoscopic versus open hernia repair in children. Pediatrics. 2009;**123**:332-337. DOI: 10.1542/peds.2007-3752

[91] Bharathi SR, Arora M, Baskaran V. Pediatric inguinal hernia: Laparoscopic versus open surgery. JSLS. 2008;**12**(03):277-281

[92] Amano H, Tanaka Y, Kawashima H, Deie K, Fujiogi M, Suzuki K, et al. Comparison of single-incision laparoscopic percutaneous extraperitoneal closure (SILPEC) and open repair for pediatric inguinal hernia: A single-center retrospective cohort study of 2028 cases. Surgical Endoscopy

and Other Interventional Techniques. 2017;**31**:4988-4995. DOI: 10.1007/s00464-017-5472-6

[93] Lin CD, Tsai YC, Chang SJ, Yang SS. Surgical outcomes of mini laparoscopic herniorrhaphy in infants. The Journal of Urology. 2011;**185**:1071-1076. DOI: 10.1016/j.juro.2010.10.044

[94] Esposito C, St. Peter SD, Escolino M, Juang D, Settimi A, Holcomb GW. Laparoscopic versus open inguinal hernia repair in pediatric patients: A systematic review. Journal of Laparoendoscopic & Advanced Surgical Techniques. 2014;**24**:811-818. DOI: 10.1089/lap.2014.0194

[95] Alzahem A. Laparoscopic versus open inguinal herniotomy in infants and children: A meta-analysis. Pediatric Surgery International. 2011;**27**:605-612. DOI: 10.1007/s00383-010-2840-x

[96] Surana R, Puri P. Iatrogenic ascent of the testis: An under-recognized complication of inguinal hernia operation in children. British Journal of Urology. 1994;**73**:580-581. DOI: 10.1111/j.1464-410x.1994.tb07648.x

[97] Nagraj S, Sinha S, Grant H, Lakhoo K, Hitchcock R, Johnson P. The incidence of complications following primary inguinal herniotomy in babies weighing 5 kg or less. Pediatric Surgery International. 2006;**22**:500-502. DOI: 10.1007/s00383-006-1695-7

[98] Jun Z, Juntao G, Shuli L, Li L. A comparative study on trans-umbilical single-port laparoscopic approach versus conventional repair for incarcerated inguinal hernia in children. Journal of Minimal Access Surgery. 2016;**12**:139-142. DOI: 10.4103/0972- 9941.169953

[99] Esposito C, Turial S, Alicchio F, Enders J, Castagnetti M, Krause K, et al. Laparoscopic repair of incarcerated inguinal hernia. A safe and effective procedure to adopt in children. Hernia. 2013;**17**:235-239. DOI: 10.1007/s10029-012-0948-8

[100] Strauch ED, Voigt RW, Hill JL. Gangrenous intestine in a hernia can be reduced. Journal of Pediatric Surgery. 2002;**37**:919-920. DOI: 10.1053/jpsu.2002.32912

Chapter 11

Management of Strangulated Inguinal Hernia

Mohamed Arif Hameed Sultan and Dayang Corieza Febriany

Abstract

Strangulated inguinal hernia occurs when part of the hernia becomes irreducible and subsequently causes bowel ischemia secondary to a reduction in blood flow to the hernia. Therefore, management strategy differs and depends on the presentation of the hernia, duration, patient, and surgical factors. One thing is for sure: conservative management is not recommended for a strangulated inguinal hernia, as it always requires surgical intervention. Among others are diagnostic laparoscopy, open hernioplasty with the hybrid technique, and laparotomy followed by inguinal herniorrhaphy. Eventually, the outcome of the surgery has to be considered while managing strangulated inguinal hernia cases. Prompt diagnosis and management are required to reduce the morbidity and mortality associated with strangulated inguinal hernias.

Keywords: hernia, herniorrhaphy, ischemia, laparoscopy, laparotomy

1. Introduction

Hernia is defined as a protrusion of the viscus or part of the viscus through an abnormal opening of the walls of its containing cavity. The incidence in full-term babies is estimated at 1–5%, and it is close to 10% in pre-term babies (bilateral hernias are more common in pre-term babies). The most commonly protruded viscus includes the small bowel, large bowel, omentum, bladder, appendix (amyand's hernia), or even gynecological organs.

An inguinal hernia happens due to the weakening of the lower abdominal wall for various reasons. Congenitally, it is due to patent processes vaginalis which is an outpouching of the peritoneum [1]. It affects both men and women of various ages. However, inguinal hernia is more prevalent in males, whereas femoral hernia is more common in females. Having said that, strangulation is seen more in the femoral hernia as opposed to the inguinal hernia due to the narrow neck of the femoral hernia. Generally, the femoral hernia will pass inferior-laterally to the pubic tubercle whereas the inguinal hernia, on the other hand, will pass superior-medially. Direct inguinal hernia involves protrusion of the viscus through the weakening of Hesslebach's triangle. The inguinal ligament, inferior epigastric vessels, and the lateral edge of the rectus sheath all encircle these triangles.

Inguinal hernias can be managed conservatively unless the patient presents with obstruction or strangulation, where surgical correction is warranted [1]. Reducible inguinal hernias can be managed expectantly with an outpatient elective hernioplasty.

Irreducible hernias, on the other hand, need further assessment and intervention. Based on a Cochrane review, it can be concluded that eventually, 54% of all inguinal hernias need surgical intervention due to complications such as incarceration or strangulation. Hence, elective surgical intervention is usually suggested for all patients with inguinal hernias. The attending surgeon should explain clearly to patients the various available options and possible complications should the patient present in an acute setting with intestinal obstruction. This is because the morbidity and mortality of hernioplasty increase in the emergency setting as opposed to the elective setting. A holistic approach needs to be taken when managing such complicated cases. Proper communication and documentation should be done in dealing with such cases to avoid any potential medico-legal issues later.

Patients with a strangulated inguinal hernia usually present with nausea and vomiting, localized abdominal pain, abdominal distention, absolute constipation or diarrhea, per-rectal bleeding in cases of bowel ischaemia and less commonly, fever. Clinically, these patients will be in pain, dehydrated and septic looking. Prompt resuscitation is needed to reverse the physiology back to normal before the operation. Chest and abdominal radiographs can be taken to look for any evidence of bowel strangulation or perforation. Fluid resuscitation, analgesia, and antibiotics should be commenced as soon as possible upon presentation in cases suspecting bowel ischaemia. Following adequate resuscitation, the patient should be brought to the operating theater for definitive surgery.

A prospective study done by Nazir Ahmad et al. found that the common operative procedure for strangulated hernia includes Darning and Bassini repair, resection and primary anastomosis of the ileum, partial omentectomy, obliteration of inguinal canal and lastly orchidectomy [2]. The treatment strategy is usually individualized depending on the patient's presentation to the emergency department. If bowels are viable, a mesh repair is recommended. However, if there is bowel ischaemia needing bowel resection, the best would be to proceed with darning or Bassini repair.

It has always been a debate about whether to apply mesh in cases where bowel resection is done. The risk of mesh infection requiring explanation as opposed to the risk of hernia recurrence later should be taken into consideration. We have to bear in mind that mesh infection can lead to severe intrabdominal sepsis and even death has been reported in some cases. Therefore, the operating surgeon must pay attention to all these potential issues when managing strangulated hernia cases.

2. Discussions on management of strangulated hernia

Irreducible inguinal hernia can either result in incarceration or strangulation. An incarcerated inguinal hernia is a hernia in which the content has become irreducible due to a narrow opening in the abdominal wall or due to adhesions between the hernia content and the sac. Intestinal obstruction may further complicate an incarcerated hernia. Usually, an incarcerated hernia can be managed electively as opposed to strangulated hernia.

A strangulated hernia on the other hand occurs when the blood supply to the contents of the hernia is compromised. This is a surgical emergency and warrants urgent surgical attention and intervention. Patients usually present with intestinal obstruction which can lead to subsequent necrosis, ischaemia and bowel perforation of the involved bowel within the hernia sac. Clinical presentations of strangulated hernia include erythema, oedema and severe pain.

Irreducible hernia can also result in testicular damage or even atrophy secondary to pressure effects in boys [1]. Taxis or manual reduction of irreducible inguinal hernia should be avoided at all times. The reason is that what if the content reduced is part of the ischemic bowel stuck within the deep ring? The strangulation of the bowel can lead to the release of many toxins formation secondary to the injured mucosal wall. This will eventually lead to intraabdominal sepsis with significant morbidity and mortality. Therefore meticulous assessment in decision-making is warranted in dealing with such cases.

Decision-making in managing such cases should not be taken lightly as the material risk associated is high. Any delay in surgical decision-making can result in serious post-operative morbidity or even mortality [3]. **Figure 1** shows summarizes the diagnosis of strangulated hernia.

The commonly encountered problems include whether the strangulated portion of the bowel is viable and can be returned to the abdomen or whether resection has to be carried out. When the bowel is deep purple color and the sac contains a hemo-serous dark fluid, the likelihood of bowel ischemia needing bowel resection is extremely high.

There are a few ways to check for normal bowel viability which include a shining peritoneal surface, deep red in color with active peristaltic movement suggestive of normal bowel viability [3]. In short, timing is of utmost essential in the management of strangulated hernia as any delay in diagnosis and subsequent delay in operative intervention can result in high morbidity and mortality. Early diagnosis of strangulated hernia can be difficult, however, missed or late intervention can result in deadly septic complications.

Figure 2 shows the description of various methods for managing strangulated inguinal hernias. No one method is superior to the other, every surgical intervention has its pros and cons. Hence, it is imperative to note that treatment strategies should be tailored accordingly. Ultimately, the outcome of the surgery is what matters. They are many ways in dealing with strangulated hernia, based on the above-mentioned figures, it can be broadly divided into open and laparoscopic surgery. However, it

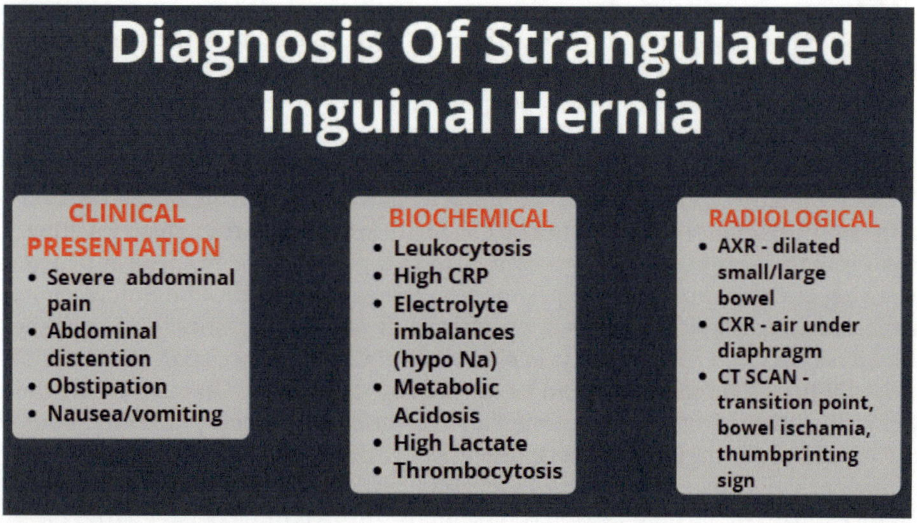

Figure 1.
Diagnosis of strangulated inguinal hernia.

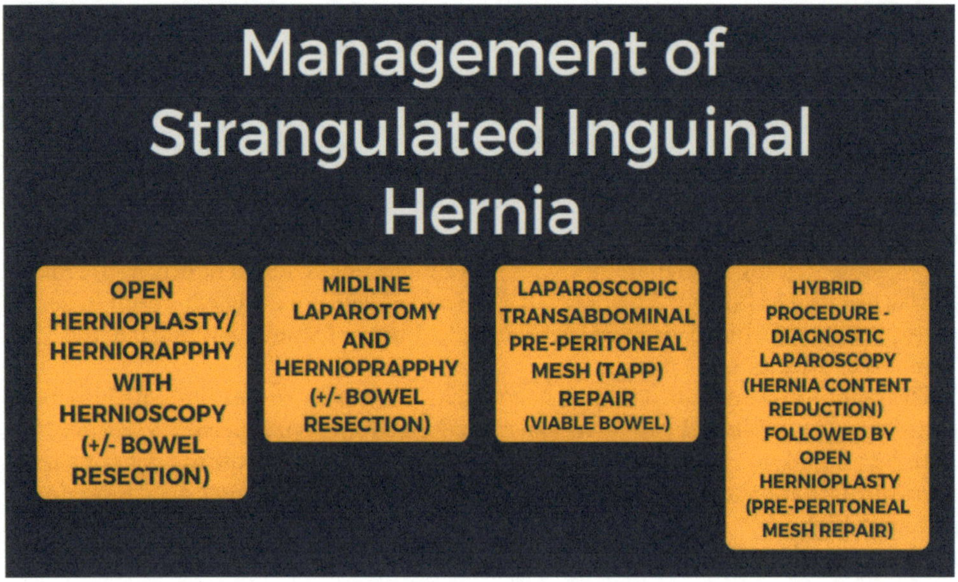

Figure 2.
Management of Strangulated Hernia.

has to be taken into consideration that laparoscopic hernia repair, especially in acute presentation with strangulation can be technically challenging. Open hernia repair closes the defects anteriorly and laparoscopic hernia repair (TAPP - transabdominal pre-peritoneal/TEP - totally extraperitoneal) closes the defects posteriorly. If the first surgery is done via open surgery, should the patient present with recurrence, a posterior approach should be advocated laparoscopically. However, if patients present under emergency as strangulated hernia, open surgery should be advocated. The role of laparoscopic hernia repair in emergency settings is debatable, depending on the availability of resources and local expertise [4].

Moving on, the following are the various available options for managing strangulated inguinal hernia. Firstly, open hernioplasty or herniorrhaphy with hernioscopy. This subset of patients includes those that can be reduced spontaneously on admission but complain of persistent pain post taxis. For this group of patients, emergency inguinal exploration can be done.

Hernioscopy is done to enable the surgeon to visualize the entire peritoneal cavity, particularly looking into any evidence of bowel ischaemia needing bowel resection and anastomosis. This technique can be challenging and requires a steep learning curve. From the hernia sac, a trocar containing a laparoscope is inserted and held in place using a stay suture, pneumoperitoneum is created, and the abdominal cavity is inspected for any evidence of bowel ischemia. If negative, the best option would be Lichtenstein mesh hernioplasty. In situations where the bowels are compromised, the feasibility of the incision should be decided by the surgeon. In cases where the bowel is dilated needing decompression and resection, midline laparotomy should be performed, and the inguinal defect closed via fascial repair.

Frequently performed techniques for fascial repair include Darning repair and Shouldice repair. In darning repair, a continuous suture is done between the conjoint tendon and the inguinal ligament without approximating the two structures.

On the other hand, in Shouldice repair, a four-layered reconstruction of the posterior inguinal region is performed, approximating conjoint tendon to transversalis fascia, transversalis fascia to the inguinal ligament and internal oblique to the inguinal ligament.

The risk of inguinal hernia recurrence following fascial repair is high. However, what remains a debate, is Lichtenstein mesh hernioplasty following bowel resection from a strangulated inguinal hernia is recommended. The risk of mesh explanation and subsequent prolonged hospital stay for sepsis secondary to mesh infection is very high. It can even result in mortality. This is assuming there is an infection of the mesh, however, if there is no risk of mesh infection, Lichtenstein mesh hernioplasty is the widely accepted surgical procedure for inguinal hernia.

Moving on to the next treatment option is laparotomy and herniorrhaphy with or without bowel resection. This subset of patients includes those with radiological, biochemical and clinical evidence of bowel ischemia. Generally, patients would have dilated bowels and distended abdomen. By performing midline laparotomy, the surgeon can easily perform bowel decompression proximally, distally or via enterotomy.

At the same time, a midline laparotomy allows closer inspection of the bowel to look for any evidence of bowel ischaemia. Proper surgical exposure facilitates surgery and improves the outcome of surgery while reducing the operating time. The inguinal defects can be closed while doing the laparotomy. However, the risk of recurrence is always there since only fascial repair is done and the patient should be well informed.

On the other hand, if no bowel resection is done, following midline laparotomy, a Lichtenstein mesh hernioplasty is strongly recommended. Another inguinal incision is usually performed once the midline laparotomy wound is closed, and Lichtenstein mesh hernioplasty is performed.

Bapurapu Raja Ram et al. published a new method called the "Window to window – one skin incision" approach. In this method, there is no division of the muscle and inguinal nerve and no ligation of the inferior epigastric artery, hence the normal anatomy is retained. Bowel resection and anastomosis are done through the same incision away from the site of the mesh repair that can be covered with a mop during operation. The incision that is used by the author is not the conventional inguinal skin crease approach, but the window-to-window – one skin incision. However, the limitation of this study is one centre and one team. Hence, it requires further multicentre study and analysis [5].

Figure 3 shows a pre-operative and intra-operative picture of a patient that presented with 3 days history of pain, progressively worsening upon presentation. Blood results revealed high lactate, leucocytosis and metabolic acidosis in blood gas. Following resuscitation, the patient was counseled for surgery and consented. Intra-operatively, noted a small bowel loop stuck at the deep inguinal ring, the bowel appeared blue and dusky with hemo-serous fluid within the hernia sac. In this case, an inguinal incision is made initially to assess for bowel viability, followed by a midline laparotomy. The Shouldice fascial repair was done for this patient.

The next treatment approach is the minimally invasive surgical (MIS) approach in managing strangulated inguinal hernia. If expertise is available, a strangulated inguinal hernia repair can be attempted laparoscopically. Laparoscopic transabdominal pre-peritoneal (TAPP) repair can be done if there is no bowel ischaemia needing bowel resection. In cases where bowel resection is needed, it can also be done laparoscopically, however, this procedure is technically challenging. Usually, these procedures are performed in high-volume hernia centres [4].

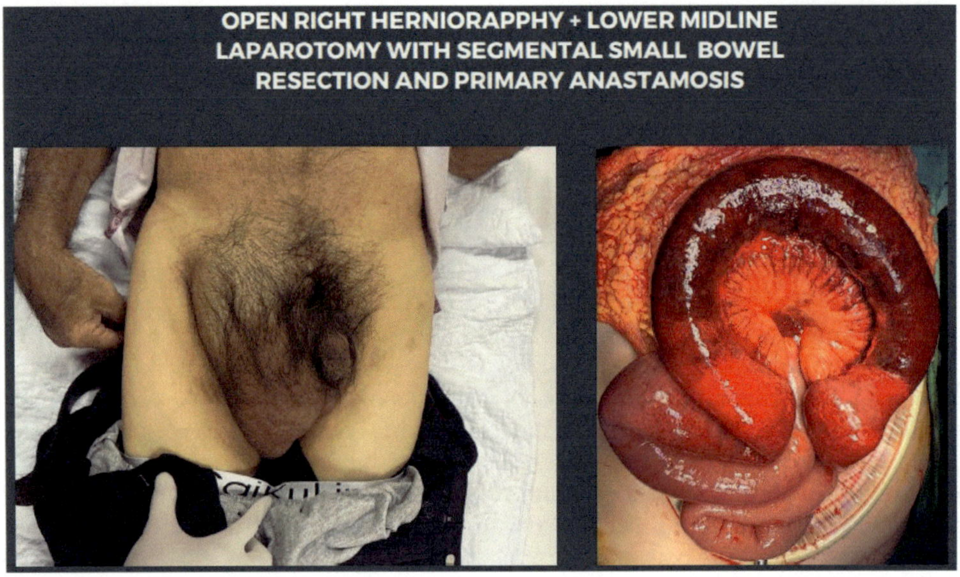

Figure 3.
Midline laparotomy, inguinal herniorrhaphy, bowel resection and primary anastomosis for strangulated inguinal hernia.

Proper patient selection is required to prevent complications later. This is because, although minimally invasive technique is advocated, we have to bear in mind that it's not without complications. However, the application of mesh especially in cases where bowel resection and anastomosis were done should be avoided as the risk of mesh infection is high in this group of patients, even though a minimally invasive technique is advocated [6].

Last but not least, a hybrid technique can be undertaken while managing strangulated inguinal hernia cases. The hernia can be reduced laparoscopically followed by Lichtenstein mesh hernioplasty in cases where there is no bowel ischaemia. If there is evidence of bowel ischaemia, following laparoscopic reduction of hernia content, bowel resection should be done, either open or laparoscopically. The principle is still the same in managing strangulated inguinal hernia. In cases where bowel resection is performed, mesh hernioplasty is not recommended. Instead, the fascial repair is preferred to prevent peritoneal protrusion through the myo-pectineal orifice.

Besides this, other pertinent issues need to be addressed when managing strangulated inguinal hernia. Among others includes, managing the co-morbidity of the patients which includes diabetes mellitus and hypertension, nutrition status, sepsis due to bowel ischemia and lastly the pain secondary to strangulated hernia itself. All these need to be addressed and patients need to be optimized medically before embarking on surgical intervention. Detailed consent-taking is indicated in managing complicated hernia cases. A detailed explanation of the complications needs to be informed to patients to avoid any potential medico-legal problems. An ideal consent for strangulated inguinal hernia cases should include open hernioplasty, keeping in view bowel resection, stoma, midline laparotomy and orchidectomy.

Next, the question about hernia repair with or without mesh or even the use of biological mesh is controversial and debatable in emergency strangulation cases.

Based on a few randomized control trials (RCTs), the usage of biological mesh for hernia repair involving large defects or recurrent hernias, especially in morbidly obese patients, is preferred [7]. There are several biological grafts available in the current market. Generally, if bowel resection is performed, herniorrhaphy is preferred rather than mesh repair as the risk of surgical site infection is high in dirty wounds, given the high recurrence rate which can be dealt with later in a more controlled environment as opposed to mesh repair that may or may not get infected. Hence, all these factors should be considered while managing strangulated inguinal hernia.

Another issue that needs to be highlighted is the occurrence of abdominal compartment syndrome following hernia repair. This subsets of patients include those with strangulated hernia with loss of domain. Assuming the hernia content can be reduced completely, the intra-abdominal pressure can be raised giving rise to abdominal compartment syndrome. If a patient presents to your clinic, then there are many ways to increase abdominal wall compliance while waiting for an elective surgery date. Among others include progressive pneumoperitoneum every week up to a few sessions and botulinum toxin injection on the anterior abdominal wall pre-operatively. Intra-operatively, to reduce the incidence of abdominal compartments, the content of the hernia can be resected to reduce the intraabdominal pressure. Post-operatively, patients at risk of abdominal compartments should be nursed in the intensive care unit and abdominal pressure can be measured constantly.

3. Conclusion

In summary, the management of strangulated inguinal hernia requires a multidisciplinary approach. Prompt diagnosis, adequate resuscitation and appropriate surgery need to be instituted soonest. Complications of bowel strangulation with regards to delayed diagnosis, misdiagnosis and delayed presentation lead to significant morbidity and even mortality. Treatment strategy should be tailored according to the patient's presentation and the best available surgical expertise.

Acknowledgements

Special thanks to Dr. Dayang Corieza Febriany, Clinical Radiologist and Medical Lecturer from the Department of Radiology, Faculty of Medicine and Health Sciences, University Malaysia Sabah for your input in radiological imaging.

Conflict of interest

No conflict of interest.

Notes

I would like to express my gratitude to my parents, wife and lecturers for their continuous support during the writing of this chapter in the hernia book.

Author details

Mohamed Arif Hameed Sultan[1*] and Dayang Corieza Febriany[2]

1 Faculty of Medicine and Health Sciences, Department of Surgery, University Malaysia Sabah, Malaysia

2 Faculty of Medicine and Health Sciences, Department of Radiology, University Malaysia Sabah, Malaysia

*Address all correspondence to: drarifhameed@ums.edu.my

References

[1] Yeap E et al. Inguinal hernia in children. Australian Journal of General Practice. 2020;**49**(1-2):38-43

[2] Ahmad N, Khan SA, Adib KJ. Management of Strangulated Inguinal Hernia. PJMHS. 2023;**8**(1):35-36

[3] MacKenzie I. Management of Strangulated Hernia. Surgical Clinics of North America. 1960;**40**:1367-1385

[4] Deeba S et al. Laparoscopic approach to incarcerated and strangulated inguinal hernia. Journal of the Society of Laparo-endoscopic Surgeons JSLS. 2009;**13**:327-331

[5] Ram BR et al. Strangulated groin hernia repair: A new approach for all. Journal of Clinical and Diagnostic Research. 2016;**10**(4):PC04-PC06

[6] Liu J et al. If laparoscopic technique can be used for treatment of acutely incarcerated/strangulated inguinal hernia? World Journal of Emergency Surgery. 2021;**16**:5. DOI: 10.1186/s13017-021-00348-1

[7] Coccoli F, Agresta F, Bassi A, et al. Italian biological prosthesis work-group (IBPWG); proposal for a decisional model in using biological prosthesis. World of Journal of Emergency Surgery. 2012;**7**(1):34. DOI: 10.1186/1749-7922-7-34

Chapter 12

Hernia Mesh Fixation

Suphakarn Techapongsatorn

Abstract

Hernia mesh fixation is an integral part of both inguinal and ventral hernia surgical repair, allowing the mesh to cover the hernia defect until the mesh-tissue fusion process is complete. There are a variety of mesh fixation methods, materials, and devices currently available. The use of mesh fixation is considered a balance between the benefit of mesh fixation or the strength of fixation to keep the mesh in place versus the adverse effect of fixing the mesh. However, there is no consensus or evidence regarding the most effective mesh fixation. This chapter will enlighten surgeons on mesh fixation, especially those who wish to implement their knowledge of hernia management.

Keywords: mesh fixation, inguinal hernia, ventral hernia, tack, suture, glue, self-gripping mesh

1. Introduction

Following the recent guideline, mesh-based hernia repair is considered the standard treatment for both inguinal hernias [1–5] and ventral hernia [4, 6, 7]. Mesh is used to reinforce the inguinal floor and can be approached using both open and laparoscopic techniques. Transabdominal preperitoneal repair (TAPP) and totally extraperitoneal repair (TEP) are commonly utilized for laparoscopic approaches, whereas Lichtenstein's hernia repair is typically utilized for an open approach. For the ventral hernia or incisional hernia, mesh is used to reinforce the hernia defect through the open or laparoscopic approach.

The purpose of the mesh used is to cover the hernia defect; subsequently, a mesh-tissue integration process will be developed. Mesh fixation is a technique used to retain the mesh in position until the mesh-tissue integration process is complete or about 2–3 weeks after surgery [8]. Presently, the mesh fixation methods are utilized in clinical practice and can be categorized as no mesh fixation or mesh fixation with a different kind of material and device such as suture, tacker, glue, or self-gripping mesh, which have different uses for both inguinal and ventral hernias. Mesh fixation is useful for keeping the mesh in position and closing the hernia defect; however, it may have adverse effects, including local tissue trauma [9], nerve injury due to entrapment [10], erosion [11], meshoma formation [12, 13], tack hernias [14], chronic pain [12, 15, 16], and infection [17].

In this chapter, we will provide updated evidence regarding various mesh fixation methods, materials, and devices for inguinal and ventral hernia repair.

2. Technique for keeping mesh in place

In clinical practice, the techniques for keeping mesh in place can be categorized as no mesh fixation and mesh fixation. No mesh fixation is the method used for laparoscopic inguinal hernias, as reported both in TEP [18–20] and TAPP [21–23]. At the end of the surgical procedure, expelling the air allows the peritoneum to attach to the mesh, while intra-abdominal pressure causes the extraperitoneal space to naturally close and constrict, allowing the mesh to be fixed in position. However, mesh fixation is still required in ventral hernia repair.

The current evidence from a recent meta-analysis comparing no mesh fixation versus mesh fixation demonstrated that no mesh fixation in laparoscopic inguinal hernia repair does not increase the risk of mesh displacement contributing to hernia recurrence [24–26], while reducing chronic groin pain and operative time is advantageous [24, 26].

However, recent guidelines for inguinal hernia repair [1, 5] still recommend mesh fixations in patients with large direct hernias (M3-EHS classification).

3. Mesh fixation methods

There is no distinct classification of mesh fixation methods. The terms "permanent versus non-permanent fixation" and "atraumatic fixation" are used in the most recent guideline [1]. However, this chapter will classify mesh fixation methods as either penetrating or non-penetrating (atraumatic) because the term can be used to designate mesh fixation mechanisms.

3.1 Penetrating mesh fixation

Penetrating mesh fixation is a method for attaching mesh to local tissue by permeating it. It includes sutures and tack. There are two types of tacks: permanent and absorbable.

3.1.1 Suture

The original Lichtenstein's inguinal hernia repair described used non-absorbable monofilament sutures for fixing mesh [27]. However, the study using

Name	Type	Loss of tensile strength	Complete absorption	Tissue reactivity
Polydioxanone (PDS)	Delayed-absorbable monofilament	Slow (45% by 3 weeks)	180 days	Minimal
Polyglyconate (Maxon)	Delayed-absorbable monofilament	Slow (31% by 6 weeks)	180 days	Minimal
Nylon (Ethilon, Dermalon)	Non-absorbable monofilament	30% at 2 years	NA	Minimal
Polybutester (Novafil)	Non-absorbable monofilament	Negligible	NA	Minimal
Polypropylene (Prolene)	Non-absorbable monofilament	Negligible	NA	Minimal

Table 1.
The characteristic of a common hernia repair suture.

delayed-absorbable monofilament sutures demonstrated a decreasing risk of postoperative inguinal pain and paresthesia (**Table 1**), [28].

3.1.2 Tack

Tack is a synthetic mesh fixation that can be subdivided by the materials into non-absorbable and absorbable tacks, and now the design of the launcher can be subdivided into an articulating and a non-articulating applier (**Table 2**).

Name	Articulation tip	Materials	Absorbable	Length (mm)	Mechanism
ProTack™	No	Titanium	No	5	Helical 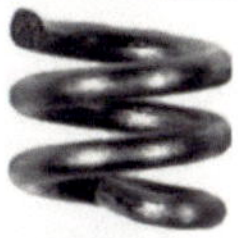
PermaFix™	No	Molded polymer	No	5	Screw 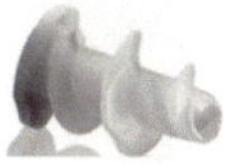
CapSure™	No	Stainless steel/PEEK	No	3.2	Helical 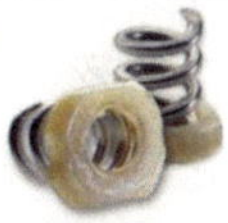
Securestrap™	No	PLG	Yes	7.2	Strap 
AbsorbaTack™	No	PGLA	Yes	5.1	Screw 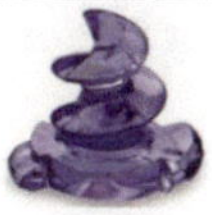
SorbaFix™	No	PLA	Yes	6	Screw 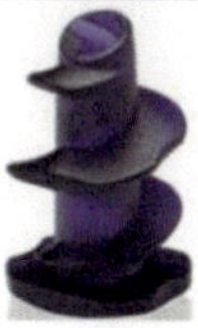
PermaSorb®	No	PLA	Yes	6.4	Screw 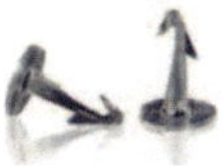
iMesh	Yes	NA	Yes	NA	Helical 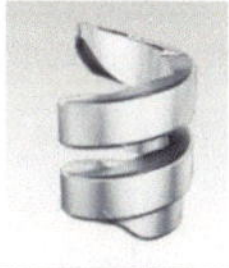
ReliaTack™	Yes	PGLA	Yes	5.1–7	Screw 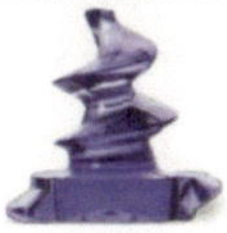

PEEK: polyetheretherketone, PLG: polydioxanone and l(−)-lactide/glycolide copolymer, PGLA: poly(glycolide-co-l-lactide), PLA: poly(d,l)-lactide.

Table 2.
The characteristic of a tacker.

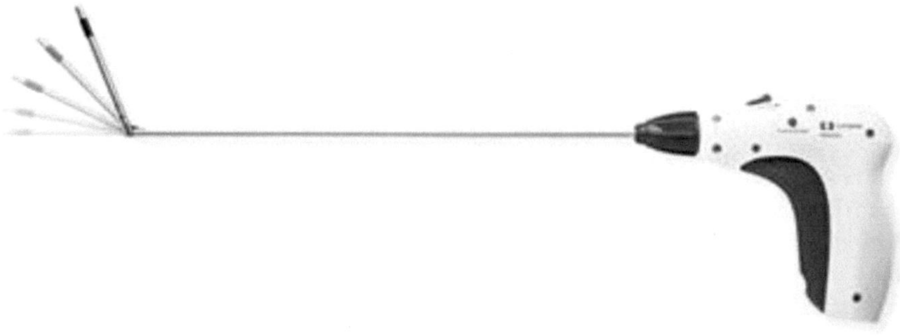

Figure 1.
Articulating mesh fixation device.

There are two varieties of tacker applicator shafts: straight and articulating (**Figure 1**). An articulating applicator has a significant benefit, as it allows the fired tacker to be at a perpendicular angle to the attachment point, resulting in a tighter fixation. This feature makes it more suitable for ventral hernias rather than inguinal hernias.

3.2 Non-penetrating (atraumatic) mesh fixation

3.2.1 Glue

Glue has been used for mesh fixation in both open and laparoscopic approaches, as it does not injure the tissue. It can be divided into fibrin glue and synthetic glue.

3.2.1.1 Fibrin glue

Fibrin glue, also known as Tisseel® or Tissucol® (Baxter Healthcare) and Evicel® (Ethicon), is a biological hemostatic agent comprised of fibrinogen and thrombin. Then activated by calcium chloride when it is added, the fibrin glue transforms into a fibrin fiber matrix, and the reaction may require 3 min to complete [29]. This not only affects hemostasis but also has strength enough to fix the mesh.

3.2.1.2 Synthetic glue

The synthetic adhesive cyanoacrylate glue is composed of n-butyl-cyanoacrylate. Histoacryl® (B-Braun), LiquiBand Fix8 (Advanced Medical Solutions), and Glubran 2® (GEM) are utilized, when available.

Polymerization occurs promptly in the presence of ionic substances like water, blood, or tissue fluids. There is a requirement for 30–45 s. The polymerized form shows excellent tensile strength and is highly effective for securing mesh.

3.2.2 Self-gripping mesh

Self-gripping mesh, ProGrip™, is a polyester monofilament mesh with a polylactic acid (PLA) microgrip or microhook. The portion of a microgrip can secure local tissue without requiring additional fixation.

4. Clinical application and evidence

4.1 Inguinal hernia

4.1.1 Open inguinal hernia repair

Open inguinal hernia repair has a mesh fixation method that involves suturing with non-absorbable monofilament sutures or the original Lichtenstein's hernia repair. While glue, self-gripping mesh, and suturing with absorbable monofilament sutures were used as alternative methods.

The effects of absorbable versus non-absorbable monofilament suture for open inguinal hernia mesh fixation were examined in a comparative study. The study evaluated the impact of delayed absorbable monofilament suture, Polyglecaprone (2-0), compared to non-absorbable monofilament suture, Polypropylene (2-0). The results indicated that the group treated with delayed absorbable sutures experienced significantly less pain after 6 months [28]. However, it is important to note that these findings were not mentioned in the recent guidelines [1].

The comparison between glue and non-absorbable monofilament suture for open inguinal hernia mesh fixation has been investigated in various study designs, such as randomized controlled trials, systematic reviews, meta-analyses [30–32], and umbrella reviews [33]. The findings consistently indicate that glue is superior to non-absorbable monofilament suture in reducing short- and medium-term postoperative pain, as well as chronic groin pain [33].

A comparison between self-gripping mesh and non-absorbable monofilament suture for open inguinal hernia mesh fixation revealed that self-gripping mesh resulted in a reduction in operative time. However, there was no significant difference observed in terms of recurrence prevention or postoperative pain [31, 33–35].

4.1.2 Laparoscopic inguinal hernia repair

The conventional method for mesh fixation in laparoscopic inguinal hernia repair involves the use of titanium or metallic tacks. However, alternative mesh fixation methods, such as glue, self-gripping mesh, and non-absorbable tacks, have been reported in clinical practice.

A study reported that a new design for the tacker mesh fixation device includes an articulation feature, allowing surgeons to adjust the angle of the device for proper

Outcome	Suggestive of mesh fixation
Hernia recurrence prevention	All techniques
Chronic groin pain prevention	Glue
Shortening of operating time	Glue, SGM
Early return to daily activities	Glue
Postoperative complication prevention	All techniques

SGM, self-gripping mesh.

Table 3.
The summarized evidence for inguinal hernia mesh fixation [33].

mesh fixation. Adjusting the angle to align with the mesh fixation point results in a better average fixation force compared to a non-articulated mesh fixation device [36].

In an *in vitro* study, it was discovered that fibrin glue provided stronger mesh fixation compared to absorbable tacks. The study involved placing the mesh on a stake and measuring the force required to detach the mesh from the stake. The applied force for the tacks was found to be 6.40 ± 1.50 N, while for the glue, it was 15.34 ± 3.93 N, indicating a significant difference between the two methods [37].

Finally, the evidence suggests that glue is beneficial compared to other methods in terms of reducing postoperative pain, but there is no significant difference observed in hernia recurrence (**Table 3**) [33, 35, 38].

4.2 Ventral hernia

The mesh fixation methods used for primary and incisional ventral hernias are similar to those employed for inguinal hernias. These methods include sutures, non-absorbable and absorbable tacks, self-gripping mesh (for open ventral hernias only), and glue. Evidence from several systematic reviews and meta-analyses indicates that there are no significant differences among these methods in terms of outcomes such as hernia recurrence and chronic pain. Therefore, the choice of method may depend on the surgeon's expertise [39–43].

5. Conclusions

The available mesh fixation techniques include sutures, tacks, self-gripping mesh, and tissue adhesive, which can be applied both openly and laparoscopically. There is no consensus for this part; the selection to be used depends on the surgeon. Mesh fixation techniques have been demonstrated to be equally safe in terms of recurrence; however, tissue adhesives are associated with a lower incidence of chronic pain.

Conflict of interest

The authors declare no conflict of interest.

Author details

Suphakarn Techapongsatorn
Faculty of Medicine Vajira Hospital, Department of Surgery, Navamindradhiraj University, Bangkok, Thailand

*Address all correspondence to: suphakarn@nmu.ac.th

References

[1] International guidelines for groin hernia management. Hernia. 2018;**22**(1):1-165

[2] Simons MP, Aufenacker T, Bay-Nielsen M, Bouillot JL, Campanelli G, Conze J, et al. European Hernia Society guidelines on the treatment of inguinal hernia in adult patients. Hernia. 2009;**13**(4):343-403

[3] Bittner R, Bain K, Bansal VK, Berrevoet F, Bingener-Casey J, Chen D, et al. Update of guidelines for laparoscopic treatment of ventral and incisional abdominal wall hernias (International Endohernia Society (IEHS))-Part A. Surgical Endoscopy. 2019;**33**(10):3069-3139

[4] Bittner R, Bain K, Bansal VK, Berrevoet F, Bingener-Casey J, Chen D, et al. Update of guidelines for laparoscopic treatment of ventral and incisional abdominal wall hernias (International Endohernia Society (IEHS)): Part B. Surgical Endoscopy. 2019;**33**(11):3511-3549

[5] Bittner R, Montgomery MA, Arregui E, Bansal V, Bingener J, Bisgaard T, et al. Update of guidelines on laparoscopic (TAPP) and endoscopic (TEP) treatment of inguinal hernia (International Endohernia Society). Surgical Endoscopy. 2015;**29**(2):289-321

[6] Henriksen NA, Montgomery A, Kaufmann R, Berrevoet F, East B, Fischer J, et al. Guidelines for treatment of umbilical and epigastric hernias from the European Hernia Society and Americas Hernia Society. The British Journal of Surgery. 2020;**107**(3):171-190

[7] Earle D, Roth JS, Saber A, Haggerty S, Bradley JF, Fanelli R, et al. SAGES guidelines for laparoscopic ventral hernia repair. Surgical Endoscopy. 2016;**30**:3163-3183

[8] Morena B, Alberto S, Luca Andrea F, Francesco G, Marco C. Mesh fixation methods in groin hernia surgery. In: Angelo G, editor. Techniques and Innovation in Hernia Surgery. Rijeka: IntechOpen; 2019 Ch. 7

[9] Delikoukos S, Fafoulakis F, Christodoulidis G, Theodoropoulos T, Hatzitheofilou C. Re-operation due to severe late-onset persisting groin pain following anterior inguinal hernia repair with mesh. Hernia. 2008;**12**(6):593-595

[10] Gossetti F, D'Amore L, Annesi E, Bruzzone P, Bambi L, Grimaldi MR, et al. Mesh-related visceral complications following inguinal hernia repair: An emerging topic. Hernia. 2019;**23**(4):699-708

[11] Liu W-Z, Qian J-H, Shen Z-J, Yang B-B, Cheng Y. Fixing tacks induced bladder erosion and recurrent stones following laparoscopic inguinal hernia repair: A case report. BMC Surgery. 2020;**20**(1):161

[12] Amid PK. Radiologic images of meshoma: A new phenomenon causing chronic pain after prosthetic repair of abdominal wall hernias. Archives of Surgery. 2004;**139**(12):1297-1298

[13] Wu JF, Chen J, Hong F. Intestinal erosion caused by meshoma displacement: A case report. World Journal of Gastrointestinal Surgery. 2023;**15**(1):114-120

[14] LeBlanc KA. Tack hernia: A new entity. JSLS : Journal of the Society of Laparoendoscopic Surgeons. 2003;**7**(4):383-387

[15] Nguyen DK, Amid PK, Chen DC. Groin pain after inguinal hernia repair. Advances in Surgery. 2016;**50**(1):203-220

[16] Nikkolo C, Lepner U. Chronic pain after open inguinal hernia repair. Postgraduate Medicine. 2016;**128**(1):69-75

[17] Johanet H, Contival N. Mesh infection after inguinal hernia mesh repair. Journal of Visceral Surgery. 2011;**148**(5):e392-e394

[18] Claus CMP, Rocha GM, Campos ACL, Paulin JAN, Coelho JCU. Mesh displacement after bilateral inguinal hernia repair with no fixation. JSLS : Journal of the Society of Laparoendoscopic Surgeons. 2017;**21**(3)

[19] Claus CM, Rocha GM, Campos AC, Bonin EA, Dimbarre D, Loureiro MP, et al. Prospective, randomized and controlled study of mesh displacement after laparoscopic inguinal repair: Fixation versus no fixation of mesh. Surgical Endoscopy. 2016;**30**(3):1134-1140

[20] Akturk R, Serinsoz S. Comparing laparoscopic totally extraperitoneal inguinal hernia repair with and without mesh fixation. Annali Italiani di Chirurgia. 2022;**92**:355-362

[21] Azevedo MA, Oliveira GBT, Malheiros CA, Roll S. Are there differences in chronic pain after laparoscopic inguinal hernia repair using the transabdominal technique comparing with fixation of the mesh with staples, with glue or without fixation? A clinical randomized, double-blind trial. Arquivos Brasileiros de Cirurgia Digestiva. 2022;**35**:e1670

[22] Qureshi S, Ghazanfar S, Leghari AA, Zubair M, Chisti S, Memon F, et al. A comparative follow up study of transabdominal preperitoneal mesh repair in inguinal hernias with or without mesh fixation. Journal of the Pakistan Medical Association. 2021;**71**(1(a)):28-30

[23] Mayer F, Niebuhr H, Lechner M, Dinnewitzer A, Köhler G, Hukauf M, et al. When is mesh fixation in TAPP-repair of primary inguinal hernia repair necessary? The register-based analysis of 11,230 cases. Surgical Endoscopy. 2016;**30**(10):4363-4371

[24] Eltair M, Hajibandeh S, Hajibandeh S, Balakrishnan S, Alyamani A, Radoi D, et al. Meta-analysis of laparoscopic groin hernia repair with or without mesh fixation. International Journal of Surgery. 2019;**71**:190-199

[25] Sajid MS, Ladwa N, Kalra L, Hutson K, Sains P, Baig MK. A meta-analysis examining the use of tacker fixation versus no-fixation of mesh in laparoscopic inguinal hernia repair. International Journal of Surgery. 2012;**10**(5):224-231

[26] Ayyaz M, Farooka MW, Malik AA, Khan A, Mansoor R, Toor AA, et al. Mesh fixation vs. non-fixation in total extra peritoneal mesh hernioplasty. The Journal of the Pakistan Medical Association. 2015;**65**(3):270-272

[27] Amid PK, Shulman AG, Lichtenstein IL. The Lichtenstein open "tension-free" mesh repair of inguinal Hernias. Surgery Today. 1995;**25**(7):619-625

[28] Subhadip S. A comparative study of mesh fixation with non-absorbable versus delayed-absorbable monofilament suture in Lichtenstein tension-free hernioplasty in a medical college. Asian Journal of Medical Sciences. 2022;**13**(7):203-207

[29] Campanelli G, Pascual MH, Hoeferlin A, Rosenberg J, Champault G,

Kingsnorth A, et al. Randomized, controlled, blinded trial of Tisseel/Tissucol for mesh fixation in patients undergoing Lichtenstein technique for primary inguinal hernia repair: Results of the TIMELI trial. Annals of Surgery. 2012;**255**(4):650-657

[30] Lin H, Zhuang Z, Ma T, Sun X, Huang X, Li Y. A meta-analysis of randomized control trials assessing mesh fixation with glue versus suture in Lichtenstein inguinal hernia repair. Medicine (Baltimore). 2018;**97**(14):e0227

[31] Rausa E, Asti E, Kelly ME, Aiolfi A, Lovece A, Bonitta G, et al. Open inguinal hernia repair: A network meta-analysis comparing self-gripping mesh, suture fixation, and glue fixation. World Journal of Surgery. 2019;**43**(2):447-456

[32] Ladwa N, Sajid MS, Sains P, Baig MK. Suture mesh fixation versus glue mesh fixation in open inguinal hernia repair: A systematic review and meta-analysis. International Journal of Surgery. 2013;**11**(2):128-135

[33] Techapongsatorn S, Tansawet A, Pattanaprateep O, Attia J, McKay GJ, Thakkinstian A. Mesh-fixation technique for inguinal hernia repair: Umbrella review. BJS Open. 2022;**6**(4)

[34] Sajid MS, Farag S, Singh KK, Miles WF. Systematic review and meta-analysis of published randomized controlled trials comparing the role of self-gripping mesh against suture mesh fixation in patients undergoing open inguinal hernia repair. Updates in Surgery. 2014;**66**(3):189-196

[35] Techapongsatorn S, Tansawet A, Pattanaprateep O, Attia J, McKay GJ, Thakkinstian A. Cost-effectiveness analysis of mesh fixation techniques for laparoscopic and open inguinal hernia surgeries. BMC Health Services Research. 2022;**22**(1):1125

[36] Elazary R, Kedar A, Abu-Gazala M, Mintz Y. Comparing laparoscopic mesh fixation strength between articulated and non-articulated tack devices. Minimally Invasive Therapy & Allied Technologies. 2013;**22**(5):288-290

[37] Hamilton D, Tan J, Chandraratna H. Fibrin glue provides stronger mesh fixation than tacks: An in-vitro study. Surgery and Rehabilitation. 2018;**2**. DOI: 10.15761/SRJ.1000150

[38] Techapongsatorn S, Tansawet A, Kasetsermwiriya W, McEvoy M, Attia J, Wilasrusmee C, et al. Mesh fixation technique in totally extraperitoneal inguinal hernia repair - A network meta-analysis. The Surgeon. 2019;**17**(4):215-224

[39] Sajid MS, Parampalli U, McFall MR. A meta-analysis comparing tacker mesh fixation with suture mesh fixation in laparoscopic incisional and ventral hernia repair. Hernia. 2013;**17**(2):159-166

[40] Mathes T, Prediger B, Walgenbach M, Siegel R. Mesh fixation techniques in primary ventral or incisional hernia repair. Cochrane Database of Systematic Reviews. 2021;**5**(5):Cd011563

[41] Baker JJ, Öberg S, Andresen K, Klausen TW, Rosenberg J. Systematic review and network meta-analysis of methods of mesh fixation during laparoscopic ventral hernia repair. The British Journal of Surgery. 2018;**105**(1):37-47

[42] Khan RMA, Bughio M, Ali B, Hajibandeh S, Hajibandeh S. Absorbable versus non-absorbable tacks for mesh fixation in laparoscopic ventral hernia repair: A systematic review and

meta-analysis. International Journal of Surgery. 2018;**53**:184-192

[43] Reynvoet E, Deschepper E, Rogiers X, Troisi R, Berrevoet F. Laparoscopic ventral hernia repair: Is there an optimal mesh fixation technique? A systematic review. Langenbeck's Archives of Surgery. 2014;**399**(1):55-63

Chapter 13

Advances in Hernia Management in Plastic Surgery

Eren Tuncer, Fatih Cınar and Percin Karakol

Abstract

Hernias represent a common surgical concern that can significantly impact patients' quality of life. In the field of plastic surgery, hernias have garnered attention due to their association with abdominal wall weakness and the potential implications for esthetic procedures such as abdominoplasty. This abstract provides an overview of the latest updates in hernia management within the context of plastic surgery.

Keywords: hernia, abdominal wall weakness, abdominoplasty, hernia repair techniques, mesh reinforcement

1. Introduction

Hernias, though commonly associated with general surgery, have emerged as a pivotal concern within the realm of plastic surgery. The pursuit of beauty, body contouring, and esthetic excellence often leads patients to consider procedures like abdominoplasty (commonly known as a tummy tuck). However, the success and safety of these esthetic surgeries are intricately intertwined with the state of the abdominal wall, which can be compromised by the presence of hernias.

In this chapter, we embark on an illuminating journey into the evolving landscape of hernia management, exploring recent advancements, cutting-edge techniques, and critical considerations that have the power to redefine patient outcomes in the context of plastic surgery.

2. Understanding hernias and their implications

Before delving into the latest developments, it's crucial to understand the nature of hernias and their implications. Hernias manifest as the protrusion of organs or tissues through weakened areas in the abdominal wall. While they may vary in location and presentation, common types include inguinal, femoral, umbilical, incisional, and ventral hernias [1]. These vulnerabilities in the abdominal wall are often attributed to factors such as pregnancy, the relentless march of time, obesity, or the consequences of prior surgical interventions. It is within this backdrop that hernias emerge as critical players in the intricate dance of plastic surgery.

2.1 Hernia types and characteristics

Inguinal hernias: Inguinal hernias, the most common type, occur in the groin area. They can be further classified as direct or indirect, depending on their anatomical location. Understanding the specific type and characteristics of inguinal hernias is essential for accurate diagnosis and treatment planning.

Femoral hernias: These hernias are less common but tend to occur more frequently in women. They protrude through the femoral canal, often presenting as a painful lump in the upper thigh.

Umbilical hernias: Umbilical hernias manifest near the navel and are commonly observed in infants. However, they can persist into adulthood, especially in cases of weakened abdominal walls.

Incisional and ventral hernias: Incisional hernias arise at the site of a previous surgical incision, while ventral hernias occur elsewhere on the anterior abdominal wall. Both types are closely associated with prior surgeries and necessitate a tailored approach to repair.

2.2 Factors leading to abdominal wall weakness

The abdominal wall serves as a protective barrier for the abdominal cavity. It comprises multiple layers of muscle and fascia, and its integrity can be compromised by various factors:

1. *Pregnancy*: The stretching of abdominal muscles during pregnancy can weaken the abdominal wall, predisposing individuals to hernias.

2. *Aging*: As we age, our muscles and connective tissues naturally lose some of their strength and elasticity, making hernias more likely.

3. *Obesity*: Excess body weight can exert pressure on the abdominal wall, increasing the risk of hernia formation.

4. *Previous surgeries*: Surgical incisions can weaken the abdominal wall, especially if not adequately closed or if there are complications during the healing process.

3. Hernias and esthetic surgery implications

In the context of plastic surgery, hernias become a significant consideration, particularly for procedures like abdominoplasty (tummy tuck). The success of these esthetic surgeries relies on the integrity of the abdominal wall. A compromised abdominal wall can impact both the functional and cosmetic outcomes of the procedure [2].

Understanding the types, causes, and implications of hernias lays the foundation for exploring the advancements and techniques that have reshaped hernia management within the field of plastic surgery. In the sections that follow, we will delve into the latest innovations in hernia repair techniques, mesh materials, combined procedures, recurrence prevention, diagnostic advances, and the promising future of hernia management.

4. Advancements in hernia repair techniques

In recent years, a wave of technological innovation and medical advancements has transformed the approach to hernia repair. Gone are the days of one-size-fits-all solutions; today's surgeons are equipped with a diverse toolkit to address hernias comprehensively. This toolkit includes traditional open repair methods, laparoscopic techniques that navigate through small incisions with the aid of cameras, and the exciting realm of minimally invasive surgery, bolstered by robotic-assisted procedures. Each of these techniques carries its unique advantages, from reduced scarring to expedited recovery, promising not only functional restoration but also improved cosmetic outcomes [3].

4.1 Traditional open repairs

Traditional open repair techniques involve making an incision near the hernia site to access and repair the weakened abdominal wall. While these methods remain effective for many cases, they often result in larger scars and longer recovery times. They continue to play a significant role, particularly in complex hernia cases where direct visualization and access are essential.

Open repairs may involve techniques such as the Shouldice repair for inguinal hernias or the Rives-Stoppa repair for ventral hernias. These procedures, performed by experienced surgeons, offer excellent outcomes with a strong focus on reinforcing the abdominal wall.

4.2 Laparoscopic techniques

Laparoscopic hernia repair represents a significant advancement in surgical approaches. This minimally invasive technique involves making small incisions through which specialized instruments and a camera are inserted. The camera provides surgeons with a magnified view of the surgical site, enhancing precision. This approach results in smaller scars, less postoperative pain, and a quicker return to daily activities.

One of the most widely adopted laparoscopic techniques for hernia repair is the totally extraperitoneal (TEP) approach for inguinal hernias. In this procedure, surgeons access the hernia from behind the abdominal wall, reducing the risk of injury to abdominal organs. The transabdominal preperitoneal (TAPP) approach is another laparoscopic option, providing a different perspective for surgeons to repair hernias safely.

4.3 Robotic-assisted surgery

Building on the advantages of laparoscopy, robotic-assisted surgery introduces the use of robotic arms controlled by the surgeon. This approach offers increased precision and control during the repair. Surgeons can manipulate the robotic arms with exceptional dexterity, allowing for complex maneuvers and suturing, even in tight spaces. Robotic-assisted surgery is gaining popularity in hernia repair due to its potential for improved outcomes.

The da Vinci Surgical System is one of the most well-known platforms for robotic-assisted hernia repair. It offers enhanced 3D visualization, tremor reduction, and a high degree of articulation, allowing surgeons to perform intricate tasks with greater ease. Patients benefit from smaller incisions, reduced pain, and faster recovery.

5. Mesh materials and techniques

Central to contemporary hernia management is the judicious use of mesh reinforcement. This critical component bolsters the weakened abdominal wall, offering the promise of long-term stability. Advances in mesh technology have ushered in a new era, with options ranging from synthetic meshes, typically composed of polypropylene or polyester, to biologic meshes derived from human or animal tissues [4]. The interplay between mesh materials and fixation techniques, including sutures and tackers, is a dynamic field where customization reigns supreme. It is this delicate balance that ensures the security of the repair while minimizing the risk of recurrence [5].

5.1 Synthetic meshes

Synthetic mesh materials, often made of polypropylene or polyester, have been a cornerstone of hernia repair for years. These meshes are known for their strength, durability, and ability to provide long-term reinforcement to the abdominal wall. They are available in various forms, including sheets, patches, and three-dimensional structures designed to fit specific hernia types.

Polypropylene meshes, such as the Marlex mesh, are widely used due to their excellent biocompatibility. They provoke minimal inflammatory responses and are suitable for most hernia repairs. Polyester meshes offer flexibility and are often chosen for their resistance to infection and tissue adhesion.

5.2 Biologic meshes

Biologic meshes represent a newer frontier in hernia repair. These meshes are derived from human or animal tissues, such as skin or intestines. Biologic meshes offer the advantage of promoting tissue ingrowth and integration, making them particularly suitable for complex hernia cases or in patients with a higher risk of infection. They are known for their reduced inflammatory responses and the potential to remodel over time.

Biologic meshes are often used in contaminated surgical fields, where the risk of infection is higher. They provide a scaffold for the patient's tissue to grow into, eventually incorporating the mesh into the body.

5.3 Mesh fixation techniques

The successful integration of mesh into the abdominal wall relies on effective fixation techniques. Surgeons employ a variety of methods tailored to each patient and hernia type. These techniques aim to provide long-term stability and reduce the risk of recurrence.

Sutures: Traditional sutures are used to secure the mesh in place. Surgeons carefully place sutures around the edges of the mesh and anchor them to the surrounding tissue. This technique provides a strong and reliable fixation.

Tackers: Tackers, or surgical staples, are another commonly used method for mesh fixation. They are applied through laparoscopic or open approaches to secure the mesh firmly in position. Tackers are known for their speed and ease of use.

Glues and sealants: Some surgeons use adhesive agents to bond the mesh to the abdominal wall. These materials can be applied during minimally invasive procedures to enhance mesh fixation. Adhesive agents offer a flexible and tissue-friendly option for mesh attachment.

Understanding these advancements in hernia repair techniques and mesh materials sets the stage for exploring combined procedures, recurrence prevention, diagnostic advances, and the future of hernia management within the context of plastic surgery. These developments hold the promise of enhancing patient outcomes and reshaping the field of plastic surgery.

6. Combined procedures: Hernia repair and esthetic surgery

The integration of function and esthetics represents a hallmark of modern plastic surgery. Patients who seek both hernia repair and cosmetic enhancements, often in the form of abdominoplasty (commonly referred to as a tummy tuck), stand at the crossroads of surgical innovation. This convergence of medical expertise presents a unique opportunity for patients to address both functional restoration and esthetic aspirations simultaneously.

6.1 Surgical planning for combined procedures

Opting for a combined hernia repair and abdominoplasty procedure necessitates meticulous surgical planning. Several key factors come into play during this crucial phase:

- *Extent of the hernia*: A comprehensive assessment of the size, location, and severity of the hernia is paramount. This evaluation informs the surgical strategy and the degree of reinforcement required to restore abdominal wall integrity.

- *Excess skin and fat*: In the context of abdominoplasty, the presence of excess skin and fat is a pivotal consideration. Surgeons must precisely determine the amount of tissue to be removed or reshaped to achieve the desired esthetic outcome while ensuring functional integrity.

- *Patient's overall health*: The patient's general health and medical history play a pivotal role in determining their suitability for combined procedures. It's essential to assess any underlying medical conditions or contraindications that might affect the surgical approach.

- *Hernia type*: Different hernia types may necessitate distinct surgical approaches. Ventral hernias, for example, often involve a larger abdominal wall defect and require specific techniques compared to inguinal or umbilical hernias.

- *Surgical expertise*: A coordinated approach involving plastic surgeons and hernia specialists is essential for optimizing outcomes. Plastic surgeons bring expertise in body contouring and esthetic enhancements, while hernia specialists focus on restoring abdominal wall integrity. This collaboration ensures that both the functional and esthetic aspects of the procedure are addressed competently.

6.2 Comprehensive care and optimized outcomes

Combined hernia repair and esthetic surgery offer patients the advantage of addressing multiple concerns in a single operation. This approach not only streamlines recovery but also yields synergistic benefits. A well-executed combined procedure can result in a stronger abdominal wall, reduced scarring, and enhanced cosmetic results.

Patients undergoing combined procedures often experience functional improvements alongside their esthetic transformations. The restoration of abdominal wall integrity not only alleviates discomfort but also contributes to a profound sense of physical well-being. This holistic approach to patient care exemplifies the evolving landscape of plastic surgery, where surgical innovation continues to enrich the lives of patients by integrating form and function seamlessly.

7. Recurrence prevention and management

Despite the promise of hernia repair surgeries, the specter of recurrence remains a legitimate concern. Modern approaches to hernia management are dedicated to mitigating this risk through a combination of innovative techniques, materials, and meticulous surgical strategies [6].

7.1 Risk of hernia recurrence

Hernia recurrence occurs when the herniated tissue re-protrudes through the repaired area, often necessitating further surgical intervention. Several factors contribute to the risk of recurrence:

- *Inadequate mesh integration*: Insufficient tissue ingrowth into the mesh can compromise the strength of the repair, increasing the risk of recurrence.

- *Tissue tension*: Excessive tension on the abdominal wall or inadequate reinforcement can strain the repair site, leading to recurrence.

- *Infection and inflammation*: Infections or chronic inflammation can interfere with the healing process, undermining the repair's long-term success.

7.2 Advances in recurrence prevention

To reduce the risk of recurrence, mesh reinforcement has become a standard practice in hernia repair. Advances in mesh technology have led to the development of lightweight, large-pore meshes that foster tissue integration while minimizing foreign body reactions.

Modern meshes, such as expanded polytetrafluoroethylene (ePTFE) meshes, offer a balance between strength and tissue-friendliness. They facilitate tissue ingrowth while resisting adhesion to the abdominal organs. These materials have demonstrated efficacy in reducing the risk of recurrence, especially in complex hernia cases where the likelihood of strain on the repair site is higher.

7.3 Meticulous surgical techniques

Surgeons employ meticulous surgical techniques to ensure proper mesh placement and secure fixation. This includes careful inspection of the abdominal wall, tension-free mesh positioning, and precise suturing or tacking to hold the mesh in place. Attention to detail during surgery is paramount in reducing the risk of recurrence.

7.4 Addressing patient-specific risk factors

Hernia recurrence prevention extends beyond surgical techniques. Surgeons work closely with patients to identify and address modifiable risk factors that could compromise the repair. These may include:

- *Obesity*: Patients are encouraged to pursue weight management strategies to reduce excess abdominal pressure, a significant risk factor for hernia recurrence.

- *Smoking cessation*: Smoking cessation programs help patients quit smoking, as smoking can impair tissue healing and increase the risk of complications.

- *Chronic cough management*: Patients with chronic cough are evaluated and treated to reduce strain on the abdominal wall, which can increase the likelihood of recurrence.

- *Infection control*: Prophylactic measures are taken to minimize the risk of surgical site infections, which can disrupt the healing process and potentially lead to recurrence.

Incorporating these strategies into the overall care plan significantly enhances the likelihood of a successful hernia repair with a reduced risk of recurrence. The comprehensive approach to recurrence prevention complements the broader landscape of hernia management within the context of plastic surgery, offering patients comprehensive care and peace of mind for their long-term well-being.

8. Hernia imaging and diagnostic advances

In the realm of hernia management, accurate diagnosis and precise characterization of hernias are fundamental prerequisites for effective surgical planning and achieving optimal patient outcomes. The past decade has witnessed remarkable progress in medical imaging and diagnostic methodologies, providing healthcare professionals with powerful tools to comprehensively evaluate hernias. These cutting-edge techniques encompass ultrasound, computed tomography (CT), magnetic resonance imaging (MRI), and more. By facilitating a more thorough understanding of hernias, these modalities enable surgeons to make informed decisions, enhance the quality of care, and ultimately improve patient well-being.

8.1 Ultrasound imaging

Ultrasound has emerged as a versatile and accessible diagnostic tool in the evaluation of hernias, particularly in outpatient settings. It offers several distinct advantages:

- *Affordability*: Ultrasound is a cost-effective imaging modality, making it widely accessible to healthcare facilities of all sizes.

- *Non-invasiveness*: Patients appreciate the non-invasive nature of ultrasound, which eliminates the need for contrast agents or ionizing radiation.

- *Real-time imaging*: Ultrasound provides real-time visualization, allowing the surgeon to assess the hernia dynamically. This is particularly valuable in cases of inguinal hernias, where the hernia's response to coughing or straining can be observed.

Furthermore, ultrasound accurately identifies the presence of a hernia, assesses its size, and evaluates its contents. In the hands of a skilled sonographer, it can play a pivotal role in the initial evaluation and follow-up of hernia patients, serving as an indispensable tool for monitoring hernia progression and postoperative outcomes.

8.2 Computed tomography (CT) scans

CT scans, characterized by their cross-sectional imaging capabilities, have long been considered a cornerstone in the diagnostic workup of hernias. The advantages of CT scans in hernia evaluation include:

- *Anatomical detail*: CT scans provide highly detailed anatomical information, allowing for precise delineation of the hernia's location, size, and its relationship with surrounding structures.

- *Complication assessment*: CT scans are invaluable in assessing complications such as bowel obstructions or strangulation, which may necessitate urgent surgical intervention. The ability to identify these complications promptly can be life-saving.

Given the comprehensive nature of CT scans, they are particularly beneficial in cases of complex hernias, recurrent hernias, or giant hernias where surgical planning demands a meticulous understanding of the hernia's unique attributes.

8.3 Magnetic resonance imaging (MRI)

MRI, with its exceptional soft tissue contrast and multiplanar imaging capabilities, has earned its place as an indispensable tool for evaluating complex hernias:

- *Soft tissue contrast*: MRI's ability to distinguish soft tissues with high fidelity makes it invaluable for assessing abdominal wall anatomy and identifying occult hernias that may elude clinical examination.

- *Complex cases*: In scenarios involving complex hernias, such as those with unusual anatomy or recurrent hernias, MRI offers a comprehensive evaluation that aids in surgical planning.

MRI's role extends to the differentiation of hernias from other conditions with similar clinical presentations, contributing to accurate diagnosis and informed decision-making.

8.4 Intraoperative assessment

Intraoperative assessment methods, including direct visualization and palpation, are pivotal in guiding surgeons during the repair process. Real-time evaluation allows for immediate adjustments to the surgical plan based on the hernia's characteristics and any unexpected findings. Surgeons rely on their extensive experience and judgment to ensure that the repair is tailored to each patient's unique anatomy and hernia type. The intraoperative phase bridges the gap between preoperative diagnostics and the surgical execution, ensuring that the repair aligns seamlessly with the patient's individual needs.

8.5 Diagnostic precision and informed decision-making

The use of advanced imaging and diagnostic techniques in hernia management significantly contributes to diagnostic precision. Accurate preoperative assessment enables surgeons to plan the most appropriate surgical approach, select the optimal mesh type, and anticipate potential challenges during surgery. This precision is particularly crucial in complex hernia cases, such as recurrent or giant hernias, where a comprehensive understanding of the hernia's anatomy and associated complications is essential for successful outcomes [7].

Moreover, these diagnostic advances have profound implications for patient engagement and education. Informed patients can actively participate in their care decisions, understand the implications of their hernia, and appreciate the rationale behind the chosen surgical approach. This collaboration between healthcare providers and patients fosters a sense of empowerment and trust, contributing to more positive surgical experiences and outcomes.

In conclusion, the continuous evolution of hernia imaging and diagnostic techniques is reshaping the landscape of hernia management within the context of plastic surgery. These advances provide healthcare professionals with the tools they need to make precise diagnoses, plan surgeries effectively, and provide patients with comprehensive care. As technology continues to advance, it is likely that hernia diagnosis and management will become even more precise and patient-centered, further enhancing the field of plastic surgery and the care provided to hernia patients.

9. Conclusion

Hernias represent a common surgical concern with significant implications for patients' quality of life. This chapter has provided a comprehensive overview of the latest updates in hernia management within the context of plastic surgery. From understanding hernias and their implications to advancements in surgical techniques, mesh materials, and combined procedures, as well as recurrence prevention, and diagnostic imaging, the field has witnessed remarkable progress.

In summary, the key takeaways are as follows:

- Hernias are characterized by the protrusion of organs or tissues through weakened areas in the abdominal wall. Abdominal wall weakness, often caused by factors such as pregnancy, aging, obesity, or previous surgeries, increases the risk of hernias. In the context of plastic surgery, hernias can impact the success and safety of esthetic procedures such as abdominoplasty due to compromised abdominal wall integrity.

- Advancements in hernia repair techniques have provided surgeons with a range of options to address different types of hernias. Traditional open repairs, laparoscopic techniques, and minimally invasive approaches like robotic-assisted surgery offer increased precision and control during the repair.

- Mesh reinforcement plays a crucial role in hernia repairs, with advances in mesh materials leading to the development of synthetic and biologic meshes. Mesh fixation techniques are tailored to each patient and hernia type, aiming to provide long-term stability and reduce the risk of recurrence.

- Combined procedures that address both hernia repair and esthetic enhancements have become increasingly popular. Surgical planning for these procedures requires careful consideration of factors such as the extent of the hernia, excess skin and fat, the patient's overall health, hernia type, and surgical expertise.

- Recurrence prevention is a key focus in hernia management. Advances in mesh technology, meticulous surgical techniques, and addressing patient-specific risk factors, such as obesity and smoking, have contributed to reducing the risk of hernia recurrence.

- Hernia imaging and diagnostic advances, including ultrasound, CT scans, MRI, and intraoperative assessment, have significantly improved the accuracy of preoperative evaluation. These techniques enable surgeons to precisely determine the hernia's size, location, and potential complications, leading to more informed surgical decisions.

In conclusion, the landscape of hernia treatment and management has evolved significantly, driven by medical advancements and technological innovation. These changes have redefined surgical practices, enhancing patient experiences and outcomes. Within plastic surgery, the integration of advanced hernia management techniques holds promise for both function and esthetics.

Minimally invasive approaches like laparoscopic and robotic-assisted surgeries have revolutionized hernia repairs, reducing pain, hastening recovery, and improving cosmetic results. Mesh reinforcement remains pivotal, with modern lightweight meshes improving tissue integration and long-term stability. Collaborative efforts between plastic surgeons and hernia specialists are key in achieving comprehensive care.

Preventing recurrence involves tailored techniques and addressing modifiable risk factors. Imaging techniques aid accurate diagnosis and real-time surgical decisions. Looking ahead, continued research and technological innovation will likely refine hernia management further, ultimately improving patient outcomes.

Patient engagement remains crucial, as informed patients can make better decisions. As hernia management progresses, a future of enhanced care and improved patient lives emerges. The dynamic field of hernia management within the context of plastic surgery continues to evolve, offering hope and holistic care to patients seeking both functional restoration and esthetic enhancement.

Author details

Eren Tuncer*, Fatih Cınar and Percin Karakol
Basaksehir Cam and Sakura Hospital, Istanbul, Turkey

*Address all correspondence to: erentuncr@gmail.com

References

[1] Kingsworth A, Le Blanc K. Hernias: Inguinal and incisional. Lancet. 2003;**362**:1561-1571

[2] Ozkaya Mutlu O, Colak O, Atay M. Abdominal wall hernias and their repair with inverse abdominoplasty. In: Tiryaki K, editor. Inverse Abdominoplasty. Cham: Springer; 2017. DOI: 10.1007/978-3-319-39310-0_9

[3] HerniaSurge Group. International guidelines for groin hernia management. Hernia. 2018;**22**:1-165

[4] Kaufmann R, Halm JA, Eker HH, et al. Mesh versus suture repair of umbilicalhernia in adults: A randomised, double-blind, controlled, multicentre trial. Lancet. 2018;**391**(10123):860-869

[5] Daniels IR, Smart NJ. In support of mesh for hernia repair. BJS. 2019;**106**(7):815-816

[6] Christoffersen MW, Helgstrand F, Rosenberg J, et al. Long-term recurrence andchronic pain after repair for small umbilical or epigastric hernias: A regionalcohort study. American Journal of Surgery. 2015;**209**:725-732

[7] Miller J, Tregarthen A, Saouaf R, Towfigh S. Radiologic reporting and interpretation of occult inguinal hernia. Journal of the American College of Surgeons. 2018;**227**(5):489-495

Chapter 14

Prehabilitation: Enhancing Recovery and Outcomes in Hernia Surgery

Gabriel Paiva de Oliveira and Carmen Maillo

Abstract

As patients get older and clinical situations become more complex, optimization before surgery is paramount. Physicians always tried to improve the pre-surgical status of patients, but they followed stochastic models. The structured intervention to improve nutritional status, cardiorespiratory and neurocognitive function and minimize frailty has been called prehabilitation. It improves functional status before and after surgery in multiple settings suggesting a possible lower length of stay, as documented by several RCTs, and improved outcomes. Hernia surgery has evolved immensely in the past decades, providing solutions for patients and situations not long ago deemed inoperable. For incisional hernia, especially if complex, the recurrence rate may increase to 60%, most of which occur in the first 2 years. The difficulty rises for each repair attempt, so teams have their best opportunity in the first intervention. Most complex hernias started as simple ones. Prehabilitation interventions may contribute to outcome optimization in hernia surgery.

Keywords: abdominal wall surgery, incisional hernia, prehabilitation, hernia recurrence, complex hernia

1. Introduction

Globally, human populations are getting older. In 2022, in Europe, one-fifth of the population was over 65. By 2030, globally, older people will outnumber children under 10; by 2050, they will double their numbers [1].

Naturally, as people get old, they accumulate numerous comorbidities, and frequently enough, they must undergo surgery for various illnesses. Surprisingly, older adults do not seem as sick as they used to [2]. Nonetheless, older people do accumulate more comorbid states than their younger counterparts. As the elderly population increases, this poses a massive concern in healthcare, most prominently surgery. How can we improve outcomes in an aged and sick population?

Every clinician, especially surgeons, always tries to improve the patient's condition after an intervention. Robert Topp and colleagues proposed, as early as 2002, the "process of enhancing functional capacity of the individual to enable them to withstand an incoming stressor" as a definition for prehabilitation [3]. As this definition points out, prehabilitation started focused on patients' physical function and

IntechOpen

consisted of a varied range of pre-surgical exercise programmes. Karin Valkenet and colleagues demonstrated, in a 2011 systematic review, that "preoperative exercise therapy" can improve postoperative outcomes [4]. Not long after, Daniel Santa Mina, in a systematic review back in 2014, identified several studies in which preoperative whole-body exercise programmes showed promise in improving post-operative outcomes such as pain, length of stay and physical function [5]. Carli and Zavorsky depicted very successfully the rationale for prehabilitation (**Figure 1**) [6].

In recent years, prehabilitation has shifted from focusing exclusively on physical conditions to entail global health improvement. Multimodal approaches include not only how fit a patient is but also how well-nourished and controlled his comorbidities are and his or her psychological status. To comprise all these dimensions, the prehabilitation definition had to evolve. The most recent and consensual definition of prehabilitation might be Durrand's: every intervention that aims at "enhancing general health and wellbeing prior to major surgery" [7].

We can only aim if we have a target. Risk assessment, especially in high-risk patients in complex hernia surgery, is part of the patient's journey and crucial to shared decision making and informed consent [8]. In potentially complex patients, the authors adopted the multidisciplinary evaluation pathway described in **Figure 2**.

The concept of enhancing recovery after surgery by minimizing surgical stress response was proposed in the early nineties by Henrik Kehlet [10]. Standard recovery protocols soon followed, focusing on various interventions implemented at or after surgery. As the preoperative period gained importance, however, some interventions were included prior to surgery as part of a truly multimodal approach to optimization of recovery and, therefore, results. These interventions resulted in savings and even reduced complications and mortality in some specific surgeries [11].

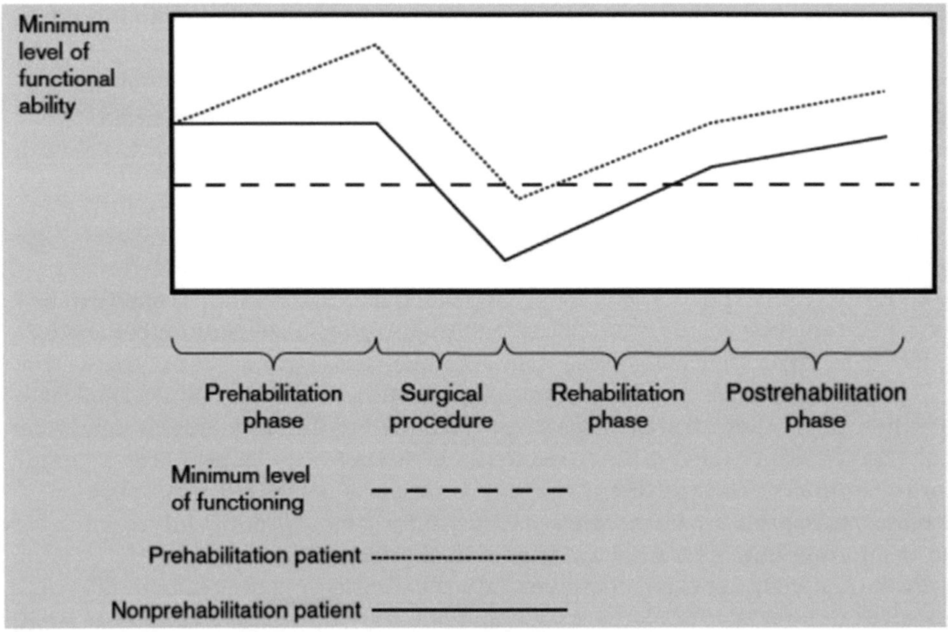

Figure 1.
Visual representation of the rationale for prehabilitation. Reproduced with permission from the lead author of Carli and Zavorsky [6].

DOI: http://dx.doi.org/10.5772/intechopen.1002367

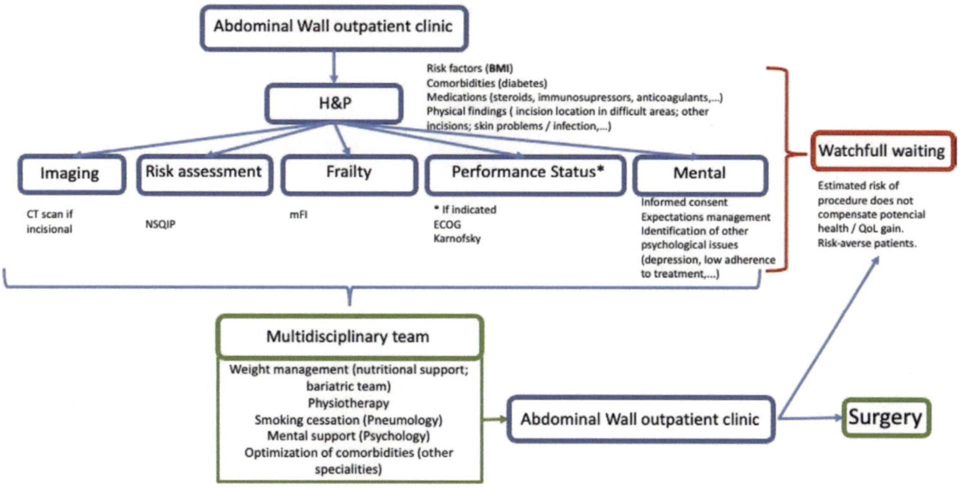

Figure 2.
Potentially complex hernia patient pathway. NSQIP—National Surgical Quality Improvement Project; mFI—Modified frailty index; ECOG—Eastern cooperative oncology group. Adapted with permission from Lages et al. [9].

The first evaluation of a patient with a hernia should include a comprehensive history and physical examination. This process should include due identification and characterization of the main problems and their valuation by the patient, based chiefly on the impact on activities of daily living or quality of life. These are paramount in a value-based healthcare paradigm. Some abdominal wall reconstructions are so complex and potentially hazardous that it is essential to discuss with the patient what he will gain by being operated on or what he might lose if so. As in finance, there are risk-averse and intrepid patients, and our joint decision must match their risk profile.

Medical and surgical history, a careful systems review and a medication review frequently identify conditions under the radar. Suppose risk factors such as obesity, diabetes, steroid use, tobacco use or undernourishment are identified. In that case, these patients are referred to the specific health professional for further evaluation and a recovery programme implementation.

In patients with highly symptomatic hernias or multiple episodes of incarceration, achievement of prehabilitation goals becomes secondary, and surgery ensues. However, patients must acknowledge the risk profile of the operation. Knowledge of a high probability of failure should prompt surgical teams to carefully choose techniques so that a later intervention is not even more difficult.

2. Weight management

Obesity poses a specific problem for abdominal wall hernia repair. Obese patients have an increased abdominal perimeter and a higher abdominal fat volume, leading to higher abdominal wall pressure [12]. Obesity patients have sarcopenia. Obesity produces a chronic low-grade inflammatory response with consequences in the immune response and alterations in the healing process [13, 14]. The overall complication rate is also higher in patients with body mass index (BMI) greater than 30, especially surgical-site infection (SSI), with an incidence of 23% for colorectal and other general surgery procedures [15].

Increased wound morbidity is tied to body mass index (BMI), as there is a linear relation between surgical-site infection (SSI) or surgical-site occurrence (SSO) and obesity. SSI also increases risk recurrence twofold; late costs will undoubtedly rise [16].

The recurrence rate at 12 months may be as high as 52% in patients with BMI higher than 30 Kg/m^2. Of these, around 30% will require surgery [17]. A systematic review of the literature in 2021 identified differences in hernia recurrences between BMI thresholds. The risk of recurrence in ventral hernia repair is 2.5-fold higher in patients with BMI greater than 25 when compared to those with BMI equal to or inferior to 25—the risk triples in patients with BMI over 40, compared with a lower BMI [18].

Even if surgery is minimally invasive, the risk still exists of trocar site hernia [TSH] formation. Early studies indicated an incidence of symptomatic TSH hernias of up to 5%, but most authors agree that this is a highly underdiagnosed problem [19].

A recent study revealed that incidence may be as high as 23%, but fewer than 50% are symptomatic. Tonouchi et al. suggest that obesity and diabetes may increase TSH, underlining the technical difficulty in closing port incisions in high BMI patients. A more recent study by Ciscar et al. determined that obesity and age over 70 constitute independent risk factors for TSH [20, 21].

There is a debate about the best pathway to treat hernia in obese patients. Obesity increases the risk of recurrence, but delaying hernia repair until the patient reaches good weight control can allow for hernia complications during this period [22]. It seems intuitive to address obesity prior to hernia surgery. The difficulty lies in setting evidence-based thresholds. It is unreasonable to expect that most patients lose enough weight to bring their BMI down to normal or even overweight, especially on their own. Maskal and colleagues found that free weight management programs can help but are insufficient to address obesity independently [23]. No patient over BMI 35 kg/m^2 should undergo elective hernia surgery before an attempt to control weight. Weight loss is an essential factor in prehabilitation before hernia surgery. The prehabilitation must include low-calorie diet and physical exercise as a first step. However, diet and physical exercise have poor long-term weight loss results in morbidly obese patients and patients with BMI higher than 35 Kg/m^2 will rarely respond to nutritional and behavioral interventions alone. Besides, patients with symptomatic hernias are at risk of hernia complications, so weight loss must be reached in the shortest possible time.

Bariatric surgery is an adequate treatment to achieve good weight loss quickly with good long-term results [24]. Morbidly obese patients [BMI > 35 kg/m^2] with symptomatic hernias must be referred to bariatric units for weight loss before elective hernia surgery. If emergent hernia surgery is warranted, obese patients should be referred to the bariatric unit as soon as possible after the hernia surgery.

3. Diabetes management

Diabetes is a well-known risk factor for SSO, especially infectious occurrences, as a higher surgical mesh infection rate in abdominal wall repair [25]. Acute glycaemic control is paramount, as infectious complications increase with blood glucose levels. Hyperglycaemia impairs neutrophil action, and the host's immune response to infection, particularly in the presence of a foreign body [mesh], will be hampered. Without hernia-specific evidence, there are strong recommendations that blood glucose levels should be kept below 200 mg/dL [26]. A meta-analysis of randomized trials showed no overall advantage in adopting a more intensive blood glucose lowering regime in studies with non-diabetic or mixed patient populations. There was, however, a reduction in SSI with intensive regime in studies involving diabetic patients. Nevertheless, the studies had considerable heterogeneity, and complications such as hypoglycemia were more significant [27].

Acute glycaemic control is essential, but chronic management of diabetes is also crucial. Based on a 2006 study by Dronge and colleagues Robert Martindale and Clifford Deveney, they proposed an HbA1c threshold of 7%, above which surgery should be postponed until better glycaemic control. Mike Liang and colleagues propose a higher threshold of 8% [28, 29]. No relevant studies show a relation between HbA1c levels and hernia surgery outcomes. Martindale and Deveney's proposal come from a study of NSQIPs non-cardiac surgery, and outcomes ranged from pneumonia to urinary tract infection, and Liang's proposal originates from a consensus. CDC guidelines on SSI, in 2017, failed to propose a recommendation on this issue based on the lack of evidence. The more recent systematic review from the European Hernia Society (EHS) Prehabilitation Project, although meeting with similar problems, did propose level 2 evidence for an HbA1c lower than 7%. That recommendation, however, comes from Liang et al.'s consensus that HbA1c higher than 6.5% increases complications in a varied array of surgeries. Participants agreed that, in diabetic patients, we should aim at a maximum of 7% preoperative HbA1c levels [30].

4. Smoking cessation

Smoking is a well-established as a risk factor for complications after surgery. Smoking cessation before surgery results in a risk reduction of 41% of postoperative complications. The longer the interval without smoking, the more significant the risk reduction [31]. After an analysis of the American College of Surgery National Surgical Quality Improvement Project (NSQIP) database, Park et al. demonstrated that obesity and smoking increased SSI incidence in ventral hernia repair. They also demonstrated smoking as a risk factor for recurrence in ventral hernia repair [32].

As far back as 2007, Lindström and colleagues demonstrated, after analysis of the Swedish inpatient register, that smoking increased complication rate even in inguinal hernia surgery. In a more recent study from NSQIP, authors concluded that, in inguinal hernia repair (both open and laparoscopic), "failure to quit smoking prior to surgical repair is associated with complications like pneumonia and return to the operating room" [33, 34]. Few high-quality studies exist on the subject. The recent systematic review from the European Hernia Society (EHS) rehabilitation project found 889 studies on smoking's effect on surgery outcomes but only selected three [30].

Smoking cessation might be one of the most frustrating endeavors for clinicians and patients. Centers for Disease Control and Prevention (CDC) states that nearly 70% of smokers want to quit, and 50% have tried in the last year, but only 7.5% of smokers succeeded [35]. Smokers that relapse begin to doubt their resolve and avoid the matter altogether. Preparing the right mindset is paramount. First, patients should be advised that smoking addiction is a chemical dependence issue. Then, it is essential to underline that few smokers succeed on their own, which is normal. The evaluation of nicotine dependence, as calculated by the Fagerström scale, might be an essential tool to understand the degree of investment and difficulty in the cessation attempt [36]. While a patient with low dependence and a regular inguinal or primary ventral hernia might be well off with basic counseling in the surgical consultation, average to high dependence patients will need specialized care and follow-up. The probability of success increases with a structured strategy that includes behavioral changes, nicotine replacement and counseling. The focus should rely on the fact that, in some cases, smoking may be a more significant health problem than the hernia itself.

Although the authors advise smoking cessation and offer help, treatment for uncomplicated hernias is not withheld if patients do not quit. Smoking cessation is essential to minimize complications, especially wound morbidity and respiratory hazards in extensive surgeries, multiple comorbidity and frailty or complex hernia repair. Following previous recommendations, the authors advise at least 4 weeks of cessation in these patients and always refer to a specific smoking cessation consultation. The authors do not, at present, perform biochemical confirmation of smoking cessation.

5. Addressing frailty

There is no uniform definition for the concept of frailty. Nonetheless, most health professionals agree that frailty includes reduced physical capacity, impaired mobility and susceptibility to hazardous outcomes [37]. Walter Joseph and colleagues proposed a modified Frailty Index [mFI] based on the NSQIP database to classify frailty and predict poor outcomes in abdominal wall reconstruction (AWR). This index includes variables such as diabetes, functional status, congestive heart failure or cerebrovascular accident with neurologic deficit. The authors successfully linked mFI to mortality and morbidity, meaning that this tool can also identify patients more likely to benefit from preoperative conditioning or prehabilitation [38].

Frailty, although not uniquely a physical impairment condition, is susceptible to improvement from physiotherapy and nutritional intervention [39]. Santa Mina and colleagues have already demonstrated that literature favors whole-body prehabilitation programs leading to improved physical functions and reduced LOS and pain [5]. Professor Francesco Carli and colleagues stated, "When exercise is undertaken on a regular basis, the body becomes more efficient in its adaptation to the stress of exercise." Combined interventions of structured physical activity and improved nutritional support prevent and treat frailty and sarcopenia [40, 41].

6. Psychological preparation of patients

Expectations matter. Psychological factors, of which expectations play an important role, can be decisive in determining surgery results. In a double-blind sham surgery involving the treatment of advanced Parkinson's disease patients, the sham procedure obtained better results than the actual procedure, again showing that the placebo effect has a role in surgery too [42].

In surgery, patient expectations concerning results may need to be revised, particularly in complex surgeries. Incisional hernia repair may have up to 30%

recurrence rates and a considerable incidence of complications. It is important to involve patients in the decision making to inform them as accurately as possible, engage them in the process and build the right expectations towards surgery. Patient expectations influence postoperative outcomes. Patient satisfaction depends on fulfilling preoperative expectations and not preoperative positive expectations [43]. Better doctor-patient communication could establish reasonable expectations, thus increasing patient satisfaction. Patient expectation management could lead to better outcomes than other measures, and it is remarkably cost-effective.

7. Implementing a prehabilitation clinic

Much of the existing literature on prehabilitation focused on cancer patients. However, many non-fit patients suffer from benign diseases, including hernia, and should be candidates for an effective improvement programme [44]. A "hernia optimization clinic" was shown to improve risk management and even increase operative yield by operating patients previously deemed inoperable. Furthermore, case discussion in a multidisciplinary team followed by a preconditioning programme could recompense the increased risk of complications associated with the presence of risk factors [9, 45].

Only a structured, documented and evidence-based programme can overcome speculative prehabilitation strategies. Prehabilitation is increasingly multimodal and involves a variety of professions, from physiotherapy to nutrition and psychological support. Patient-centered care in hernia surgery, similarly to cancer surgery, should be tailored to specific patient needs and referral to a speciality should reflect those needs. Also, implementing a prehabilitation programme should consider the circumstances in which the patient is included [46].

8. Conclusion

Prehabilitation has demonstrated clear benefits in some, but not all, surgeries. In colorectal cancer surgery, several recent RCTs proved the positive effect of multimodal interventions. In thoracic surgery for lung cancer, it also demonstrated a positive, however more heterogeneous, effect [47, 48]. The mechanism through which prehabilitation contributes to potential outcome improvement is very intuitive. Nonetheless, evidence of its actual efficacy is lacking in many areas, especially for benign conditions [30]. On the other hand, improving patient function before surgery serves not for the surgery alone. Weight management strategies like bariatric surgery in morbidly obese patients improve health outcomes and QoL in itself. Better diabetes control or smoking cessation not only allows for fewer SSIs but also contributes to patients' overall health. Reverting frailty through exercise programs and nutritional support improves people's lives. Mindfulness about expectations and their management and identification of psychological barriers or misconceptions might improve doctor-patient communication and contribute to increased patient satisfaction. The authors believe the implementation of a structured multimodal preoperative intervention is essential to improve hernia care outcomes in patients with identifiable risk factors and potentially complex hernias.

Acknowledgements

We want to thank Prof Dr. Nuno Figueiredo, Hospital Lusíadas Lisboa and Hospital Lusíadas Amadora for their invaluable support of the abdominal wall team and patient pathway. We also thank Dr. Patrícia Lages for her input and support. Their insights and expertise were instrumental in shaping this manuscript.

Conflict of interest

The authors declare no conflict of interest.

Acronyms and abbreviations

RCT	randomized control trial
BMI	body mass index
SSI	surgical-site infection
SSO	surgical-site occurrence
TSH	trocar site hernia
NSQIP	National Surgical Quality Improvement Project
EHS	European Hernia Society
CDC	Centers for Disease Control and Prevention
mFI	modified Frailty Index
AWR	abdominal wall reconstruction

Author details

Gabriel Paiva de Oliveira[1*] and Carmen Maillo[2]

1 Hospital Garcia de Orta, Almada, Portugal

2 Hospital dos Lusíadas Lisboa, Lisbon, Portugal

*Address all correspondence to: gp.oliveira@outlook.com

References

[1] World Health Organization. Decade of Healthy Ageing: Baseline Report. World Health Organization; 2020. Available from: https://apps.who.int/iris/handle/10665/338677. License: CC BY-NC-SA 3.0 IGO

[2] Chang AY, Skirbekk VF, Tyrovolas S, Kassebaum NJ, Dieleman JL. Measuring population ageing: An analysis of the global burden of disease study 2017. The Lancet Public Health. 2019;**4**(3):e159-e167

[3] Topp R, Ditmyer M, King K, Doherty K, Hornyak J. The effect of bed rest and potential of prehabilitation on patients in the intensive care unit. AACN Clinical. 2002;**13**:268

[4] Valkenet K, van de Port IG, Dronkers JJ, de Vries WR, Lindeman E, Backx FJ. The effects of preoperative exercise therapy on postoperative outcome: A systematic review. Clinical Rehabilitation. 2011;**25**(2):99-111

[5] Santa Mina D, Clarke H, Ritvo P, Leung YW, Matthew AG, Katz J, et al. Effect of total-body prehabilitation on postoperative outcomes: A systematic review and meta-analysis. Physiotherapy. 2014;**100**(3):196-207

[6] Carli F, Zavorsky GS. Optimizing functional exercise capacity in the elderly surgical population. Current Opinion in Clinical Nutrition & Metabolic Care. Jan 2005;**8**(1):23-32

[7] Durrand J, Singh SJ, Danjoux G. Prehabilitation. Clinical Medicine. 2019;**19**(6):458-464

[8] Matthews L, Levett DZH, Grocott MPW. Perioperative risk stratification and modification. Anesthesiology Clinics. 2022;**40**(1):e1-e23

[9] Delaney LD, Howard R, Palazzolo K, Ehlers AP, Smith S, Englesbe M, et al. Outcomes of a Presurgical optimization program for elective Hernia repairs among high-risk patients. JAMA Network Open. 2021;**4**(11):e2130016

[10] Kehlet H. The surgical stress response: Should it be prevented? Canadian Journal of Surgery. 1991;**34**(6):565-567

[11] Golder HJ, Papalois V. Enhanced recovery after surgery: History, key advancements and developments in transplant surgery. Journal of Clinical Medicine. 2021;**10**(8):1634

[12] Liang MK, Bernardi K, Holihan JL, Cherla DV, Escamilla R, Lew DF, et al. Modifying risks in ventral Hernia patients with Prehabilitation: A randomized controlled trial. Annals of Surgery. 2018;**268**(4):674-680

[13] Alma A, Marconi GD, Rossi E, Magnoni C, Paganelli A. Obesity and wound healing: Focus on mesenchymal stem cells. Life. 2023;**13**(3):717

[14] Khanna D, Khanna S, Khanna P, et al. Obesity: A chronic low-grade inflammation and its markers. Cureus. 28 Feb 2022;**14**(2):e22711, 1-2

[15] The Ventral Hernia Group Tilburg, van Silfhout L, LAM L, Heisterkamp J, Ibelings MS. Recurrent incisional hernia repair: Surgical outcomes in correlation with body-mass index. Hernia. 2021;**25**(1):77-83

[16] Tastaldi L, Krpata DM, Prabhu AS, Petro CC, Rosenblatt S, Haskins IN, et al. The effect of increasing body mass index on wound complications in open ventral hernia repair with mesh. American Journal of Surgery. 2019;**218**(3):560-566

[17] Wehrle CJ, Shukla P, Miller BT, Blake KE, Prabhu AS, Petro CC, et al. Incisional hernia rates following midline laparotomy in the obese patient: A retrospective review. Hernia. 2022;**27**(3):557-563

[18] Parker SG, Mallett S, Quinn L, Wood CPJ, Boulton RW, Jamshaid S, et al. Identifying predictors of ventral hernia recurrence: Systematic review and meta-analysis. BJS Open. 2021 52):zraa071.

[19] Helgstrand F, Rosenberg J, Bisgaard T. Trocar site hernia after laparoscopic surgery: A qualitative systematic review. Hernia. 2011;**15**(2):113-121

[20] Ciscar A, Badia JM, Novell F, Bolívar S, Mans E. Incidence and risk factors for trocar-site incisional hernia detected by clinical and ultrasound examination: A prospective observational study. BMC Surgery. 2020;**20**(1):330

[21] Tonouchi H, Ohmori Y, Kobayashi M, Kusunoki M. Trocar site hernia. Archives of Surgery. 2004;**139**:1251, 1253

[22] Maia R, Salgaonkar H, Lomanto D, Shabbir A. Ventral hernia and obesity: Is there a consensus? Annals of Laparoscopic and Endoscopic Surgery. 2019;**4**:17-17

[23] Maskal SM, Boyd-Tressler AM, Heinberg LJ, Montelione KC, Petro CC, Krpata DM, et al. Can a free weight management program "move the needle" for obese patients preparing for hernia surgery?: Outcomes of a novel pilot program. Hernia. 2022;**26**(5):1259-1265

[24] Courcoulas AP, Yanovski SZ, Bonds D, Eggerman TL, Horlick M, Staten MA, et al. Long-term outcomes of bariatric surgery: A National Institutes of Health symposium. JAMA Surgery. 2014;**149**(12):1323

[25] Quiroga-Centeno AC, Quiroga-Centeno CA, Guerrero-Macías S, Navas-Quintero O, Gómez-Ochoa SA. Systematic review and meta-analysis of risk factors for mesh infection following abdominal wall hernia repair surgery. American Journal of Surgery. 2022;**224**(1):239-246

[26] Berríos-Torres SI, Umscheid CA, Bratzler DW, Leas B, Stone EC, Kelz RR, et al. Centers for disease control and prevention guideline for the prevention of surgical site infection. JAMA Surgery. 2017;**152**(8):784

[27] Lai J, Li Q, He Y, Zou S, Bai X, Rastogi S. Glycemic control regimens in the prevention of surgical site infections: A Meta-analysis of randomized clinical trials. Frontier in Surgery. 2022;**9**:855409

[28] Novitsky YW. Hernia Surgery Current Principles [Internet]. 2016 [Cited April 4, 2019]. DOI: 10.1007/978-3-319-27470-6

[29] Liang MK, Holihan JL, Itani K, Alawadi ZM, Gonzalez JRF, Askenasy EP, et al. Ventral hernia management: Expert consensus guided by systematic review. Annals of Surgery. 2017;**265**(1):80-89

[30] Jensen KK, East B, Jisova B, Cano ML, Cavallaro G, Jørgensen LN, et al. The European Hernia Society Prehabilitation project: A systematic review of patient prehabilitation prior to ventral hernia surgery. Hernia. 2022;**26**(3):715-726

[31] Mills E, Eyawo O, Lockhart I, Kelly S, Wu P, Ebbert JO. Smoking cessation reduces postoperative complications: A systematic review and meta-analysis.

The American Journal of Medicine. 2011;**124**(2):144-154

[32] Park H, De Virgilio C, Kim DY, Shover AL, Moazzez A. Effects of smoking and different BMI cutoff points on surgical site infection after elective open ventral hernia repair. Hernia. 2021;**25**(2):337-343

[33] Lindström D, Sadr Azodi O, Bellocco R, Wladis A, Linder S, Adami J. The effect of tobacco consumption and body mass index on complications and hospital stay after inguinal hernia surgery. Hernia. 2007;**11**(2):117-123

[34] Landin M, Kubasiak JC, Schimpke S, Poirier J, Myers JA, Millikan KW, et al. The effect of tobacco use on outcomes of laparoscopic and open inguinal hernia repairs: A review of the NSQIP dataset. Surgical Endoscopy. 2017;**31**(2):917-921

[35] Centers for Disease Control and Prevention. Smoking Cessation: Fast Facts [Internet]. 2023. Available from: https://www.cdc.gov/tobacco/data_statistics/fact_sheets/cessation/smoking-cessation-fast-facts/index.html

[36] Ferreira PL, Quintal C, Lopes I, Taveira N. Teste de dependência à nicotina: validação linguística e psicométrica do teste de Fagerström. Revista Portuguesa de Saúde Pública. 2009;**2009**:27

[37] Xue QL. The frailty syndrome: Definition and natural history. Clinics in Geriatric Medicine. 2011;**27**(1):1-15

[38] Joseph WJ, Cuccolo NG, Baron ME, Chow I, Beers EH. Frailty predicts morbidity, complications, and mortality in patients undergoing complex abdominal wall reconstruction. Hernia. Apr 2020;**24**(2):235-243

[39] Puts MTE, Toubasi S, Andrew MK, Ashe MC, Ploeg J, Atkinson E, et al. Interventions to prevent or reduce the level of frailty in community-dwelling older adults: A scoping review of the literature and international policies. Age and Ageing. 2017;**2017**:afw247v1

[40] Carli F, Scheede-Bergdahl C. Prehabilitation to enhance perioperative care. Anesthesiology Clinics. 2015;**33**(1):17-33

[41] Cruz-Jentoft AJ, Woo J. Nutritional interventions to prevent and treat frailty. Current Opinion in Clinical Nutrition and Metabolic Care. 2019;**22**(3):191-195

[42] McRae C, Cherin E, Yamazaki TG, Diem G, Vo AH, Russell D, et al. Effects of perceived treatment on quality of life and medical Outcomesin a double-blind placebo surgery trial. Archives of General Psychiatry. 2004;**61**(4):412

[43] Auer CJ, Glombiewski JA, Doering BK, Winkler A, Laferton JAC, Broadbent E, et al. Patients' expectations predict surgery outcomes: A Meta-analysis. International Journal of Behavioral Medicine. 2016;**23**(1):49-62

[44] Lages P, Oliveira G, Simões J, Costa PM. The time has come for a community and home-based prehabilitation: Narrative of an implementation process. Revista Portuguesa de Cirurgia. Feb 2022;**3**:115-123

[45] De Jong DLC, Wegdam JA, Berkvens EBM, Nienhuijs SW, De Vries Reilingh TS. The influence of a multidisciplinary team meeting and prehabilitation on complex abdominal wall hernia repair outcomes. Hernia. 2023;**27**(3):609-616

[46] Fernandes ADV, Gonçalves D, Come J, Rosa NC, Costa V, Lopes LV, et

al. Prehabilitation program for African sub-Saharan surgical patients is an unmet need? The Pan African Medical Journal. 2020;**2020**:36. Available from: https://www.panafrican-med-journal.com/content/article/36/62/full/

[47] Molenaar CJL, Minnella EM, Coca-Martinez M, Ten Cate DWG, Regis M, Awasthi R, et al. Effect of multimodal prehabilitation on reducing postoperative complications and enhancing functional capacity following colorectal Cancer surgery: The PREHAB randomized clinical trial. JAMA Surgery. 2023;**158**(6):572

[48] Voorn MJJ, Franssen RFW, Hoogeboom TJ, et al. Evidence base for exercise prehabilitation suggests favourable outcomes for patients undergoing surgery for non-small cell lung cancer despite being of low therapeutic quality: A systematic review and meta-analysis. European Journal of Surgical Oncology. 2023;**49**(5):879-894

Chapter 15

Male Fertility Following Inguinal Hernia Repair

Krzysztof Balawender and Anna Pliszka

Abstract

Tension-free mesh hernia repair has become the standard procedure in inguinal hernia repair. The incidence of inguinal hernias has steadily decreased following mesh and laparoscopic techniques, but the potential risk of fertility disorders after surgery remains a controversial issue. The aim of this chapter was to establish the clinical impact of open (mesh and/or without mesh) and laparoscopic hernia repair on male fertility. The results of the research published to date do not allow clear conclusions and guidelines in hernia surgery for young patients of reproductive age. Evidence is inevitably difficult to find because of the wide range of causes of infertility and their complexity. However, the choice of method and the possible impact on fertility should be discussed with the patient before surgery. Additionally, preoperative and postoperative semen analysis will help exclude or confirm its impact on patient fertility in the future.

Keywords: inguinal hernia, inguinal hernia repair, inguinal hernia surgery, infertility, fertility disorders, vas deferens obstruction

1. Introduction

The World Health Organisation (WHO) has determined the common definition of infertility as the inability to achieve spontaneous pregnancy during at least 1 year of regular, unprotected sexual intercourse. It can affect both women and men, while the male factor is approximately 20–30%, the female factor 50% and a combination of both around 20–30%; therefore, the correct factor that causes categorisation is required to be investigated in both partners simultaneously, which enables a proper management. According to the WHO publication from 2022, related to global prevalence of infertility, one in six people has experienced infertility in their lifetimes. In general, the male factor (including the 'both' group) is approximately 50% globally (Western Europe (EU) 50%, Central EU 56% and Eastern EU 37%) [1, 2]. Infertility can be divided into primary—when spontaneous conception never occurred during the patient's life despite regular attempts at conceiving a child for at least 1 year, and secondary—in case of pregnancy in the past with the same or a different partner as present. The aetiology of this disease is compounded, while the main causes can be divided into lifestyle, genetic, hormonal, systemic disease and varicocele. Idiopathic male infertility defined by disorder without identifiable cause, arising spontaneously, reaches 50% of all cases. Azoospermia is a condition in which there are no spermatozoa in the ejaculate, and it is one of the most frequent symptoms in semen analysis paired with the infertility. It can be divided into obstructive (when testes have the ability to produce normal sperm but there is obstruction of the ejaculatory route at the epididymal, vas deferens or ejaculatory duct level) and non-obstructive (when there is a clear problem with the spermatogenesis process). According to the European Association of Urology (EAU) 2023 Guidelines infertility among male patients can be the result of: varicocele in the mechanism of increased scrotal temperature (with an incidence of 14.8% of all infertility causes in unselected vs. 10.9% in patients with azoospermia), cryptorchidism (8.4% vs. 17.2% with azoospermia), vasectomy (0.9% vs. 5.3% with azoospermia), cystic fibrosis (0.5% vs. 3% with azoospermia) and idiopathic infertility (30% vs. 13.3% with azoospermia). Apart from previously presented disorders, fertility disorders may be the result of, underestimating among men, genitourinary tract infections that are not always manifested symptomatically, but sometimes only as abnormal semen parameters in sperm analysis, concomitant with positive semen culture and elevated inflammatory markers [3, 4]. The interest of this chapter is certainly the theory of possible formation of fertility disorders due to hernia repair surgery.

2. Patient evaluation

The medical interview focusing on fertility disorders contains an investigation of potential risk factors and lifestyle patterns, including partner fertility, family history of oncological and systemic diseases, coexisting diseases (such as especially hypertension, diabetes mellitus, obesity and genitourinary tract infections), the presence of erectile and ejaculatory dysfunctions, previous surgical interventions (together with testicular trauma or torsion), congenital anomalies (mainly cryptorchidism), exposure to gonadotoxins (e.g. anabolic drugs, chemotherapeutics) and radiation [4].

On medical examination, attention is paid to the presence/absence of gonads in the scrotum, size, consistency, abnormal masses of the testes (thick, cohesive ones suggest cancer), penis (including strictures negatively affecting ejaculation, due, for example, to phimosis, hypospadias, epispadias and other abnormalities such as acquired curvature of the penis—Peyronie's disease) as well as the presence of gynaecomastia, female pattern hair, fat and muscle distribution, possibly indicating hormonal disorders. Visible varicoceles (abnormal enlargement of the pampiniform plexus veins greater than 2–3 mm in diameter) are also observed at this stage of evaluation as one of the main known causes of fertility disorders. They are examined using the Valsalva manoeuvre in both the supine and standing positions and look like a bag of worms above the gonad [4, 5]. Varicoceles are more common on the left side due to anatomical conditions, but in an advanced stage they can occur bilaterally. Only the manifestation on the right side of this disease may indicate the tumour of the retroperitoneal site, which causes pressure on the testicular vein that disrupts the flow of testicular blood to the inferior vena cava [6].

Male infertility is strictly associated with abnormal semen parameters. Semen analysis is an important first-line test for guiding the clinician to identify the cause of fertility disorders. The semen parameters have been standardised by the WHO in the sixth edition of the WHO Manual for the Examination and Processing of Human Semen and published in 2021. Semen analysis standards have been lowered in recent years not only due to the decrease in semen quality due to the greater amount of stress among men related to pollution and lifestyle changes, but also partly as a consequence

Parameter of semen analysis	WHO 2021 reference limit (95% CI)
Semen volume (mL)	1.4 (1.3–1.5)
Total number of sperm (106/ejaculate)	39 (35–40)
Sperm concentration (106/ml)	16 (15–18)
Total motility (PR + NP, %)	42 (40–43)
Progressive motility (PR, %)	30 (29–31)
Vitality (live spermatozoa, %)	54 (50–56)
Sperm morphology (normal forms, %)	4 (3.9–4.0)

Table 1.
Basic semen examination standards according to WHO 2021. CI- confidence interval.

of the development of testing technology that allows the detection of increasingly subtle sperm disorders. The basic examination includes total sperm number, sperm concentration, semen volume, total motility, progressive motility, vitality (live spermatozoa) and sperm morphology (normal forms) (**Table 1**). Extended semen examination additionally consists of tests aimed at counting peroxidase positive leukocytes, markers of genitourinary tract inflammations (for example, pH), antibodies of sperm, mixed antiglobulin reaction (MAR) test (motile spermatozoa with bound particles), immunobead test (motile spermatozoa with bound beads), zinc, fructose, neutral α-glucosidase and fragmentation of sperm DNA. The advanced semen examination has also been differentiated and contains tests such as reactive oxygen species (ROS), acrosome reaction and sperm chromatin stability and structure. Consonant with WHO in the case of normal semen analysis, there is no need to perform re-test, while if the test is abnormal, the second confirmational one should be performed. Two basic tests with abnormal semen parameters qualify the patient for further extended (and advanced if needed) semen examinations and their evaluation by an andrologist [7, 8].

In the management of fertility disorders, the imaging test, which is ultrasound (US), also plays the crucial role. Due to its accessibility and non-invasive character, it allows to visualise abnormalities in the genitourinary tract at an early stage of the diagnostic process. It also allows the measurement of testicular volume, detection of abnormalities in epididymis, hydrocele, testicular neoplasms and non-optically visible varicoceles with the ability to measure its diameters. Moreover, it illustrates the vascularity in Colour Doppler Mode strictly correlating with testicular blood perfusion, which is enhanced in orchitis, epididymitis, and in some neoplasms, and reveals echotexture and calcifications related to testicular tumours. Research data show that there is a higher risk of testicular cancer among infertility sufferers than among fertile men; therefore, every patient with infertility disorders is examined in scrotal US in relation to the presence of neoplasia. Additionally, the scrotal US may expose the distal and proximal part of the vas deferens (the median part cannot be visualised). The extension of the distal section of vas deferens indicates obstruction at some level, while the absence of vas deferens indicates the presence of the cystic fibrosis transmembrane regulator (CFTR) gene and should prompt the physician to perform a kidney ultrasound to look for other defects or agenesis. Transrectal ultrasound (TRUS) can reveal abnormalities in the ejaculatory ducts such as stricture due to the median cyst of the prostate and allows one to count the volume of the seminal vesicles, where their dilatation suggests obstruction in the ejaculatory ducts. Seminal vesicles agenesis, similar to vas deferens agenesis, indicates the presence of the CFTR gene and further investigation is needed in such cases [4, 9, 10].

The evaluation of the full infertile patient also includes hormonal level tests (e.g. high levels of follicle stimulating hormone (FSH) and luteinising hormone (LH) with a low testosterone level refer to hypergonadotropic hypogonadism suggesting gonadal dysgenesis) and genetic testing (chromosomal abnormalities—sex chromosome as well as autosomal, cystic fibrosis gene mutations—e.g. the most common microdeletions of F508 'Y' spermatogenesis gene—AZFa, AZFb, AZFc, aneuploidy in sperm or particularly sex chromosome aneuploidy) [11–14].

3. Treatment options

The management of fertility disorders depends on their cause. As previously mentioned, the aetiology of infertility is complex, therefore only a correct, precise evaluation of the patient and extended diagnostic process is needed. Generally, treatment options can be divided into invasive and conservative.

The conservative approach first includes lifestyle changes. Male fertility is undoubtedly positively correlated with a healthy lifestyle and overall human well-being. There is some evidence in the literature that increased body mass index (BMI), excessive alcohol consumption and smoking have a negative impact on semen quality [15, 16]. Observational studies report that men with obesity, after loss of 17.2–25.4% of body weight, have an improvement in semen volume, total sperm count, testosterone level and sperm morphology than before [17]. Moreover, moderate physical activity has a positive effect on sperm concentration and progressive motility [18]. Moderate swimming exercises in the pool can not only lower the scrotal temperature (especially in the case of varicoceles) and thus positively influence spermatogenesis, but also reduce the species of oxidative stress in the testes, which was confirmed experimentally [19]. The most effective obesity treatment is bariatric surgery, which, on the one hand, provokes a 6-month lasting reduction in sperm concentration and, on the other, normalises the levels of reproductive hormones and improves general quality of life [20, 21]. In summary, lifestyle changes should be promoted in all male patients with fertility disorders regardless of the cause.

When it comes to conservative treatment, apart from lifestyle changes, hormonal therapy should be considered. Fertility problems may reflect the malfunction of the hypothalamic–pituitary-gonadal (HPG) axis, which is responsible for the regulation of the main testicular functions: spermatogenesis and testosterone production. The HPG axis controls FSH and LH secretion and maintains the proper level of testosterone in male gonads. LH acts on Leydig cells that release testosterone. Intratesticular testosterone, together with FSH, stimulates Sertoli cells to demarcate the wall of the seminiferous tubules, which allows the development of male germ cells. However, in men with normal levels of reproductive hormones, exogenous administration of testosterone and other androgens has a negative impact on spermatogenesis because it inhibits negative feedback of lower testosterone levels, which normally enhances LH secretion on the HPG axis. In this situation, through suppression of LH, endogenous intratesticular testosterone production is reduced [22, 23]. HPG axis disorders can also be a result of different systemic or neoplastic diseases along with pharmaceutical therapies. Depending on which level of HPG axis secretion we want to boost or suppress, different hormonal treatments are implemented. In the treatment of male infertility caused by the inability of hypothalamus hormones to secrete (hypogonadotropic hypogonadism), the agents used primarily are gonadotropin-releasing hormone (GnRH), gonadotropins. The other group, dopamine agonists, is administered to patients with hyperprolactinaemia as a result of pituitary gland prolactinoma [23]. Aromatase inhibitors, which lower oestrogen levels, are used especially in obese infertile men with oligozoospermia or azoospermia. In such patients, peripheral hormonal conversion from androgens to oestrogens in fatty tissue is enhanced, leading to HPG axis malfunction. Selective oestrogen receptor modulators (SERMs) are drugs that act as agonist or antagonist. For example, clomifene citrate increases hypophysical LH and FSH secretion, which also contributes to an improvement in testosterone level. SERMs are one of the applicable treatment options for idiopathic fertility [23, 24].

There are some suggestions in the literature that ROS formation and sperm DNA fragmentation can be reduced by antioxidants. It seems that they can be useful in patients with abnormally high ROS levels and DNA fragmentation. However, according to the EAU 2023 Guidelines, the role played by both of them is still unclear, because there are not sufficient data to demonstrate their therapeutic effect [4, 23].

Invasive management of male infertility comprises procedures that improve semen parameters (like varicocele correction) together with direct sperm collection from the testicle on biopsy (in case of obstructive azoospermia). Few methods of sperm retrieval evolved over the years. The retrieved sperm from this procedure can be used, after special preparation, for intracytoplasmic sperm injection (ICSI). Testicular fine-needle aspiration (TfNA) is a percutaneous insertion of the needle into the gonad under local anaesthesia. It is characterised by low costs and less tissue injury. In testicular sperm aspiration (TESA), sperm retrieval is also performed percutaneously but with a large needle (40 × 12 mm). Sperm are aspirated with the use of negative pressure created by the syringe. This procedure usually requires intravenous anaesthesia and a longer recovery (up to 24 h) but has low complication rates. Conventional testicular sperm extraction (c -TESE) is single or multiple open testicular biopsies. Samples are examined immediately after the procedure under the microscope in the laboratory. The c-TESE is fast, relatively inexpensive, and has a higher retrieval rate than the previously presented ones, but it injures testicular vascularisation and testicular tissue that may permanently or temporarily lower testosterone level. Unlike c-TESE that is performed without magnification, microdissection testicular sperm extraction (micro-TESE) is a similar procedure but carried out with the use of a microscope and a microsurgical technique during preparation to detect seminiferous tubules with greater probability of sperm in their lumen. Micro-TESE is recommended in men with non-obstructive azoospermia with an unfavourable prognosis. It has a high retrieval rate and microscopic dissection minimises testicular tissue damage. However, it is characterised by the highest costs among all sperm retrieval techniques. Open testicular mapping (OTEM) is the newest technique that involves a scrotal incision and multiple testicular punctures with a 19-G needle and syringe aspiration. The samples are then analysed under the microscope with 400× magnification to check the spermatozoa presence. If there is a lack of them in the samples, the next punctures are made. The advantage of OTEM is that there is no need for a surgical microscope and microsurgical skills along with not as extensive tissue damage as in c-TESE. This approach is a combination of two methods; it incorporates minimal invasion of micro-TESE and low costs of c-TESE [25–27].

4. Possible impact of inguinal hernia repair on fertility

Possible fertility problems after inguinal hernia repair surgery can be divided into iatrogenic vas deferens damage and inflammatory due to mesh placement.

Injury related to vas deferens may be the result of ligation, cauterisation, interruption of continuity by accidental intersection or microdamage due to intense pulling of the sperm cord. Vas deferens can also be exposed to compression and tension from tight non-mesh herniorrhaphy or scars formed by mesh insertions in hernioplasty. These factors contribute to vas deferens obstruction (or discontinuation in the case of incision), which could be reflected as oligozoospermia or azoospermia in semen analysis. The obstruction seems not only to appear early after surgery and expand to normal lumen as a result of tissue recovery after direct vas deferens damage but can also be late-onset due to the formation of adjacent tissue scars. In addition, early-onset obstruction due to severe and extensive vas deferens damage may be permanent. Paediatric and infant patients are more susceptible to vas deferens damage due to its immature tissues, which results in less strength of its wall.

Mesh inserted in hernioplasty involves an inflammatory fibroblastic reaction of the monofilaments of the foreign body with adjacent tissue, strengthening the inferior wall of the inguinal canal to prevent future inguinal hernias. When the spermatic cord adheres strictly to the mesh, vas deferens and its vascularization can be involved in scar formation, which can lead to damage due to its wall inflammation and hyperplasia, as well as impaired blood perfusion. Visible vas deferens injury can be corrected during surgery, but most damages do not appear to be detectable during herniorrhaphy or hernioplasty and this could be a reason for underestimation and underdiagnosis.

In case of postoperative suspicion of obstruction, the check of vas deferens patency and the level of eventual narrowing can be done by vasography, which is, however, an invasive examination. The patient could choose, under favourable anatomical conditions and a high probability of success of the procedure, whether to undertake an attempt at his vas deferens reconstruction by a surgeon or to immediately opt for a testicular biopsy to obtain sperm for ICSI. Reconstruction of vas deferens in injuries due to inguinal hernia repair performed in childhood and manifesting later as oligo/azoospermia in adulthood is possible, but not always successful in more extended defects with impaired blood supply and secondary epididymal loss of patency, which developed over years in such cases. Sperm should be collected during reconstruction surgery. Among these men, the reconstruction attempt of vas deferens, in case of its failure, is paired with direct sperm aspiration and then cryopreservation for future ICSI [28–32].

The impact of inguinal hernia surgery on male fertility is one of the controversial issues concerning the implications of surgical intervention within the inguinal canal on the quality of sperm and male sexual activity. The potential impact of hernioplasty on fertility was first reported at the end of the twentieth century and the beginning of the twenty-first century. To date, published research results have analysed a wide variety of aspects of fertility assessment and external genitalia function. An additional aspect that makes an unambiguous assessment difficult is the development of surgical techniques (non-mesh versus mesh surgery, open versus laparoscopic approach and different types of materials used in tension-free surgery). Authors investigating the impact of inguinal hernia surgery on male fertility have hitherto evaluated various parameters, including testicular volume, testicular perfusion based on vascular resistive index values, sex hormone values, semen analysis and anti-sperm antibody (ASA) level.

4.1 Animal study

Few experimental studies in animals have shown that polypropylene mesh used in hernia repair stimulates a foreign body reaction that can lead to the encapsulation of spermatic cord structures and is postulated to cause symptoms of dysejaculation and genital pain during sexual activity with deleterious effects on patient sexual functions and quality of life [33]. Peiper et al. based on the results of experimental studies in the pig and rabbit reported that implantation of a polypropylene mesh in the inguinal region induces a major response of the structures of the spermatic cord, which may also influence spermatogenesis [34]. Uzzo et al. reported the effect of mesh implantation on the spermatic cord structures in a canine model including histological evaluation of the spermatic cord following surgery. The authors found dysfunction in the external genitalia in three out of six dogs operated with mesh; furthermore, the size of the vessel lumen in the cross-sectional section was significantly reduced with a marked foreign-body reaction of the soft tissue identified after mesh repair. A post-traumatic neuroma was identified suggesting nerve entrapment in the fibrous branch of the mesh, which may be the culprit in the postoperative pain observed in some patients [35]. In another animal model study, a histopathological alteration of the vas deferens was evaluated in rats exposed to polypropylene mesh. The authors reported that polypropylene mesh induces a foreign-body reaction, with histological changes in the vas deferens that cause functional obstruction, with dilatation and spermatozoid repression [36]. Contrary to these results, Damous et al. published results of an experimental study in rats after surgery with the use of bilateral polypropylene mesh. On the basis of the results, the mesh placement did not alter the morphology of the vas deferens in any of the analysed segments. The authors concluded that surgery, with or without mesh placement, did not alter morphology, wall thickness or lumen area [37]. A separate issue related to the consequences of mesh implantation in the region of the spermatic cord on an animal model was the evaluation of the effect of mesh bioprosthesis in inguinal hernia repair on testicular nitric oxide metabolism and apoptosis in rat testis. The authors reported that long-term polypropylene mesh implantation has no effect on testicular hormonal function and only a limited effect on nitric oxide levels and this effect is not sufficient to cause apoptosis in the testis that could lead to infertility [38].

4.2 Human study

4.2.1 Laparoscopic versus open surgery hernia repair

Singh et al. in randomised controlled trial (RCT) compared testicular dysfunction, incidence and factors that influence chronic groin pain, and quality of life after open mesh and laparoscopic repair. A significant decrease in testicular volume was observed and less improvement in blood flow after open repair. There was also a significant reduction in serum testosterone level with a significant increase in FSH and LH level; however, there was no testicular atrophy. The incidence and severity of chronic groin pain were significantly lower after laparoscopic repair during normal and strenuous activities, although they were similar to those after open repair during rest after 3 months postoperatively [39]. In another trial, Abkulut et al. compared changes in testis volume and sex hormone levels after inguinal hernia repair (Lichtenstein vs. laparoscopic totally extraperitoneal (TEP) hernia repair techniques). Neither the Lichtenstein nor the TEP method could affect LH, FSH, and testosterone values, but TEP could lead to a decreasing effect on testis volume, but within normal limits [40]. Immunological factor is considered another potential factor that may affect fertility after mesh hernia surgery. In the general male fertile population, the positivity of ASAs is estimated to be between 0.9 and 4% [41]. Eight to ten percentage of infertile patients have immunological infertility. The effect that autoimmunization causes on the various passages of fertility is still under discussion. First of all, ASAs are supposed to cause poor penetration into cervical mucus. The conception rate in infertile couples with antibodies is almost 40% lower than in the group without antibodies. Damage to the vas deferens, testicular ischemia, and inflammatory reaction to the mesh may be possible causes of sperm antigen intolerance. In the study by Stula et al., the quantitative value of antisperm antibodies (ASA) in serum was analysed after hernia repair. After the operation, the ASA increased in most of the patients but remained in the normal range. The ASA value increased significantly by an average of 13.5% in the group of patients who were operated with the open technique. In the group of patients who underwent laparoscopic surgery, no significant change in the value of ASA was found postoperatively. In the concluding study, inguinal hernia mesh repair does not have a clinically significant influence on the immunological response [42]. Goupta et al. presented suitable results in a randomised three-arm study comparing open mesh hernioplasty, laparoscopic totally extraperitoneal (TEP) and transabdominal preperitoneal (TAPP) repair of the groin hernia and antisperm antibodies (ASA) levels increased after surgery in the study population, which reached statistical significance. On the contrary, patients undergoing open mesh hernioplasty showed a significant increase in ASA compared to preoperative values. In the TAPP and TEP groups, there was no significant increase in ASA in the postoperative period after 3 months. However, all these values were within the normal range of antisperm antibodies [43]. Negri et al. in their study investigated the influence of inguinal hernia repair on sperm autoimmunity. This retrospective study includes all infertile male patients with a history of unilateral or bilateral inguinal hernia surgery repair who underwent mixed antiglobulin reaction tests. Antisperm antibodies would appear to increase in patients who performed groin hernia surgery 2.45 (95% confidence interval: 1.01–5.99; $p < 0.05$) times more than in the unselected infertile population. The authors concluded that the MAR test could be useful in patients who have undergone previous hernia surgery, to avoid false unexplained infertility diagnoses and to direct the couple to assisted reproductive technology procedures [44].

4.2.2 Laparoscopic totally extra peritoneal (TEP) versus transabdominal preperitoneal (TAPP) hernia repair

Bansal et al. suggested no changes in testis and sexual function after TAPP compared to TEP. According to the report, changes in male fertility are not related to the techniques used in TAPP or TEP. However, the authors considered that hands-on ligation of spermatic cord structures during the procedure may alter the aetiology of testicular dysfunction after open mesh repair [45]. A prospective randomised study of sexual function and semen analysis following TEP and TAPP inguinal hernia repair showed that both methods are comparable in terms of sexual function and effect on semen analysis. Antisperm antibody levels were insignificant both preoperatively and 3 months postoperatively in the study population and there was no significant difference between the two methods [46]. Based on the study by Gupta et al., most of the parameters of semen analysis improved significantly from preoperative to post-TEP or post-TAPP period. Semen volume, total sperm concentration, sperm count, and vitality improved significantly during the postoperative period at 3 months. However, progressive motility decreased slightly. Non-progressive motility did not show any change from the preoperative to postoperative period. On comparison of the laparoscopy approach (TAPP + TEP) vs. open, no parameter showed any statistically significant difference [43].

4.2.3 Lightweight versus heavyweight mesh for inguinal hernia repair

Patients operated on with a lightweight mesh (VyproII® or TiMesh®) exhibited a decreased sperm motility compared with heavyweight mesh (Marlex®) patients, respectively −9.5% and − 5.5% versus +2%. When the results after uni- and bilateral hernia repair were analysed separately, this difference only remained significant in the bilateral hernia subgroup: −10% for VyproII® and − 17% for TiMesh® versus +1% for Marlex®. The authors concluded that the use of lightweight meshes for laparoscopic inguinal hernia repair in male patients negatively influences sperm motility, without any benefit on quality of life [47]. Peeters et al. in a forthcoming study analysed the effects of lightweight meshes on laparoscopic repair of inguinal hernia on male fertility aspects, at 3-year follow-up. They did not report significant differences between the percentage of lightweight mesh (VyproII® and TiMesh®) versus Marlex® patients with a decreased sperm motility or concentration at 3 years of follow-up (−8.5% and −8% vs. −2.8%, respectively). Furthermore, no significant changes were observed in the number of patients with decreased sperm motility or concentration 3 years after surgery compared to 1 year after operatively [48].

4.2.4 Non-mesh versus mesh inguinal hernia repair

Based on Kordzadeh et al. pooled analysis, sperm motility could be affected following the inguinal hernia repair technique, but this is limited to the immediate postoperative period (<48 h). Obstructive azoospermia was observed in 0.03% of open hernia and 2.5% of bilateral mesh laparoscopic hernia repair. Male infertility was detected in 0.8% of open hernia repair (mesh) with no correlation to the type of mesh. The authors concluded that the repair of the inguinal hernia without mesh has no impact on male fertility and obstructive azoospermia [49].

Dong et al. in systemic review investigated 29 related trials with a total of 36,552 patients, including 7 randomised controlled trials (RCTs) with 616 patients and 10 clinical trials (1230 patients) with mesh or non-mesh repairs. They suggested that mesh hernia repair in an open or laparoscopic procedure has no significant effect on male fertility [50].

5. Conclusions

Undoubtedly, infertility, due to the increase in its prevalence in the population in recent years, has become one of the civilisation diseases. Therefore, of great importance is the identification of the causes of this disease.

There were theories of a negative impact on male fertility by inguinal hernia repair surgery. However, most of the research results available so far have not confirmed that hernioplasty procedures contribute to male infertility. Evidence is inevitably difficult to reach because of a wide range of causes of infertility and their complexity. However, the choice of method and the possible impact on fertility are worth discussing with the patient before surgery. Furthermore, preoperative and postoperative semen analysis will help exclude or confirm its impact on patient fertility in the future.

The role of surgeon during procedure is to raise awareness of the possibility of vas deferens injury and obstruction formation, which can be avoided by delicate and careful mobilisation of the spermatic cord without grasping, exposure to coagulation and any additional compression. Although there is no proof of whether any kind of mesh negatively impacts male fertility, obstruction of the vas deferens due to fibroblastic scar formation may be taken into account in follow-up in case of poor results of the semen analysis. Prevention may be achieved by avoiding excessive spermatic cord compression by the mesh to reduce the development of pathologic tissue adhesions.

Conflict of interest

The author declares no conflict of interest.

Author details

Krzysztof Balawender[1,2*] and Anna Pliszka[1,2]

1 Clinical Department of Urology and Urological Oncology, Municipal Hospital in Rzeszow, Rzeszów, Poland

2 Department of Normal and Clinical Anatomy, Institute of Medical Sciences, Medical College of Rzeszow University, Rzeszów, Poland

*Address all correspondence to: balawender82@gmail.comx

References

[1] Infertility Prevalence Estimates, 1990-2021. Geneva: World Health Organization; 2023 Licence: CC BY-NC-SA 3.0 IGO

[2] Agarwal A, Mulgund A, Hamada A, Chyatte MR. A unique view on male infertility around the globe. Reproductive Biology and Endocrinology. 2015;**13**:37. Published 2015 Apr 26. DOI: 10.1186/s12958-015-0032-1

[3] Agarwal A, Parekh N, Panner Selvam MK, et al. Male oxidative stress infertility (MOSI): Proposed terminology and clinical practice guidelines for Management of Idiopathic Male Infertility. World Journal of Men's Health. 2019;**37**(3):296-312. DOI: 10.5534/wjmh.190055

[4] EAU Guidelines. Edn. presented at the EAU Annual Congress Milan 2023. ISBN 978-94-92671-19-6

[5] Pozzi E, Ramasamy R, Salonia A. Initial Andrological evaluation of the infertile male. European Urology Focus. 2023;**9**(1):51-54. DOI: 10.1016/j.euf.2022.09.012

[6] Li R, Liu J, Li Y, Wang Q. Effect of somatometric parameters on the prevalence and severity of varicocele: A systematic review and meta-analysis. Reproductive Biology and Endocrinology. 2021;**19**(1):11. Published 2021 Jan 20. DOI: 10.1186/s12958-021-00695-3

[7] WHO Laboratory Manual for the Examination and Processing of Human Semen. sixth ed. Geneva: World Health Organization; 2021 Licence: CC BY-NC-SA 3.0 IGO

[8] Campbell MJ, Lotti F, Baldi E, et al. Distribution of semen examination results 2020 - a follow up of data collated for the WHO semen analysis manual 2010. Andrology. 2021;**9**(3):817-822. DOI: 10.1111/andr.12983

[9] Lotti F, Maggi M. Ultrasound of the male genital tract in relation to male reproductive health. Human Reproduction Update. 2015;**21**(1):56-83. DOI: 10.1093/humupd/dmu042

[10] Schurich M, Aigner F, Frauscher F, Pallwein L. The role of ultrasound in assessment of male fertility. European Journal of Obstetrics, Gynecology, and Reproductive Biology. 2009;**144** (Suppl. 1):S192-S198. DOI: 10.1016/j.ejogrb.2009.02.034

[11] Martin-du-Pan RC, Bischof P. Increased follicle stimulating hormone in infertile men. Is increased plasma FSH always due to damaged germinal epithelium? Human Reproduction. 1995;**10**(8):1940-1945. DOI: 10.1093/oxfordjournals.humrep.a136211

[12] Krausz C, Hoefsloot L, Simoni M, Tüttelmann F, European Academy of Andrology; European Molecular Genetics Quality Network. EAA/EMQN best practice guidelines for molecular diagnosis of Y-chromosomal microdeletions: State-of-the-art 2013. Andrology. 2014;**2**(1):5-19. DOI: 10.1111/j.2047-2927.2013.00173.x

[13] Jensen CFS, Fode M, Østergren PB, Sønksen J. A refined view on the association between Y-chromosome microdeletions and sperm concentration. European Urology. 2019;**76**(5):637-638. DOI: 10.1016/j.eururo.2019.08.015

[14] Savant A, Lyman B, Bojanowski C, Upadia J. Cystic fibrosis. In: Adam MP,

Mirzaa GM, Pagon RA, et al., editors. GeneReviews®. Seattle (WA): University of Washington, Seattle; 2001

[15] Sharma A, Minhas S, Dhillo WS, Jayasena CN. Male infertility due to testicular disorders. The Journal of Clinical Endocrinology and Metabolism. 2021;**106**(2):e442-e459. DOI: 10.1210/clinem/dgaa781

[16] Fedder J, Carlsen E, Jørgensen N, Jensen CFS. Ugeskrift for Laeger. 2021;**183**(48):V05210402

[17] Håkonsen LB, Thulstrup AM, Aggerholm AS, et al. Does weight loss improve semen quality and reproductive hormones? Results from a cohort of severely obese men. Reproductive Health. 2011;**8**:24. Published 2011 Aug 17. DOI: 10.1186/1742-4755-8-24

[18] Ibañez-Perez J, Santos-Zorrozua B, Lopez-Lopez E, Matorras R, Garcia-Orad A. An update on the implication of physical activity on semen quality: A systematic review and meta-analysis. Archives of Gynecology and Obstetrics. 2019;**299**(4):901-921. DOI: 10.1007/s00404-019-05045-8

[19] Osváth P, Szűcs M, Börzsei D, et al. Andrological aspects of exercise: Moderate swimming protects against isoproterenol induced testis and semen abnormalities in rats. Antioxidants (Basel). 2022;**11**(3):436. Published 2022 Feb 22. DOI: 10.3390/antiox11030436

[20] Wei Y, Chen Q, Qian W. Effect of bariatric surgery on semen parameters: A systematic review and Meta-analysis. Medical Science Monitor Basic Research. 2018;**24**:188-197. Published 2018 Nov 12. DOI: 10.12659/MSMBR.910862

[21] Legro RS, Kunselman AR, Meadows JW, et al. Time-related increase in urinary testosterone levels and stable semen analysis parameters after bariatric surgery in men. Reproductive Biomedicine Online. 2015;**30**(2):150-156. DOI: 10.1016/j.rbmo.2014.10.014

[22] Oduwole OO, Huhtaniemi IT, Misrahi M. The roles of luteinizing hormone, follicle-stimulating hormone and testosterone in spermatogenesis and Folliculogenesis revisited. International Journal of Molecular Sciences. 2021;**22**(23):12735. DOI: 10.3390/ijms222312735

[23] Dabaja AA, Schlegel PN. Medical treatment of male infertility. Translational Andrology and Urology. 2014;**3**(1):9-16. DOI: 10.3978/j.issn.2223-4683.2014.01.06

[24] Wheeler KM, Sharma D, Kavoussi PK, Smith RP, Costabile R. Clomiphene citrate for the treatment of hypogonadism. Sexual Medicine Reviews. 2019;**7**(2):272-276. DOI: 10.1016/j.sxmr.2018.10.001

[25] Vieira M, Bispo de Andrade MA, Santana-Santos E. Is testicular microdissection the only way to retrieve sperm for non-obstructive azoospermic men?. Front. Reproductive Health. 2022;**4**:980824. Published 2022 Aug 23. DOI: 10.3389/frph.2022.980824

[26] Vieira M, Glina FPA, Mizrahi FE, Mierzwa TC, Glina S. Open testicular mapping: A less invasive multiple biopsy approach for testicular sperm extraction. Andrologia. 2020;**52**(4):e13547. DOI: 10.1111/and.13547

[27] Rosellen J, Steffens J, Kranz J. Testikuläre Spermienextraktion bei männlicher Infertilität : Indikationen, Erfolgsraten, praktische Durchführung und mögliche Komplikationen [testicular sperm extraction in male infertility : Indications, success rates, practical implementation,

and possible complications]. Urologe A. 2021;**60**(7):921-931. DOI: 10.1007/s00120-021-01480-1

[28] Bouchot O, Branchereau J, Perrouin-Verbe MA. Influence of inguinal hernia repair on male fertility. Journal of Visceral Surgery. 2018;**155**(Suppl 1):S37-S40. DOI: 10.1016/j.jviscsurg.2018.04.008

[29] Yamaguchi K, Ishikawa T, Nakano Y, Kondo Y, Shiotani M, Fujisawa M. Rapidly progressing, late-onset obstructive azoospermia linked to herniorrhaphy with mesh. Fertility and Sterili. 2008;**90**(5):2018.e5-2018.e7. DOI: 10.1016/j.fertnstert.2008.04.062

[30] Shin D, Lipshultz LI, Goldstein M, et al. Herniorrhaphy with polypropylene mesh causing inguinal vasal obstruction: A preventable cause of obstructive azoospermia. Annals of Surgery. 2005;**241**(4):553-558. DOI: 10.1097/01.sla.0000157318.13975.2a

[31] Flechner L, Smith J, Treseler P, Maa J. Vasal injury during inguinal herniorrhaphy: A case report and review of the literature. The Permanente Journal. 2014;**18**(4):85-88. DOI: 10.7812/TPP/14-073

[32] Zhao J, Zhai XQ, Li HC, Chong T. High ligation of the hernia sac in open nonmesh inguinal herniorrhaphy is an important cause of iatrogenic vas deferens injury [published online ahead of print, 2023 Apr 28]. Asian Journal of Andrology. 2023;**25**:1-5. DOI: 10.4103/aja202312

[33] Tekatli H, Schouten N, van Dalen T, Burgmans I, Smakman N. Mechanism, assessment, and incidence of male infertility after inguinal hernia surgery: A review of the preclinical and clini- cal literature. American Journal of Surgery. 2012;**204**(4):503-509

[34] Peiper C, Junge K, Klinge U, Strehlau E, Ottinger A, Schumpelick V. Is there a risk of infertility after inguinal mesh repair? Experimental studies in the pig and the rabbit. Hernia. 2006;**10**(1):7-12. DOI: 10.1007/s10029-005-0055-1

[35] Uzzo RG, Lemack GE, Morrissey KP, Goldstein M. The effects of mesh bioprosthesis on the spermatic cord structures: A preliminary report in a canine model. The Journal of Urology. 1999;**161**(4):1344-1349

[36] Maciel LC, Glina S, Palma PC, Nascimento LF, Netto NR Jr. Histopathological alterations of the vas deferens in rats exposed to polypropylene mesh [published correction appears in BJU Int. 2007 Aug;100(2):481. Costa, Nascimento F C [corrected to Nascimento, Luiz F C]]. BJU International. 2007;**100**(1):187-190. DOI: 10.1111/j.1464-410X.2007.06782.x

[37] Damous SHB, Damous LL, Miranda JDS, Montero EFS, Birolini C, Utiyama EM. Does a bilateral polypropylene mesh alter the duct deferens morphology, testicular size and testosterone levels? Experimental study in rats. Acta Cirúrgica Brasileira. 2020;**35**(2):e202000201. DOI: 10.1590/s0102-865020200020000001

[38] Taneli F, Aydede H, Vatansever S, Ulman C, Ari Z, Uyanik BS. The long-term effect of mesh bioprosthesis in inguinal hernia repair on testicular nitric oxide metabolism and apoptosis in rat testis. Cell Biochemistry and Function. 2005;**23**(3):213-220. DOI: 10.1002/cbf.1139

[39] Singh AN, Bansal VK, Misra MC, et al. Testicular functions, chronic groin pain, and quality of life after laparoscopic and open mesh repair of inguinal hernia: A prospective randomized controlled trial. Surgical

Endoscopy. 2012;**26**(5):1304-1317. DOI: 10.1007/s00464-011-2029-y

[40] Akbulut G, Serteser M, Yücel A, et al. Can laparoscopic hernia repair alter function and volume of testis? Randomized clinical trial. Surgical Laparoscopy, Endoscopy & Percutaneous Techniques. 2003;**13**(6):377-381. DOI: 10.1097/00129689-200312000-00006], 10.1097/00129689-200312000-00006]

[41] Bronson RA. Antisperm antibodies: a critical evaluation and clinical guidelines. Journal of Reproductive Immunology. 1999;**45**:159-183

[42] Stula I, Družijanić N, Sršen D, et al. Influence of inguinal hernia mesh repair on testicular flow and sperm autoimmunity. Hernia. 2012;**16**(4):417-424. DOI: 10.1007/s10029-012-0918-

[43] Gupta S, Krishna A, Jain M, et al. A three-arm randomized study to compare sexual functions and fertility indices following open mesh hernioplasty (OMH), laparoscopic totally extra peritoneal (TEP) and transabdominal preperitoneal (TAPP) repair of groin hernia. Surgical Endoscopy. 2021;**35**(6):3077-3084. DOI: 10.1007/s00464-020-07697-

[44] Negri L, Romano M, Cirillo F, et al. Influence of inguinal hernia repair on sperm autoimmunity: The largest single center experience. Andrology. 2022;**10**:105-110. DOI: 10.1111/andr.1308

[45] Bansal VK, Krishna A, Manek P, Kumar S, Prajapati O, Subramaniam R, et al. A prospective randomized comparison of testicular functions, sexual functions and quality of life following laparoscopic totally extra-peritoneal (TEP) and trans-abdominal pre- peritoneal (TAPP) inguinal hernia repairs. Surgical Endoscopy. 2017;**31**(3):1478-1486

[46] Asuri K, Mohammad A, Prajapati OP, et al. A prospective randomized comparison of sexual function and semen analysis following laparoscopic totally extraperitoneal (TEP) and transabdominal pre-peritoneal (TAPP) inguinal hernia repair. Surgical Endoscopy. 2021;**35**(6):2936-2941. DOI: 10.1007/s00464-020-07733-y

[47] Peeters E, Spiessens C, Oyen R, et al. Laparoscopic inguinal hernia repair in men with lightweight meshes may significantly impair sperm motility: A randomized controlled trial. Annals of Surgery. 2010;**252**(2):240-246. DOI: 10.1097/SLA.0b013e3181e8fac5

[48] Peeters E, Spiessens C, Oyen R, et al. Sperm motility after laparoscopic inguinal hernia repair with lightweight meshes: 3-year follow-up of a randomised clinical trial. Hernia. 2014;**18**(3):361-367. DOI: 10.1007/s10029-012-1028-9

[49] Kordzadeh A, Liu MO, Jayanthi NV. Male infertility following inguinal hernia repair: A systematic review and pooled analysis. Hernia. 2017;**21**(1):1-7. DOI: 10.1007/s10029-016-1560-0

[50] Dong Z, Kujawa SA, Wang C, Zhao H. Does the use of hernia mesh in surgical inguinal hernia repairs cause male infertility? A systematic review and descriptive analysis. Reproductive Health. 2018;**15**(1):69. DOI: 10.1186/s12978-018-0510-y

Chapter 16

Parastomal Hernia – Latest Knowledge and Approach

Omar Alhafidh

Abstract

Parastomal hernia is developed after the creation of a stoma which happens after bowel resection or diversion. With the developed screening program for bowel cancer and its related surgeries, a lot of stomas have been done and its complications including parastomal hernias appeared. At the same time, its diagnosis is well developed with the advancement of imaging techniques, but unfortunately, there is no standard treatment for the repair. It is noticed that each surgeon deals with the PSH with their own experience as there is no strong evidence or standard approach, with most of the PSH patients treated conservatively till they reach a big size or develop other complications. A lot of effort was spent on the primary prevention of PSH and still under trial. Considering evidence-based medicine, the best way to deal with PSH is to be tailored to the patient's extent of complaint, which is determined by the surgeon's experience. It is estimated that third of these patients are treated surgically, and this is due to the high recurrence rate that makes surgeons try to avoid surgical correction. In this chapter, we will try to cover the latest update about the diagnosis, complications and repair techniques.

Keywords: parastomal hernia, colorectal surgery, fascial repair, stoma relocation, mesh repair

1. Introduction

Parastomal hernia is a form of incisional hernia because it happens in a surgical incision and is considered one of the most complications that happen after stoma formation [1]. In this complication, part of the intraabdominal viscera protrudes through the same opening of the stoma surrounded by a hernia sac [2].

Earlier in 1973 Devlin put a classification based on four types of hernia [3]:

type I—integumentary (the so-called true parastomal hernia); type II—subcutaneous; type III—intra-stomal; and type IV—pseudo-pre-stomal.

From this classification, we notice that not all parastomal deformities are PSH and this makes it difficult in treating different abnormalities and made this classification weak and difficult to implement [4].

As a result, two more classifications had been proposed with the aid of the CT scan by Moreno-Matias in 2009 [5] and Seo in 2011 [6] and another one by Szczepkowski in 2011 based on clinical examination of the hernia [6, 7].

Moreno-Matias in 2009 and Seo in 2011	Szczepkowski 2011
0—CT image normal, peritoneum follows the wall of the bowel forming the stoma, with no formation of a sac	I—isolated, small parastomal hernia
Ia—bowel forming the colostomy with a sac of under 5 cm	II—small parastomal hernia with coexisting midline incisional hernia without any significant front abdominal wall deformity
Ib—bowel forming the colostomy with a sac of over 5 cm	III—isolated, large parastomal hernia with front abdominal wall deformity
II—sac containing omentum	IV—large parastomal hernia with coexisting midline incisional hernia, with front abdominal wall deformity
III—sac containing an intestinal loop other than the bowel forming the stoma	

Table 1.
Moreno-Matias and Seo vs. Szczepkowski classification.

None of these classifications had been used in clinical trials so they lack the evidence and because only Szczepkowski considered the presence of an incisional hernia which is needed for the repair together with the PSH but requires more accurate measure than the clinical examination which can be achieved by the CT scan; for this reason, the European Hernia Society (EHS) in 2014 had published a new classification based on Szczepkowski classification to be the standard for evidence-based therapeutic guidelines (**Table 1**). The European Hernia Society Subclasses of classification were defined as follows:

- type I—PSH is less than 5 cm in diameter without coexisting incisional hernia.
- type II—PSH is less than 5 cm in diameter with coexisting incisional hernia.
- type III—PSH is larger than 5 cm in diameter without coexisting incisional hernia.
- type IV—PSH is larger than 5 cm in diameter with coexisting incisional hernia.

The coexisting incisional hernia is in the previous scar.

Additionally, in each type of PSH one should note whether it is primary (labelled P) or recurrent (labelled R), This classification should be aided with a CT scan to help for accurate measurement of the defect [8].

2. Epidemiology

PSHs usually develop in the first year after its creation; however, the incidence increases in the following years up to twenty years. It has been noticed that in colostomy the incidence in the first year is 30%, becoming 40% in two years and 50% in three years to reach 76% in twenty years [9, 10].

The hernia development is influenced by the ageing process of the muscles with increasing risk each year by 4% [Odds ratio—1.04; $p = 0.4$] [11].

Global data shows that the incidence of PSH is related to the specific type of stomas is as follows:

- end colostomy—4.0–48.1% (mean: 15.3%),
- loop colostomy—0.0–30.8% (mean: 4.0%),
- end ileostomy—1.8–28.3% (mean: 6.7%),
- loop ileostomy—0.0–6.2% (mean: 1.3%) [11–13].

The risk factors for developing PSH are as follows:

1. Age: Above 60 years. The most important factor is statistically significant.
2. Obesity (BMI > 30 kg/m^2).
3. Waist size (>10 cm).
4. ASA classification (>2).
5. Smoking.
6. Diabetes mellitus.
7. Physical labour.
8. Chronic cough.
9. COPD (chronic obstructive pulmonary disease).
10. Immune disorders.
11. Steroid therapy.
12. Cancer.
13. Ischaemia.
14. Crohn's disease.
15. Disorders involving collagen metabolism.

All these apart from age are non-statistically significantly linked to PSH [14–17].

The site of the stoma was claimed to be a risk factor for the development of PSH but there is a meta-analysis of 24 publications shows that the incidence of PSH is not affected by the relation to the rectus abdominis muscle; for example, the percentage of stomas formed through the rectus abdominis muscle versus adjacent to the muscle is as follows: 3% vs. 22% [18], 37% vs. 33% [19], 52% vs. 46% [20].

Another problem that most of surgeons are worried about is the high recurrence rate after corrective surgery, and it can be summarised as follows:

- after surgery with stoma transposition—0–76.2% (mean: 24.3%),
- after mesh plasty—0–33.3% (mean: 2.9%),
- simple tissue plasty—46–100% (mean: 64.9%) [17]

After corrective surgery, the risk of recurrence is [21]:
radiological recurrence ($p = 0.05$):

- with mesh—22%,
- without mesh—45%;

clinical recurrence ($p < 0.001$):

- with mesh—13%,
- without mesh—80%

As PSH is associated with a high incidence of development, there are certain measures that can be implemented to reduce the risk, these include [22, 23]:

- Good preoperative assessment.
- Identification of the risks that had been mentioned above.
- Checking for any collagen metabolism disorders.
- Weight reduction programme.
- Stop smoking for at least 2 months prior to elective procedures.
- Encourage physical activities.
- Counselling with the stoma nurse and marking the area that is suitable for the patient.

3. Clinical presentation

The most common presentation for PSH is a deformity, lack of symmetry and bulging of the abdominal wall especially on straining. However, the main bothering symptoms are discomfort and poor fitting of the stoma appliance that makes it leak especially at night [22, 23].

Another important complaint is the psychological problem as the patient starts to have accidents and is afraid of ongoing enlargement of the hernia [23].

As with other hernias, acute complications like strangulation or obstruction can be encountered but are rare, and it usually started with obstruction and then develops into strangulation, which is difficult to diagnose and treat [1].

4. Diagnosis and indications of interventions

In most patients, clinical examination is enough to establish the diagnosis, although some hernias are easily missed because of obesity and tenderness to palpate. In these situations and in order to get a clear classification, a CT scan or ultrasound is needed [24].

Most of the surgeons adopt watchful waiting because of the high risk of recurrence making the surgical intervention limited to those with severe symptoms or complications that happen in 30% of the patients.

The indications for surgery can be divided into absolute and relative.

Absolute indications (acute complications)

- obstruction, when a patient develops intestinal obstruction due to an obstructed loop of the bowel within the hernia.
- Strangulation, when a segment of viscera within the hernia develops ischaemia due to a cut of the blood supply.
- Incarceration, which is the irreducibility of the hernia.
- Parastomal fistula,
- Perforation, when perforation of the bowel happens within the hernia sac.
- Stomal ischaemia.

Of course, a full assessment of the patient's condition needs to be done as sometimes the decision of palliation in severe frailty is made and sometimes repair of local complications such as obstruction and perforation is done within the hernia sac without repair of the hernia especially in a comorbid patient with loss of domain.

Relative indications:

- Recurrent admission with incarceration.
- Recurrent temporary obstruction, treated conservatively in the past.
- Difficulty in caring for the stoma bag, with recurrent leaks.
- Problems with irrigation in patients with constipation.
- Painful hernia.
- Pressure-related erosion or erosion of the adjacent skin.
- Social or aesthetic unacceptance.

- Irreducibility of the hernia.
- Other associated complications that need fixing, like stenosis or prolapsed.

However, it is absolutely contraindicated to repair the PSH in end-stage cancer and relatively in unresectable malignant tumours and severe comorbidity.

5. Management

5.1 Watch and wait

The widest approach adopted by most surgeons as we see only a third of the PSH is repaired, the reasons behind that are that the patients are asymptomatic, fail to report their problems, are afraid of recurrence or have other comorbidities that make the repair risky [11].

The EHS (European Hernia Society) Guidelines published in 2018 considered the watch and wait policy has no specific recommendations as it lacks evidence. In an asymptomatic hernia patient with no risk of strangulation, a watch-and-wait policy with regular monitoring is recommended [25].

5.2 Surgical repair

5.2.1 Indications of surgical intervention

It can be divided into two categories:

I. Emergency repair.

1. Strangulation.
2. Obstruction.
3. Incarceration.
4. Ischaemia of the stoma.

II. Elective repair:

1. Previous complications had been successfully treated with conservative measures like obstruction or incarceration.
2. Parastomal fistula.
3. Difficulty to take care of the stoma including placing the collecting bag.
4. Difficult irrigation.
5. Pain and difficulty in wearing the clothes.
6. Skin erosion.

7. Prolapse.

8. Patient preference.

It is worth knowing that it is contraindicated to repair the PSH in terminal malignant conditions, metastatic cancer, and serious comorbidities [13, 16].

5.2.2 Before surgery

- A computerised tomography scan (CT scan) is needed to plan the type of surgery.

- It is better to have a period of three months after the last abdominal surgery.

Smoking should be stopped at least 4 weeks before the operation.

- Weight reduction for high BMI >30.

- Full anaesthetic assessment including CPET is needed.

- Antibiotics are needed before the operation.

- VTE prophylaxis.

These points are general for all abdominal wall hernias including PSH [26, 27].

6. Surgical options

There are different approaches for PSH repair, and the choice of each technique depends on the surgeon's experience and the patient's condition.

6.1 Suture repair

This is the oldest technique that had been described in 1965 by Thorlakson. It is used mainly in emergency repair when other techniques are not suitable and sometimes as a step for other definitive procedures.

It has a high failure rate with recurrence ranging from 45 to 100%.

It is done by an incision around the stoma by about 5 cm, dissection of the sac and suturing the defect under tension.

6.2 Relocation

Simple relocation of the stoma is not a wise option for different reasons: It needs a midline laparotomy wound which carries its own complications such as incisional hernia and wound dehiscence, the old stoma wound may develop a hernia (52%) and the new stoma may develop a new parastomal hernia [13, 28].

Current practice by most surgeon that they choose relocation for the stomas that had been placed wrongly and they use a non-absorbable mesh primarily in the new stoma site to reduce the recurrence [29, 30].

The relocation of the stoma should be avoided unless the fascia adjacent to the original site is really week and cannot hold it [31].

6.3 Mesh repair

6.3.1 Open mesh repair

Onlay mesh repair is achieved with a semicircular incision on the lateral edge of the stoma and then, the mesh can be placed in a keyhole technique or stove pipe hat technique when the stoma is passed through the opening of the mesh and another mesh is then attached to the bowel circumference on the onlay mesh [32].

The recurrence rate is 25.9% at 48 months, with 1.9% infection of the wound and 2.6% mesh infection.

Retro muscular mesh repair is by placing the mesh beneath the rectus abdominis muscle using the Sugarbaker technique, keyhole, or midline incision. The associated incisional hernia can be repaired with mesh, or the stoma can be relocated [33].

These several techniques have an average pooled recurrence rate of 6.9%, while the incidence rate of wound infection is 4.8% in the absence of mesh infection.

Intraperitoneal placement of the mesh makes it less prone to infection [33].

A systematic review in 2014 concluded no sufficient evidence about which mesh repair is more successful, but the overall recurrence rate is 7.9–14% compared to suture repair which is 57% [34]. The lowest recurrence rate is for neuromuscular repair at 6.9%, while the Sugarbaker technique is 11.6% and the onlay mesh is 17.2%. The worst is the intraperitoneal keyhole with 34.6% [35].

In conclusion, if contamination happens, the biological mesh is the best option but has a high recurrence rate. While using medium weight or lightweight, large-pore polypropylene placed in the retro-muscular fashion is acceptable regarding infection and recurrence for PSH repair where there is a risk of contamination [34, 35].

6.3.2 Laparoscopic repair

Similar to the open repairs that had been mentioned above, laparoscopic techniques had been applied like retro muscular mesh placement or intraperitoneal mesh placement (Lap IPOM), performed using any of the keyhole, Sugarbaker, or sandwich approaches.

Compared to the open technique, the laparoscopic approach has less morbidity by 60% [36].

Regarding the recurrence rate, it is found that the recurrence is less in laparoscopic repair with no increase in wound infection rate, which is at 3.3%, mesh infection at 2.7% and morbidity at 17.2% [37].

In 2018, the EHS indicates no preference for laparoscopic or open repair with mesh for elective surgery [25].

6.3.3 Laparoscopic intraperitoneal only mesh: Keyhole technique

This was done first by Hanson as a keyhole approach. The abdomen is entered through the contralateral side of the stoma with the working port away from the stoma, and adhesiolysis is performed clearing 5 cm away from the defects in the abdominal wall.

One piece of the bilayer is cut in the centre forming a slit that results in a hole of 2 cm which houses the stoma in the middle, and the rest of the mesh is used to make a keyhole shape by wrapping it on the stoma, and then fixed in position using sutures or tacks [38].

The keyhole technique is suitable when the mesentery length is inadequate [39].

6.3.4 Laparoscopic intraperitoneal only mesh: Modified Sugarbaker technique

This was done first by Votik when he combined laparoscopic and Sugarbaker techniques.

In this technique, the non-slit bilayer or coated-non-absorbable meshes are used to cover the stoma and the hernia [40].

The hernia was reduced first; then, the defect is covered with the mesh centred over the site of the stoma, and the mesh was then extended to 5 cm or more. It is optimum for the lateralized colon up to the abdominal wall to form a tunnel of not less than 5 cm for the bowel before entering the enterocutaneous junction. Then, the mesh is fixed with tacks or sutures [41].

For this method, the rate of recurrence was found to be 10.2%compared to the keyhole of 27.9% [42].

This method is recommended and optimum if the mesentery has a good length [39].

6.3.5 Laparoscopic intraperitoneal only mesh: Sandwich or two-patch technique

The sandwich technique was made by LeBlanc and Bellanger when two meshes used one to cover the opening of the stoma and the second mesh patch in the opposite direction to the first mesh patch; for this, DualMesh Plus TM was employed and positioning the slit is used to cover the defect which has been created in the previous mesh.

Berger et al. [43] create a modification in this technique by combining the Sugarbaker and the keyhole method and employing a pair of mesh pieces. The first mesh is 15 × 15 cm, which is positioned using a keyhole technique with a central hole of 1.5 cm in size, and this mesh is placed around the stoma to wrap it and cover the defect in the same time and then closing the incised mesh using spiral tacks and two transracial sutures, and fixing the mesh at the same time with the tacks to make it secure in its place. Another non-absorbable mesh is used to cover the first mesh and the whole anterior abdominal wall. The stoma loop is then positioned between the two meshes with lateralization of more than 5 cm. Fixing is with spiral tacks and transracial sutures [43].

6.3.6 Laparoscopic transversus abdominis release (TAR) and modified retro rectus Sugarbaker

In this technique, component separation is through the TAR to create a retro rectus space and positioning of the mesh in this space without touching the intestine. Paulie et al. [44] first describe open TAR in combination with Sugarbaker technique [4].

The mesh is usually placed in the retro rectus space in a manner that is similar to the Sugarbaker technique and laterally in a sling around the bowel, medially it extends to the contralateral Linea semilunaris, so can strengthen the Medline.

The advantage of this technique is that there is no need to take down the mesh and lower wound problems, skin necrosis and subcutaneous seroma if compared with the ant component separation. Also, it is a cost-effective method as we can use by using non-coated non-absorbable mesh and allow integration of the mesh on both sides, one side with the anterior abdominal wall and the other side with the post-facial layers. This provides superior tensile strength [43, 44].

7. What type of mesh to use

As the parastomal hernia has a high rate of recurrence and failure, there were a lot of controversies about the type of mesh and its effect on recurrence and other post-operative morbidities especially the presence of mesh making the operation a clean contaminated not like strictly clean operations.

A post hoc analysis of a multicentre randomised controlled trial done in the United States comparing biologic versus synthetic mesh in a contaminated ventral hernia concluded that there is no difference in wound morbidity, reoperation, two-year hernia recurrence rate and the quality of life in PSH repair, so the cost should be taken in consideration in operation [45].

8. Which technique is the best for the outcome and long-term follow-up?

Although we mentioned earlier that the best technique is the technique that the surgeon is confident to do, still continuously improving the techniques is needed in PSH hernia repair given the high morbidity and failure rate.

A retrospective cohort study done in Finland across five university hospitals and 4 central hospitals: it showed that the recurrence rate is as follows:

- Keyhole 35.1%
- Sugarbaker 21.5%
- Sandwich method 13.5%
- Specific funnel-type mesh 15%
- Other techniques 26.3%

From this, we find that the recurrence is high in all types of repair of PSH and this is the cause that PSH repair is low in volume [45].

9. Prevention

Once a stoma is created, there will be a risk of the development of PSH and prevention of its development is better than repair.

The reduction of the risk can be achieved by good patient preparation, patient education with the stoma nurse, prior marking of the stoma and treating the modifiable risk factors like smoking and obesity and encouraging exercise.

During the technique, it is advised to use a small trephine less than 3 cm as it is associated with a higher risk of development of PSH [4]. Although it still lacks solid evidence.

There is growing evidence about prophylactic mesh use during the creation of the stoma to prevent recurrence. A study comprised an analysis of 12 systematic reviews and meta-analyses, including the Cochrane review, for a period covering 2010–2018. The analysed studies included 451–844 participants. The study found that the rate of PSH is reduced when a prophylactic mesh is used compared to the standard stoma formation.

Now, the EHS strongly recommends the use of prophylactic mesh for PSH prevention. However, because of poor evidence, it is now advised to use prophylactic mesh for a cancer patient when planned end permanent colostomy and this needs to be discussed with the patient.

The post-operative instructions to reduce the recurrence after the repair are generally similar to other ventral hernia repairs which include: avoidance of heavyweight lifting for three weeks, use of abdominal binder for three to six months and after that the binder used during heavy exercise [39].

10. Conclusions

PSH is a common complication after stoma surgery and its incidence rises with time after surgery. Numerous approaches are adopted by surgeons ranging from the watch and waiting to extensive big surgery. Only a third of the patients with PSH are treated surgically with a significant recurrence rate which made the surgeons try to find different techniques to reduce the risk of recurrence. The most popular now is intraperitoneal onlay fashion using the Sugarbaker technique as it has a favourable outcome. Moreover, the two-pouch mesh repair is gaining popularity. In elective cancer patients when an end stoma is adopted, it is recommended now to use a prophylactic mesh. Further studies are ongoing now to determine the best technique with regard to the recurrence and other complications.

Conflict of interest

The author has no conflict of interest.

Thanks

For My parents who always pray for my success.

For My wife and children: Alyaa the most supportive and loving person and Ola, Sama and the little Misk, who give the joy of life.

Author details

Omar Alhafidh
Royal Bolton Hospital, Bolton, UK

*Address all correspondence to: omar.alhafidh@boltonft.nhs.uk

References

[1] Tadeo-Ruiz G, Picazo-Yeste JS, Moreno-Sanz C, Herrero-Bogajo ML. Parastomal hernias: Background, current status and future prospects. Cirugía Española. 2010;**87**:339-349

[2] Carne PW, Robertson GM, Frizelle FA. Parastomal hernia. The British Journal of Surgery. 2003;**90**:784-793

[3] Israelsson LA. Preventing and treating parastomal hernia. World Journal of Surgery. 2005;**29**:1086-1089

[4] Arumugam PJ, Bevan L, Macdonald L, et al. A prospective audit of stomas-analysis of risk factors and complications and their management. Colorectal Disease. 2003;**5**:49-52

[5] Moreno-Matias J, Serra-Aracil X, Darnell-Martin A, et al. The prevalence of parastomal hernia after formation of an end colostomy. A new clinico-radiological classification. Colorectal Disease. 2009;**11**:173-177

[6] Seo SH, Kim HJ, Oh SY, Lee JH, Suh KW. Computed tomography classification for parastomal hernia. Journal of the Korean Surgical Society. 2011;**81**:111-114

[7] Gil G, Szczepkowski M. A new classification of parastomal hernias: From the experience at Bielanski hospital in Warsaw. Polski Przeglad Chirurgiczny. 2011;**83**:430-437

[8] Śmietański M, Szczepkowski M, Alexandre JA, et al. European hernia society classification of parastomal hernias. Hernia. 2014;**18**:1-6

[9] Jänes A, Cengiz Y, Israelsson LA. Preventing parastomal hernia with a prosthetic mesh: A 5-year follow-up of a randomized study. World Journal of Surgery. 2009;**33**:118-121

[10] Sohn YJ, Moon SM, Shin US, et al. Incidence and risk factors of parastomal hernia. Journal of the Korean Society of Coloproctology. 2012;**28**:241-246

[11] Shah NR, Craft RO, Harold KL. Parastomal hernia repair. The Surgical Clinics of North America. 2013;**93**:1185-1198

[12] Cheung MT. Complications of an abdominal stoma: An analysis of 322 stomas. The Australian and New Zealand Journal of Surgery. 1995;**65**:808-811

[13] Aquina CT, Iannuzzi JC, Probst CP, et al. Parastomal hernia: A growing problem with new solutions. Digestive Surgery. 2014;**31**:366-376

[14] Andersen RM, Klausen TW, Danielsen AK, et al. Incidence and risk factors for parastomal bulging in patients with ileostomy or colostomy: A register-based study using data from the Danish stoma database capital region. Colorectal Disease. 2018;**20**:331-340

[15] Malik T, Lee MJ, Harikrishnan AB. The incidence of stoma related morbidity - a systematic review of randomised controlled trials. Annals of the Royal College of Surgeons of England. 2018;**100**:501-508

[16] Styliński R, Alzubedi A, Rudzki S. Parastomal hernia - current knowledge and treatment. Wideochirurgia I Inne Techniki Maloinwazyjne. 2018;**13**:1-8

[17] Shabbir J, Britton DC. Stoma complications: A literature overview. Colorectal Disease. 2010;**12**:958-964

[18] Sjödahl R, Anderberg B, Bolin T. Parastomal hernia in relation to site of the abdominal stoma. The British Journal of Surgery. 1988;**75**(4):339-341. DOI: 10.1002/bjs.1800750414

[19] Williams JG, Etherington R, Hayward MW, Hughes LE. Paraileostomy hernia: A clinical and radiological study. The British Journal of Surgery. 1990;**77**(12):1355-1357. DOI: 10.1002/bjs.1800771212

[20] Ortiz H, Sara MJ, Armendariz P, de Miguel M, Marti J, Chocarro C. Does the frequency of paracolostomy hernias depend on the position of the colostomy in the abdominal wall? International Journal of Colorectal Disease. 1994;**9**(2):65-67. DOI: 10.1007/BF00699414

[21] Cingi A, Solmaz A, Attaallah W, Aslan A, Aktan AO. Enterostomy closure site hernias: A clinical and ultrasonographic evaluation. Hernia. 2008;**12**:401-405

[22] Pearl RK. Parastomal hernias. World Journal of Surgery. 1989;**13**:569-572

[23] Krogsgaard M, Pilsgaard B, Borglit TB, et al. Symptom load and individual symptoms before and after repair of parastomal hernia: A prospective single Centre study. Colorectal Disease. 2017;**19**:200-207

[24] Thompson MJ. Parastomal hernia: Incidence, prevention and treatment strategies. The British Journal of Nursing. 2008;**17**:18-20

[25] Antoniou SA, Agresta F, Garcia Alamino JM, et al. European hernia society guidelines on prevention and treatment of parastomal hernias. Hernia. 2018;**22**:183-198

[26] Earle D, Roth JS, Saber A, et al. SAGES guidelines for laparoscopic ventral hernia repair. Surgical Endoscopy. 2016;**30**:3163-3183

[27] Silecchia G, Campanile FC, Sanchez L, et al. Laparoscopic ventral/incisional hernia repair: Updated consensus development conference based guidelines. Surgical Endoscopy. 2015;**29**:2463-2484

[28] Rubin MS, Schoetz DJ Jr, Matthews JB, Parastomal hernia. Is stoma relocation superior to fascial repair? Archives of Surgery. 1994;**129**:413-418

[29] Allen-Mersh TG, Thomson JP. Surgical treatment of colostomy complications. The British Journal of Surgery. 1988;**75**:416-418

[30] Riansuwan W, Hull TL, Millan MM, et al. Surgery of recurrent parastomal hernia: Direct repair or relocation? Colorectal Disease. 2010;**12**:681-686

[31] Mäkäräinen-Uhlbäck E, Vironen J, Falenius V, Nordström P, Välikoski A, Kössi J, et al. Parastomal hernia: A retrospective Nationwide cohort study comparing different techniques with long-term follow-up. World Journal of Surgery. 2021;**45**(6):1742-1749. DOI: 10.1007/s00268-021-05990-z

[32] Berger D. Prevention of parastomal hernias by prophylactic use of a specially designed intraperitoneal onlay mesh (Dynamesh IPST®). Hernia. 2008;**12**:243-246

[33] Al Shakarchi J, Williams JG. Systematic review of open techniques for parastomal hernia repair. Techniques in Coloproctology. 2014;**18**:427-432

[34] Guzmán-Valdivia G, Guerrero TS, Laurrabaquio HV. Parastomal hernia-repair using mesh and an open technique. World Journal of Surgery. 2008;**32**:465-470

[35] Colvin J, Rosenblatt S. Surgical Management of Parastomal Hernias. The Surgical Clinics of North America. 2018;**98**:577-592

[36] Halabi WJ, Jafari MD, Carmichael JC, et al. Laparoscopic versus open repair of parastomal hernias: An ACS-NSQIP analysis of short-term outcomes. Surgical Endoscopy. 2013;**27**:4067-4072

[37] Hansson BM, Slater NJ, van der Velden AS, et al. Surgical techniques for parastomal hernia repair: A systematic review of the literature. Annals of Surgery. 2012;**255**:685-695

[38] Tastaldi L, Haskins IN, Perez AJ, et al. Single center experience with the modified retromuscular Sugarbaker technique for parastomal hernia repair. Hernia. 2017;**21**:941-949

[39] Smith JM, Kapur SK, Mericli AF, Baumann DP, Butler CE. Parastomal hernia repair. Plastic and Aesthetic Research. 2022;**9**:10. DOI: 10.20517/2347-9264.2021.48

[40] Voitk A. Simple technique for laparoscopic paracolostomy hernia repair. Diseases of the Colon and Rectum. 2000;**43**:1451-1453

[41] Stelzner S, Hellmich G, Ludwig K. Repair of paracolostomy hernias with a prosthetic mesh in the intraperitoneal onlay position: Modified Sugarbaker technique. Diseases of the Colon and Rectum. 2004;**47**:185-191

[42] DeAsis FJ, Lapin B, Gitelis ME, Ujiki MB. Current state of laparoscopic parastomal hernia repair: A meta-analysis. World Journal of Gastroenterology. 2015;**21**:8670-8677

[43] Berger D, Bientzle M. Laparoscopic repair of parastomal hernias: A single surgeon's experience in 66 patients. Diseases of the Colon and Rectum. 2007;**50**:1668-1673

[44] Pauli EM, Juza RM, Winder JS. How I do it: Novel parastomal herniorrhaphy utilizing transversus abdominis release. Hernia. 2016;**20**:547-552

[45] Miller Benjamin T, KrpataDavid M, PetroClayton C, Beffa Lucas RA, Carbonell Alfredo M, Warren Jeremy A, et al. Biologic vs synthetic mesh for Parastomal hernia repair: Post hoc analysis of a Multicenter randomized controlled trial. Journal of the American College of Surgeons. 2022;**235**(3):401-409. DOI: 10.1097/XCS.0000000000000275

Chapter 17

Treatment of Low-Back Pain with Oxygen-Ozone Therapy

Matteo Bonetti, Gian Maria Ottaviani, Luigi Simonetti, Giannantonio Pellicanò, Francesco Bonetti and Mario Muto

Abstract

Oxygen-ozone therapy for the treatment of low back pain was introduced for the first time in 1985. Over the years, numerous case studies have been presented in the literature reporting positive results ranging from 75% up to almost 90% in the treatment of low back pain, whether or not complicated by sciatica due to disc-radicular impingement caused by disc herniation. The authors have been carrying out these treatments for over 25 years, and in this chapter, they report their experience in the treatment with oxygen-ozone therapy, first examining the biochemical bases and the mechanisms of action of the gaseous mixture of oxygen and ozone, the various infiltrative techniques, then moving on to evaluate the therapeutic results obtained in the treatment of patients suffering from both discogenic and non-discogenic low back pains caused by pathology of the posterior compartment (facet synovitis, Baastrup syndrome, spondylolysis and spondylolisthesis, facet degeneration).

Keywords: oxygen ozone, ozone therapy, herniated disc, low back pain, root pain, facet synovitis, Baastrup syndrome, spondylolysis, spondylolisthesis, facet degeneration

1. Introduction

Low back pain—with or without sciatic nerve involvement—affects roughly 80% of the population at least once in a lifetime and is the leading cause of lost working days, with a major impact on national health organization and cost.

The treatment of choice for LBP sciatica, up to 20 years ago, was surgery, but conservative measures are now preferred in the wake of unsatisfactory surgical outcomes in around 15–20% of the cases. Among the techniques adopted in the last decade for the treatment of pain in the sciatic nerve caused by disc herniation or non-discal spine diseases (osteophytosis, spondylolysis, facet joint syndrome, etc.), the use of the treatment of back pain with targeted infiltration of O_2-O_3 has increasingly gained a foothold in many countries.

In recent years, several studies have demonstrated the utility of oxygen-ozone therapy in the treatment of herniated disc-related sciatica with its reduction in size on follow-up imaging examination (**Figure 1a-b**).

Oxygen-ozone therapy for the treatment of herniated discs was introduced for the first time in 1985. Over the years numerous cases have been presented in the literature

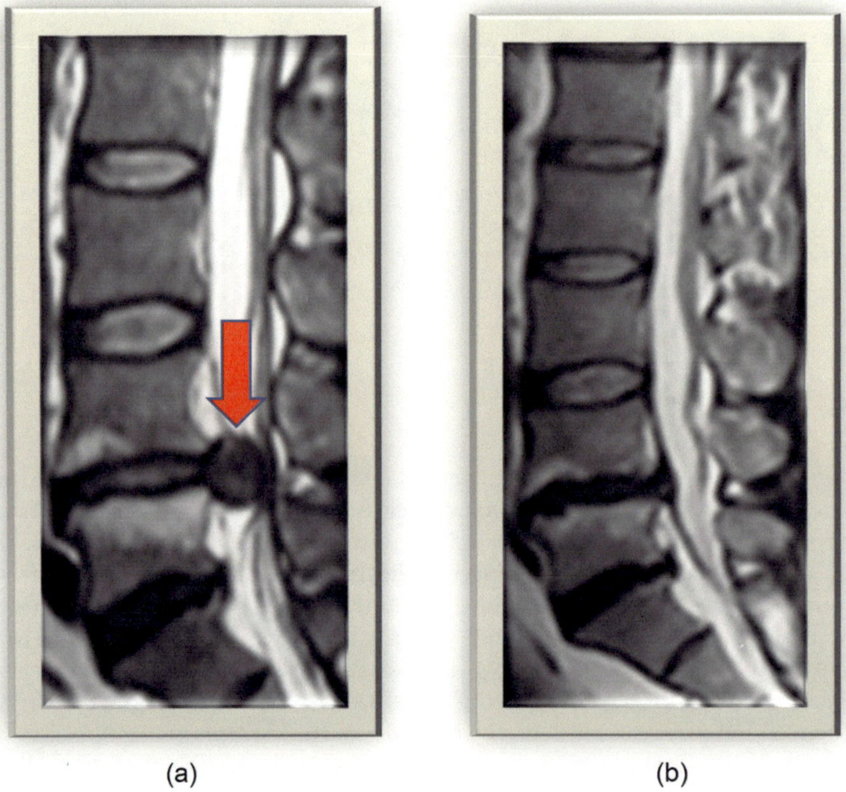

Figure 1.
a-b: (a) Large L4-L5 disc herniation (arrow), (b) completely resolved by oxygen-ozone therapy.

reporting positive results ranging from 75% to almost 90% in the treatment of low back pain, also complicated by sciatica due to disc-radicular impingement, determined by the presence of a herniated intervertebral disc [1–16].

Low back pain and sciatica are pathologies, which can be identified as highly disabling, increasingly widespread in every social category. In recent years, they have also constantly manifested themselves at an earlier age, in the population. They arise acutely, following unusual effort or movement, or slowly, often with progressive aggravation.

They can be sustained by numerous and different vertebral pathologies, often concomitant: discopathies, facet joints, spondylolysis (with or without listhesis), somatic and interapophyseal arthrosis, spinal canal stenosis, root and synovial cysts, meningiomas, primary or metastatic neoplastic pathology, etc.

To choose the best therapy, in cases of low back pain and/or sciatica, a precise diagnosis—formulated after a careful objective clinical examination supported by adequate diagnostic tools—is therefore essential. It is very important to exclude the presence of a motor neurological deficit, which may represent an indication for surgical treatment. In particular, in addition to standard radiograms of the spine, computed tomography (CT) and/or magnetic resonance imaging (MRI) offer important information about the nature and etiology of the clinical situation associated with the symptoms encountered.

2. Pharmacological mechanisms of action of oxygen-ozone therapy for herniated disc

An analysis of pain caused by nerve root compression is a prerequisite for understanding the mechanisms underlying the effect of ozone on pain in patients with herniated discs [16]. Root pain is commonly related to nerve compression (disc root impingement or spinal impingement). However, there is a lot of evidence in clinical practice that the cause-and-effect relationship of radicular pain is not as simple as generally thought. For example, we know that many people are asymptomatic despite an incidental disc herniation during spinal neuroimaging for reasons other than disc disease. In two well-known published articles, only 3% of 98 and 116 asymptomatic patients showed a normal MRI finding. Furthermore, patients with known disc herniation live with the lesion between pain attacks, even though the morphology of the disc lesion and subsequent nerve root compression remain unchanged on CT and MRI scans.

Successful medical management of medical management or micro-invasive surgery such as intramuscular or intradiscal injection of oxygen-ozone is commonly found in a fair number of patients, in resolution pain without altering the morphology of the hernia, i.e., without changing the structure of the disc lesion.

Lastly, even though disc compression is surgically corrected, many patients continue to experience pain, relieved or even exacerbated, regardless of the herniated disc structural changes seen on neuroimaging scans after surgery, related to inflammation of neural structures and perineural. These results led us to investigate the mechanisms responsible for radicular pain related to pharmacological mechanisms of ozone action on herniated disc.

3. Pathogenesis of root pain

Reviewing the state of the art, we can distinguish two broad categories of pathogenetic mechanisms: mechanical and inflammatory, to which pain exacerbation linked to chronic illness should be added pain exacerbation linked to chronic illness [17, 18].

1. *Pathogenetic components of root pain:*

Mechanical pressure

The mechanical factors responsible for pain are related to the mass effect of the herniated disc material.

In turn, these can be divided into:

- *Direct mechanical factors:* considering the absence of nociceptors located in the nerve bundle, these factors are associated, in order of importance, to:
    - Compression of the spinal ganglion, possible intraforaminal and extraforaminal herniation;
    - Deformation and flattening of the ligaments and annulus, location of the afferent nociceptors to Luschka's nerve of the posterior root of the spinal nerve;
    - Deformation and flattening of nerve fibers disrupting the myelin nerve sheath with possible major conduction abnormalities.

- *Indirect mechanical factors I* (also known as "vasculomediated")*:*
  - o "Ischemic" vasculomediated factors. Characterized by trophic nerve impairment caused by compression of the arterial afferents and microcirculation of the nerve bundle and secondary anoxic demyelination of the nerve fibers;
  - o Vasculomediated factors due to venous stasis with edema and trophic nerve impairment caused by partial or total blockage of venous reflux (especially in intraforaminal herniations). This factor appears to be the most important mechanical factor responsible for root pain because of its effects on the spinal ganglion (considering the anatomical relations between the intraforaminal vessels and spinal ganglion).

2. *Pathogenetic components of root pain:*

Inflammation

A major role in the origin of root pain is to be found in neural and perineural inflammation [19, 20]. Some evidence, though speculative, concerning the importance of inflammatory factors suggests that higher levels of antibodies anti-pso P27 (markers for inflammatory process, particularly of autoimmune origin) can be found in CSF from patients with low back pain and sciatica [21].

They include:

- *Immune-mediated inflammatory reaction:* evidence demonstrates that disc protrusion can be the cause of immune inflammatory events.

The hypothesis (even if not universally accepted) regarded as most likely to account for this behavior may be the fact that the adult intervertebral disc, from a humoral standpoint, is segregated with respect to the immune system as long as it is confined within the fibrocartilaginous structure of the annulus. Once herniated, the disc is recognized as "non-self" by the immunocompetent system, and this factor triggers a cell-mediated reaction in other tissues. The presence of peridiscal inflammatory tissue is confirmed by the CT and MR finding of peripheral enhancement of the disc fragment after i.v. contrast administration [22].

Additional experimental findings of the autoimmune component of peridiscal inflammation underline the action macrophages with expression of the IL 1β gene—characteristic of autoimmune reactions—and the reduction of mechanical hyperalgesia following drug-induced leucopenia under experimental conditions [23].

- *Inflammatory reaction due to biohumoral factors linked to disc tissue*. Experimental evidence in this field includes the following:
  - o Phospholipase A2 (PLA2): The herniated disc material contains increased levels of PLA2 enzyme activity. PLA2 plays the role of powerful inducer of the inflammatory reaction for its enzymatic activation to arachidonic acid causes to the production of major chemical mediators of inflammation, like prostaglandins and leukotrienes. Moreover, PLA2 may damage nerve fibers by attacking perineural and neural membrane phospholipids [24];

- Matrix metalloproteinases (MMPs): There is a significant production of this enzyme that enhances the inflammatory reaction by attacking disc tissue;

- Prostaglandin E2 (PGE2): The disc tissue and the enzymatic intervention of PLA2 (a powerful inducer of inflammation) produce PGE2. The same factors are applied to interleukin 6 (IL6) [25];

- Evidence investigating a recently identified glycoprotein, YKL-40, is undergoing, at the moment. This glycoprotein is produced in abundance following joint lesions, including degenerative disease, which could be one of the main mediators of the inflammatory reaction in disc disease [26].

3. *Pathogenetic components of root pain: Symptoms exacerbated by chronic pain:*

By exacerbation of symptoms caused by chronic pain we mean the mechanism by which the chronic mechanical and inflammatory stimulation of the nerve root stimulates the ganglionic and periganglionic nociceptors (mainly polymodal type C) responsible for hyperalgesia, a condition presenting allodynia, i.e., a lowering of the pain threshold and an increase in pain intensity also following subliminal stimuli, in some cases also activating spontaneous pain discharges [20].

3.1 Pharmacological mechanisms underlying the effect of ozone on the various components of root pain

1. *Effect of ozone on direct mechanical pressure*

The effect ozone is thought to have on the herniated disc as such is based on biochemistry composition of the intervertebral disc, mainly composed of proteoglycans and collagen [26, 27]. Cartilage proteoglycans [28] comprise a series of copolymers consisting of a protein core, called the "core protein," bound to about 100 unbranched side chains of chondroitin sulfate and up to 50 keratan sulfate chains. Chondroitin sulfate chains are strongly polyanionic and bind large amounts of water, while keratan sulfate chains are less so.

Collagen forms a solid fibrous armor that supports and neutralizes traction and shear forces due to joint movement. Of the 14 known collagen types, the outermost part of the annulus fibrosus mainly belongs to type I. Type II collagen predominates in the innermost part of the annulus, and type IV is mainly found in the "nucleus pulposus" [29].

Thus, the nucleus pulposus and herniated disc are complex macromolecular structures containing water bound to various hydrophilic matrices.

How does ozone attenuate direct mechanical compression?

Due to its solubility and pressure, once injected into the disc, ozone dissolves into the intradiscal water and decomposes immediately generating a cascade of reactive oxygen species (ROS) [25]. Because intradiscal water contains a minimal amount of fatty acids, lipoperoxides are unlikely to form. The oxidation of the various substrates present in the disc, in particular glucose, galactose, N-acetylglycosamine, glucuronic acid, glycine, and 4-hydroxyproline, breaks the intra- and intermolecular ligands leading to the collapse of its three-dimensional structure. These events can occur in both the nucleus pulposus and disc herniation and are thought to lead to fluid reabsorption and fibrosis [30–32].

2. *Effect of ozone on the indirect mechanical factors*

Indirect mechanical factors are largely mediated by vessels. In this case, oxygen-ozone exerts one of its best-known pharmacological effects, namely the increase of intra- and trans-tissue oxygenation, thus improving hypoxia and venous and lymphatic stasis.

3. *Effect of ozone on the cell-mediated inflammatory response*

Ozone influences the cell-mediated inflammatory response to hernia by two main pharmacological mechanisms [25]:

- inhibition of proteinase release by macrophages and polymorphonuclear neutrophils;

- enhance the release of immunosuppressive cytokines (interleukin 10, TGF beta 10) which inhibit any cytotoxic clones [33].

4. *Effect of ozone on the biohumoral inflammatory response*

The possible effect of ozone on the biohumoral component of the inflammatory response is more complex. Taking into account the biohumoral factors involved in the inflammatory response, ozone could carry out its action as follows:

- inhibiting the synthesis of pro-inflammatory prostaglandins;

- inhibiting the release of bradykinin or pain-inducing compounds;

- neutralizing the endogenous ROS and stimulating the local production of antioxidant enzymes;

- increasing the release of antagonists and the pro-inflammatories cytokines such as interleukin 1, 2, 8, and 15 [33].

5. *Effect of ozone on symptoms exacerbated by chronic pain*

Ozone is thought to relieve symptoms exacerbated by chronic pain as a type of "chemical acupuncture" or "reflex therapy." This depends on the counter-irritant effect of the needle-gas combination, which would have a bending action on the antinociceptor system. The insertion of the needle and the subsequent injection of positive pressure ozone stimulate the nociceptors of the paravertebral muscles. This in turn can inhibit nociceptive neurons in the spinal cord by releasing opioid peptides. In other words, stimulation by pressure and chemoreceptors and muscle spindle fibers at the site of disc disease can give rise to a kind of local lateral inhibition. Last but not least, any direct nociceptive stimulation is known to relieve pain through the mechanism of diffuse noxious inhibitory control [25].

3.2 Conclusive remarks

In light of current knowledge, radicular pain from nerve root compression is to be considered a symptom of multifactorial origin in which the neural and perineural inflammatory reaction and its biohumoral mediators play a preponderant role, flanked by venous stasis from mass effect on the circulation perineural. Nerve compression seems to play an adjuvant role by generating nerve conduction abnormalities due to demyelination of the fibers with a direct or indirect anoxic-ischemic mechanism.

Since pain is multifactorial, ozone can also have a multifactorial pharmacological effect by relieving disc compression through narrowing and triggering pro-fibrous mechanisms in disc herniation, thus counteracting the inflammatory cascade of biohumoral and cell-mediated components and improving the hypoxic state related to artery compression and venous stasis. Finally, ozone can have a reflexotherapy effect ("chemical acupuncture") by breaking the chain of chronic pain that stimulates the anti-nociceptor analgesic mechanisms [32, 33].

4. Application methods

4.1 Ozone therapy in the paravertebral muscle bundles: "Classic" technique

The patient is placed on the bed in the prone position. The disc space to be treated is identified through anatomical cutaneous landmarks: line of the spinous process with recognition of the spinous process of L4 at the level of the trans-iliac line and then positioned 2÷2.5 cm bilaterally to the interspinous spaces (**Figure 2**). Thorough skin disinfection is carried out in the area to be infiltrated, skin anesthesia with ethyl chloride spray, needle insertion, generally 23G (Gauge) for lumbar treatment, and 25G for the cervical.

Following the correct insertion of the needles into the muscles, aspiration occurs, and we proceed with the injection of the oxygen-ozone mixture with an optimal

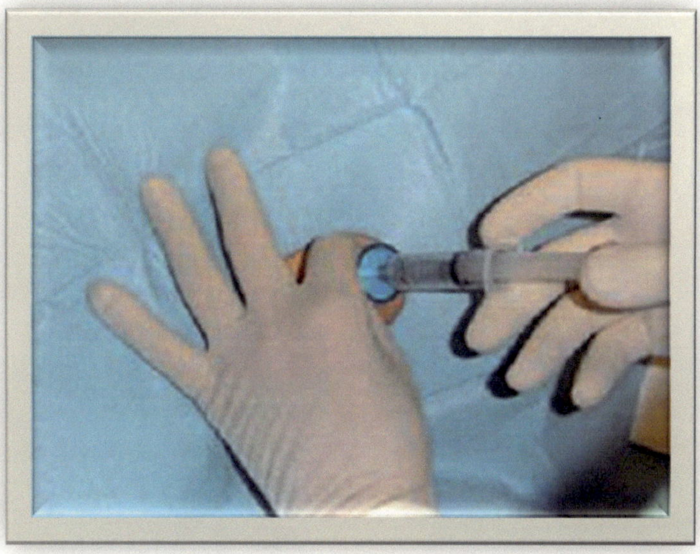

Figure 2.
Paravertebral intramuscular infiltration of O_2-O_3.

therapeutic window using doses at a concentration of 20/25 μg/ml. and volume: 5 ml. by injection, the entire therapeutic cycle consists on average of 8–10 infiltrations, 2 infiltrations every week.

4.2 CT-guided intraforaminal technique

The treatment is carried out in day hospital and the infiltration technique is the same that is used for discographies; in fact, a preliminary CT examination is foreseen to establish the infiltration point at the skin level and subsequently, the distance of this is measured last from the conjugation foramen. Local anesthesia with ethyl chloride spray is performed. The needle used is always a 22G needle of variable length, and usually, we use 9-cm Terumo needles. Proper needle placement is then verified using CT scans. The tip of the needle must be approximately 4–5 mm from the foraminal region; 3 cc of oxygen-ozone mixture at 25 μg/ml are injected. After that, the needle is withdrawn a few mm and another 5–6 cc. of gaseous mixture are injected into the mass of the joint. We then proceed by carrying out a CT check of the correct distribution of the oxygen-ozone mixture (**Figure 3**). The patient remains under clinical supervision for about 30 minutes before being discharged. The clinical benefit of the treatment is almost immediate. The patient is then clinically re-evaluated after 10 days, and if the result has not been satisfactory a second treatment is carried out, this operation can be repeated once or twice. Three months after the end of treatment, a CT scan of the treated disc herniation is performed in

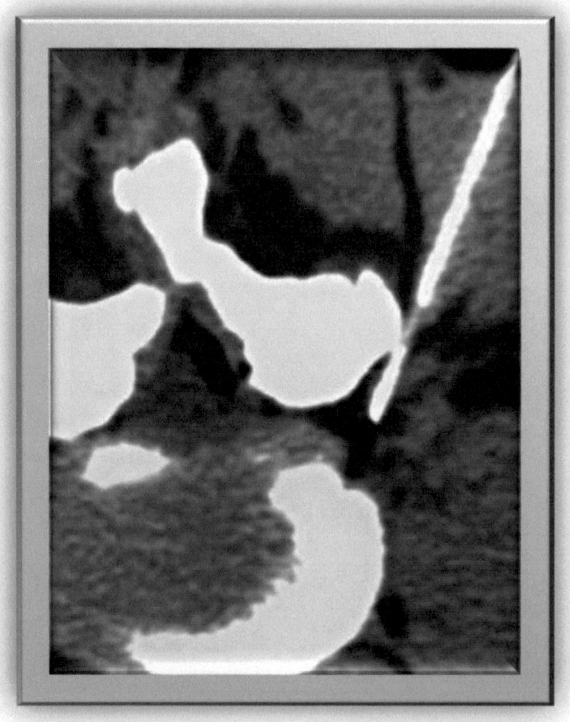

Figure 3.
Correct positioning of the needle under CT guidance.

all treated patients. There are no contraindications, and no side effects have ever been reported.

The intraforaminal administration of ozone CT guided with the proposed modality combines the precision in the control of the needle path with the curative possibility of all the O_2-O_3 infiltration techniques used up to now. Improvement of local circulation with eutrophic effect in the both vicinity of the compressed and suffering nerve root and at the level of muscle spasm; the normalization of the level of cytokines and prostanglandins with anti-inflammatory and pain-relieving effect; the increase in the production of superoxide dismutase (SOD) with minimization of oxidizing reagents (ROS); and finally the close proximity to the herniated material that determines accelerated dehydration or destruction of a non-vascularized tissue that justifies the good final result.

The rapid resolution of painful symptoms with no complications, the ease of execution of the method, and complete control of the infiltration *via* CT allow, today, to propose oxygen ozone therapy with CT-guided intraforaminal technique as a valid alternative to surgical treatment of herniated disc if the latter is not considered essential and therefore a method of choice among conservative therapies.

4.3 Intradiscal technique

Percutaneous treatment of discolysis with oxygen-ozone (O_2-O_3) can be performed subcutaneously fluoroscopically or under CT guidance. In both cases the oxygen-ozone mixture is injected into the intervertebral disc, along the postero-lateral, extra-articular route.

The procedure can be performed in Day Hospital or One Day Surgery.

4.4 Fluoroscopic guide

It is necessary to observe some pretreatment recommendations also concerning the X-ray room for the surgery.

The X-ray room must in fact have instruments suitable for anesthesiological assistance. Compliance with asepsis must be guaranteed, a fluoroscopic apparatus must be available (preferably isocentric) with a "C" arm that allows direct scopic control, and, finally, peripheral venous access to the patient must be guaranteed.

Thorough skin disinfection and a sterile field must be carried out before the puncture.

The patient lies on the X-ray bed in lateral decubitus (access is ipsilateral to the site of the symptoms). Under fluoroscopic guidance, the puncture of the intervertebral disc is performed with a 22 G needle.

The intradiscal position (the needle tip must be in the center of the interbody space) is documented by acquiring radiographic images in the A-P and L-L projections (**Figure 4a-b**). After placing a millipore filter on the syringe, proceed with the injection of 7–8 cc of O_2-O_3 mixture at a concentration of 25 μg/ml, of which 3–4 ml intradiscally and, once the needle has been withdrawn with the apex projecting at the interapophyseal joint, another 4 cc is injected in the periradicular and paravertebral soft tissues.

For higher interbody spaces, disc access is more direct than the L5-S1 space. Once the patient has been placed in lateral decubitus position and the nucleus pulposus has been positioned in the center of the interbody space, a lateral rotation of the arc of about 35° is performed, which allows recognition of the ipsilateral joint at the level of

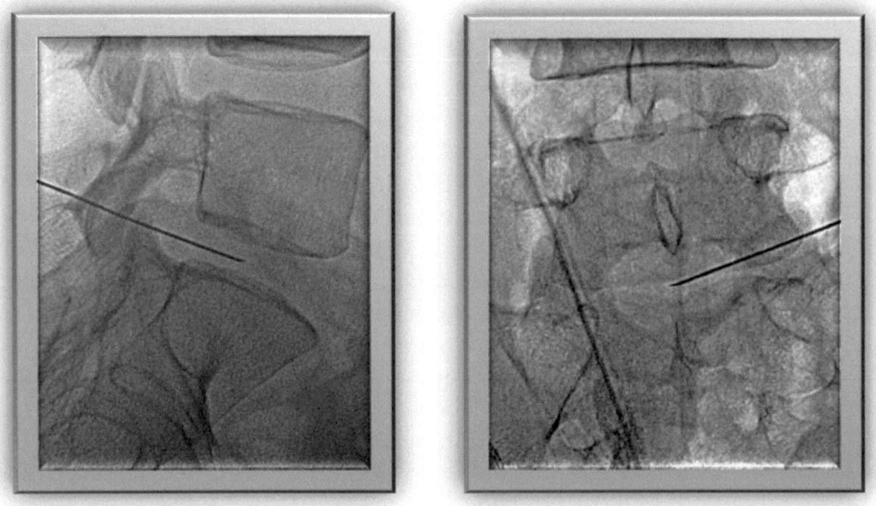

Figure 4.
a-b. (a) Latero-lateral view, (b) antero-posterior view. Correct needle placement.

the posterior third of the interbody space. The needle is inserted in the middle third of the interbody space, and its path must be followed in the lateral projection. During the procedure under fluoroscopic guidance, radiographic documentation of the final position of the needle in the main radiological projections is performed.

As mentioned, the approach to the L5-S1 space under fluoroscopic guidance differs from that of the higher disc spaces: Once the patient is positioned in lateral decubitus position and the nucleus pulposus of L5-S1 in the center of the radiographic image, rotation is performed of the arc of about 35°, which allows recognition of the intervertebral joint thus projected at the level of the posterior third of the disc space.

Access to the disc, masked by the ipsilateral iliac wing, is possible, at this level, only with a further inclination of the arch in the cranio-caudal direction. An area of access to the disc is thus obtained, delimited inferiorly by the superior somatic limiter of S1, posteriorly by the anterior profile of the superior articular process of S1 and anteriorly by the superior profile of the ipsilateral iliac wing. At the end of the procedure, the patient must maintain the lateral decubitus position for about 30 minutes; bed rest on the first day after treatment and chair rest on the second day are also indicated. For the following period, a gradual resumption of activities without loading the lumbosacral region should be recommended.

4.5 CT guide

The patient must be positioned in prone decubitus with devices that reduce the physiological lumbar lordosis. A targeted CT examination is carried out on the level to be treated and the distance from the spinous process to the cutaneous entry point of the needle is calculated, which allows an easy puncture of the central part of the disc (preferably the nucleus pulposus) with an angle of 45°.

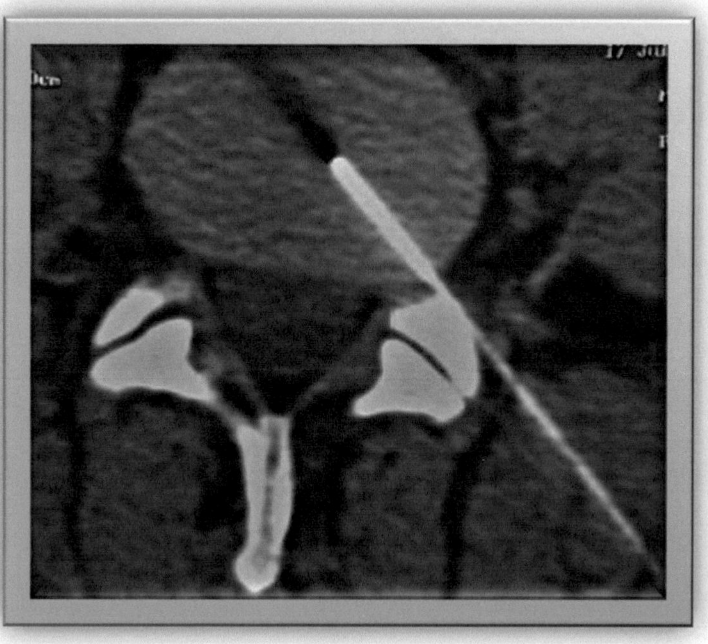

Figure 5.
Correct positioning of the needle in the heart of the disc.

Metal landmarks are placed on the skin and, once the entry point has been identified, it is traced with a demographic pencil.

Once you reach the level of the disc you will feel the sensation of yielding of a tense structure due to the entry of the needle into the disc itself (**Figure 5**).

This is followed by the intradiscal injection of the O_2-O_3 mixture in quantities of 3–4 ml at a concentration of about 25 μg/ml.

Finally, a CT control of the distribution of the mixture is performed. At the end of the treatment, the patient will have to switch from prone to supine position and keep the latter for about 2 hours.

5. What to treat

5.1 Disc herniation

Several studies have demonstrated the utility of oxygen-ozone therapy in the treatment of herniated discs with the result of herniated discs reduced in size [1–16, 34–36].

In our experience, which dates back to 1993, we carry out treatments of both lumbar and cervical disc herniation with CT-guided intraforaminal technique with therapeutic results in complete agreement with what is reported in the international literature, ranging from 75% up to almost 90% of success therapeutic in the treatment of low back pain complicated or not by sciatica due to disc-radicular impingement due to disc herniation (**Figure 6a-b**).

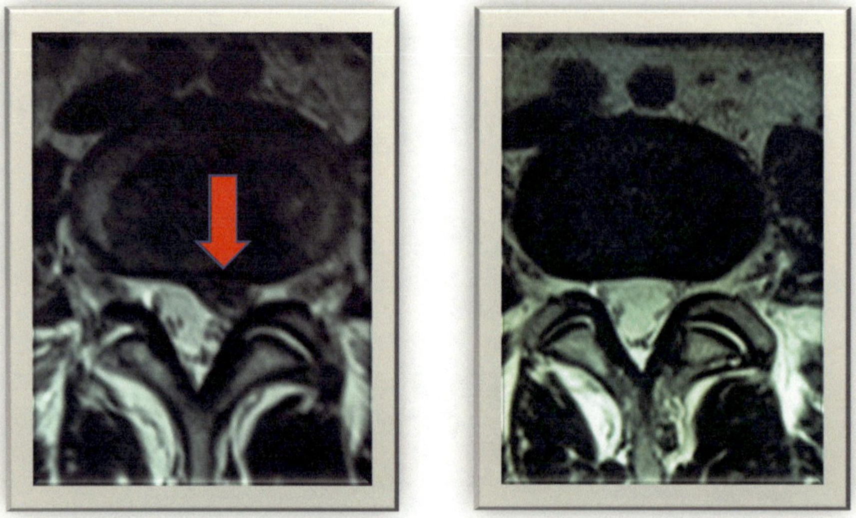

(a) (b)

Figure 6.
a-b: (a) L4-L5 paramedian left preforaminal disc herniation (arrow). (b) Complete dehydration after treatment with oxygen-ozone.

6. Infiltration technique: Our experience

Treatments are performed under CT guidance, using the deep intraforaminal-paravertebral infiltration technique. Based on the neuroradiological documentation and the patient's clinical symptoms, it is decided to treat the patient and at what level. After being informed about the procedure and possible complications, the patient signs the informed consent. Preliminary CT scans are performed in the prone patient to confirm the pathology and level to be treated. At this point, the skin is disinfected using special preparations for general skin antisepsis (Citro jod 100 registration n° 1805 of the Ministry of Health based on polyvinylpyrrolidone iodine). A preliminary CT scan is performed to locate the skin approach point. Local anesthesia is carried out with ethyl chloride spray and subsequently, always using the CT guide, the spinal needle is positioned; normally, needles of variable caliber between 22 and 25 G are used. The perfect positioning of the needle is checked with a CT scan. Fill a 10-ml syringe in polyethylene with the gas mixture at a concentration of 25 μg/ml. The gaseous mixture is then injected. Generally injecting a variable volume from 3 to 5 cc of O_2-O_3 gaseous mixture in relation to the pathology to be treated. After the infiltration, further CT scans are performed to document the correct distribution of the gaseous mixture. All materials used must be sterile and disposable.

In recent years, especially thanks to the introduction of MR sequences with Fat Saturation and gadolinium in patients with degenerative disease of the lumbar spine and low back pain, diagnostic imaging has become even more helpful to the clinician in making diagnoses to decide the best therapeutic strategy to adopt based on the pathology to be treated.

In particular, in patients with non-radicular low back pain, this syndrome may arise from changes of the posterior elements of the lumbar spine (the "posterior vertebral compartment").

In fact, in most cases, good patient selection allows striking clinical results; with reference to our case studies in all the different applications selected we have found optimal therapeutic results in a percentage of about 75% of the cases treated considering the various pathologies overall.

The rapid resolution of pain, with no complications, the ease of performing the method and complete control of infiltration under TC control allow today to propose the CT-guided oxygen ozone therapy as a viable alternative to the various treatments currently being proposed for the various pathologies of the posterior compartment so much that it can be proposed as a method of choice between conservative therapies.

Emphasizing how this type of therapy does not contraindicate other infiltrative or surgical therapies.

It is also possible to treat selected frameworks with oxygen-ozone such as:

Facet synovitis

Intra and/or interapophyseal synovitis is an inflammatory disease of the synovial membrane, at the base there is usually a micro- or macro-traumatic event, sometimes it can also arise in young adults as a result of excessive stress on the spine, a typical finding in sportsmen who practice extreme sports with considerable spinal stresses.

The onset, in most cases, is acute with low back pain, and the symptoms can be unilateral if only one joint is involved or "bar" in case of involvement of both massive joints [37].

Diagnosis is often not easy and it is essential to perform an MR with contrast media injection to have a clear diagnosis ([38–42]; **Figures** 7 and **8**).

Baastrup syndrome

Baastrup syndrome, described by the Danish radiologist Christian Baastrup in 1933 and also known by the Anglo-Saxon term of "kissing spines," is characterized

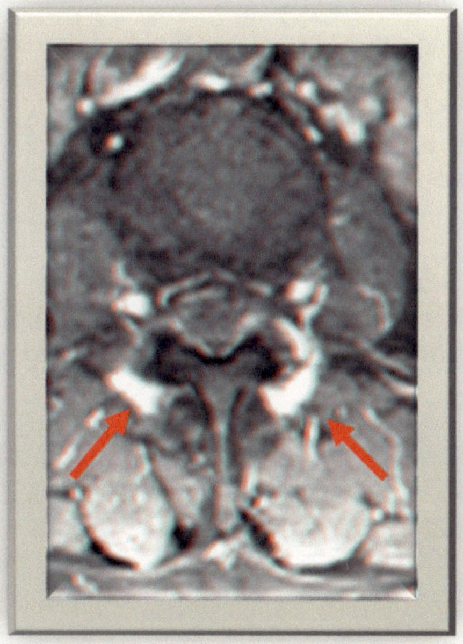

Figure 7.
Axial lumbosacral MRI after gadolinium administration: Bilateral post-traumatic apophyseal synovitis (arrows).

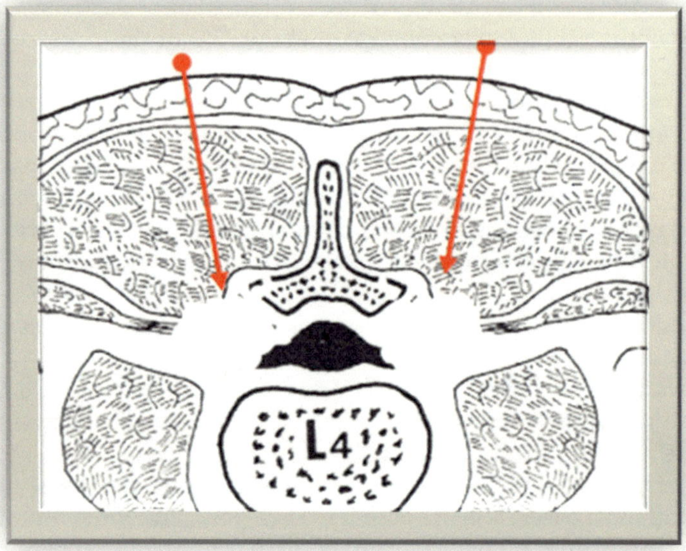

Figure 8.
In the treatment of interapophyseal synovitis, the needle is positioned under CT guidance at the level of the joint.

by the presence of arthrosis between the spinous apophyses of the vertebral column, which leads to the formation of real "neo-joints" and is often the cause of low back pain that is refractory to common treatments with anti-inflammatory and pain-relieving drugs. It predominantly affects the female sex with an F:M = 4:1 ratio and is usually diagnosed in the third decade of age.

The diagnosis is radiological: The standard Rx shows an extreme hyperlordosis of the lumbar tract up to the mutual contact of the spinous processes and a degeneration of the same.

The course of the disease is progressive and in the face of an accentuation of the low back pain, it is indicated to complete the investigations with an MRI with Fat/Sat sequences and possible administration of gadolinium in order to highlight any inflammatory focal points in the acute phase ([43–49]; **Figures 9** and **10a-b**).

Spondylolysis and spondylolisthesis

Spondylolysis is a bony defect of the neural arch. If the bony defect results in a forward shift of one vertebral body on another, this is called spondylolisthesis (a term coined by Kilian in 1854).

Spondylolisthesis is classified according to the Meyerding classification in relation to the degree of sliding of the overlying vertebral body compared to the underlying one (**Figure 11**).

7. Meyerding's classification

The degree of forward shift of one vertebral body on another is measured as a percentage according to Meyerding's classification:

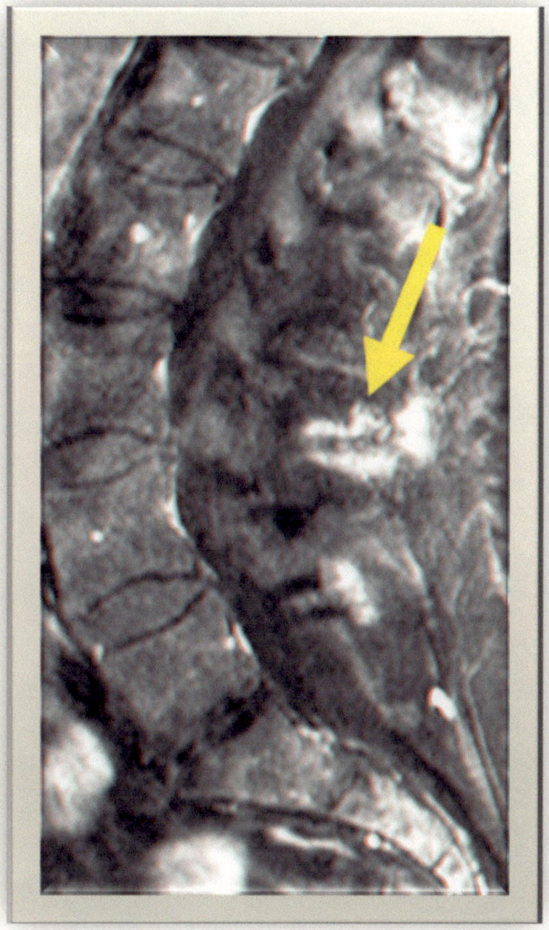

Figure 9.
Sagittal MRI after contrast medium administration: Pathological impregnation at the interspinous ligament at L3-L4.

Grade I 0-33%

Grade II 34-66%

Grade III 67-99%

Grade IV 100% and spondyloptosis

First-degree spondylolisthesis is asymptomatic in most cases and is often an occasional finding; however, in a small percentage of patients it can manifest itself with back pain complicated or not by sciatica.

Most patients with symptomatic grade I spondylolisthesis and spondylolysis do not require surgery and the treatment approach is physiokinesitherapy in nature, but

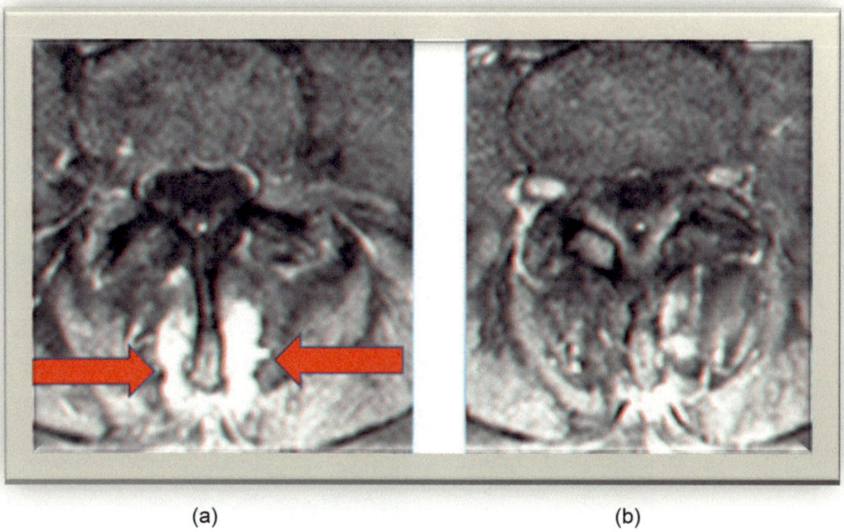

Figure 10.
a-b: (a) axial MRI intense and homogeneous impregnation of the interspinous ligament at L3-L4 (Baastrup syndrome) (arrows), (b) resolution of the picture after infiltration with oxygen-ozone.

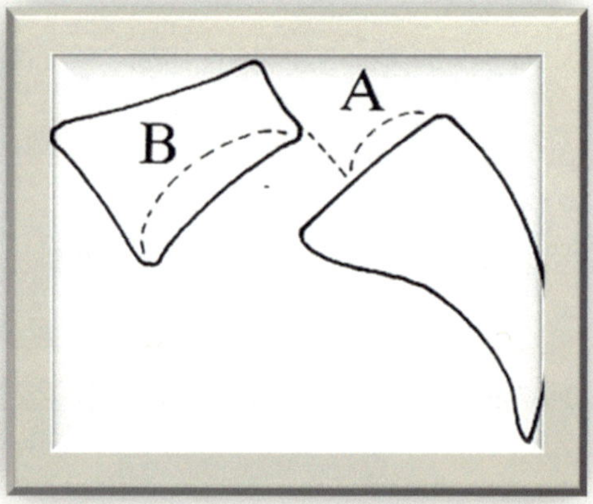

Figure 11.
Meyerding's classification uses as a criterion the degree of sliding of the overlying vertebra (B) with respect to the underlying one (A).

when symptoms do not resolve with physical therapy, they may require spinal stabilization surgery.

Based on our experience, we carry out treatments in patients with first-degree spondylolisthesis (less than 33% anthelisthesis), bilateral isthmic lysis, and associated discopathy (disc herniation or protrusion).

All patients are treated by CT-guided bilateral periganglionic infiltration of O_2-O_3 and O_2-O_3 injection into the lysis points in the neural arch ([12]; **Figures 12** and **13a-b**).

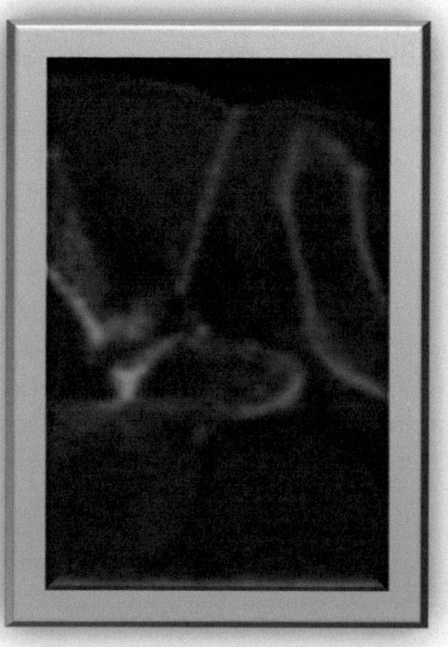

Figure 12.
Positioning of the spinal needle in the lysis point. CT check.

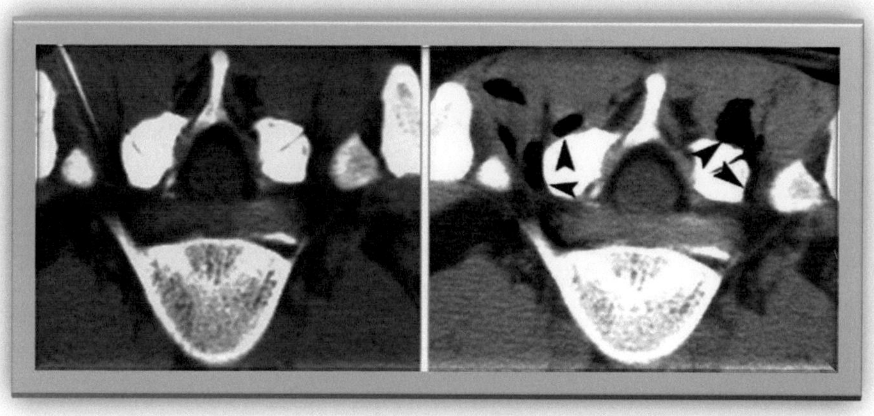

Figure 13.
a-b. (a) Placement of the spinal needle at the intraforaminal level. (b) Control of the distribution of the post-infiltration gaseous mixture.

8. Facet degeneration

Twenty-five to 45% of chronic low back pain is due to facet joint syndrome. Obviously, this syndrome can be accompanied by other problems contributing, mainly or partially, to pain and disability. Facet degeneration commonly occurs in the elderly. There are many conditions capable of generating facet symptoms, and among these, osteoarthritis is the most frequently encountered. This condition results in the reduction or disappearance of articular cartilage, erosion of the adjacent bone margin, abnormal bone growth of the facet and articular processes, and ultimately joint instability, which can lead to vertebral subluxation. The sensitive nerve endings of the facet joints and surrounding tissues undergo irritation resulting in the sensation of spinal pain. The selection of patients eligible for interventional treatment makes use of both clinical-anamnestic data and data derived from the use of Diagnostic Imaging. Conventional radiographic examination and computed tomography are used to highlight joint relationships, anomalous growths of the joint bone component, and the reduction of joint spaces, an indirect index of cartilage remodeling; but MRI is mainly used, in particular in T2-weighted fast spin echo with fat suppression and T1-weighted fast spin echo with fat suppression and administration of paramagnetic contrast medium, to identify the active inflammatory process within or surrounding the facet joint.

Several types of treatment have been proposed for the pain of facet syndrome: intra-articular injection, nerve blocks, and radiofrequency thermos-neurolysis [12].

At a clinical level, to select patients afflicted by this pathology, we use a series of now well-codified criteria. The diagnosis is suspected from the description of the pain and by making the patient practice both passively and actively movements that set the facets in motion:

- Deep low back pain, often more on one side than the other;
- Pain referred to the groin, thigh, buttock, and iliac crest;
- Pain on acupressure of the facets themselves;
- Increased pain with movement of extension (bending back) of the spine;
- Pain on rotation of the trunk toward the affected side;
- Aggravation of pain after prolonged standing and sitting position;
- Improvement with bed rest;
- Stiffness of the column;
- Absence of lower limb neurological deficits in sensation and movement;
- X-ray picture on plain X-ray, CT scan, and typical MRI.

All patients are treated with CT-guided technique, positioning the 22G spinal needle near or inside the facet joint and injecting 2–3 cc of O_2-O_3 gas mixture at 25 μg/ml (**Figure 14**).

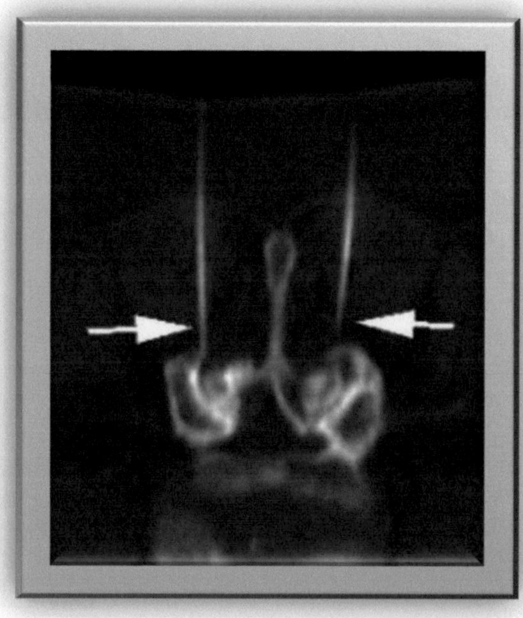

Figure 14.
CT check of the correct positioning of the needles at the level of the massive joints.

Author details

Matteo Bonetti[1]*, Gian Maria Ottaviani[2], Luigi Simonetti[3], Giannantonio Pellicanò[4], Francesco Bonetti[5] and Mario Muto[6]

1 Department of Neuroradiology, Istituto Clinico Città di Brescia, Brescia, Italy

2 Department of Emergency Urgency, Spedali Civili di Brescia, Brescia, Italy

3 Operational Unit of Neuroradiology, Ospedale Maggiore IRCCS ISNB Bologna, Bologna, Italy

4 Neuroradiology Service A.O.U.C. Azienda Ospedaliera-Universitaria Careggi, Firenze, Italy

5 Vita-Salute San Raffaele University, Milan, Italy

6 Dept of Neuroradiology Ospedale Cardarelli Napoli, Napoli, Italy

*Address all correspondence to: dottorbonetti@gmail.com

References

[1] Andreula CF, Simonetti L, De Santis F, Agati R, Ricci R, Leonardi M. Minimally invasive oxygen-ozone therapy for lumbar disk herniation. AJNR. American Journal of Neuroradiology. 2003;**24**:996-1000

[2] Bonetti M, Fontana A, Cotticelli B, Dalla Volta G, Guindani M, Leonardi M. Intraforaminal O_2-O_3 versus periradicular steroidal infiltrations in lower back pain: Randomized controlled study. American Journal of Neuroradiology. 2005;**26**:996-1000

[3] Bonetti M, Cotticelli B, Raimondi D, Valdenassi L, Richelmi P, Bertè FA. Ossigeno-ozono terapia vs infiltrazioni epidurali cortisoniche. Rivista di Neuroradiologia. 2000;**13**:203-206

[4] Gallucci M, Limbucci N, et al. Sciatica: Treatment with Intradiscal and Intraforaminal injections of steroid and oxygen-ozone versus steroid only. Radiology. 2007;**242**(3):907-913

[5] Lehnert T, Naguib NN, Wutzler S, Nour-Eldin NE, Bauer RW, Kerl JM, et al. Analysis of disk volume before and after CT-guided intradiscal and periganglionic ozone-oxygen injection for the treatment of lumbar disk herniation. Journal of Vascular and Interventional Radiology: JVIR. 2012;**23**(11):1430-1436

[6] Leonardi M, Albini Riccioli L, Battaglia S, de Santis F, Cenni P, Raffi L, et al. Oxygen-ozone chemonucleolysis for herniated disc with sciatica. A comparison of treatments in patients with subacute and chronic symptoms. Rivista Italiana di Ossigeno-Ozonoterapia. 2006;**5**:33-36

[7] Leonardi M, Simonetti L, Agati R. Neuroradiology of spine degenerative disease. Best Practice & Research Clinical Rheumathology. 2002;**16**:59-88

[8] Leonardi M, Simonetti L, Raffi L, Cenni P, Barbara C. Mini-invasive treatment of herniated disc by oxygen-ozone injection. Interventional Neuroradiology. 2003;**9**(Suppl.2):75

[9] Magalhaes FN, Dotta L, Sasse A, Teixera MJ, Fonoff ET. Ozone therapy as a treatment for low back pain secondary to herniated disc: A systematic review and meta-analysis of randomized controlled trials. Pain Physician. 2012;**15**(2):115-119

[10] Muto M, Andreula C, Leonardi M. Treatment of herniated lumbar disc by intradiscal and intraforaminal oxygen-ozone (O_2-O_3) injection. Journal de Neuroradiologie. 2004;**31**:183-189

[11] Bonetti M, Zambello A, Leonardi M, Princiotta C. Herniated disks unchanged over time: Size reduced after oxygen-ozone therapy. Interventional Neuroradiology. 2016;**22**(4):466-472

[12] Bonetti M, Zambello A, Princiotta C, Pellicanò G, Della Gatta L, Muto M. Non-discogenic low back pain treated with oxygen-ozone: Outcome in selected applications. Journal of Biological Regulators and Homeostatic Agents. 2020;**34**(4 Suppl. 1):21-30

[13] Rimeika G, Saba L, Arthimulam G, Della Gatta L, Davidovic K, Bonetti M, et al. Metanalysis on the effectiveness of low back pain treatment with oxygen-ozone mixture: Comparison between image-guided and non-image-guided injection techniques. European Journal of Radiology Open. 2021;**8**:1-6

[14] Zhang Y, Ma Y, Jiang J, Ding T, Wang J. Treatment of the lumbar disc

herniation with intradiscal and intraforaminal injection of oxygen-ozone. Journal of Back and Musculoskeletal Rehabilitation. 2013;**26**(3):317-322

[15] Bonetti M, Lauritano D, Ottaviani GM, Fontana A, Frigerio M, Zambello A, et al. New approach to chronic Back pain treatment: A case control study. Biomedicine. 2022;**11**(1):73

[16] Muto M, Avella F. Percutaneous treatment of herniated lumbar disc by intradiscal oxygen-ozone injection. Interventional Neuroradiology. 1998;**4**:279-286

[17] Simonetti L, Agati R, et al. Mechanism of pain in disc disease. Rivista di Neuroradiologia. 2001;**14**:171-174

[18] Simonetti L, Agati R. Why does disc-root conflict generate pain? Rivista di Neuroradiologia. 1998;**11**:403-404

[19] Guerne PA, Carson DA, Lotz M. IL-6 production by human articular chondrocytes. Modulation of its synthesis by cytokines, growth factors, and hormones in vitro. Journal of Immunology. 1990;**144**:499-505

[20] Saal J. The role of inflammation in lumbar pain. Spine. 1995;**20**:1521-1527

[21] Hawkins CL, Davies MJ. Direct detection and identification of oxidative radicals generated during the hydroxyl radical induced degradation of hyaluronic acid and related materials. Radical Biology and Medicine. 1996;**133**:321-325

[22] Oystein PN, Svein IM, Osterud B. The inflammatory properties of contained and noncontained lumbar disc herniation. Spine. 1997;**22**:2484-2488

[23] Zwart JA, Ivernes OJ, et al. Higher levels of antibodies against the psoriasis-associated antigen pso p27 in cerebrospinal fluid from patients with low back pain and sciatica. Spine. 1999;**24**(4):373-377

[24] Kang JD, Georgescu HI, et al. Herniated lumbar IntervertebraI discs spontaneously produce matrix metalloproteinases, nitric oxide, InterIeukin-6, and prostaglandin E2. Spine. 1996;**21**:271-2771

[25] Bocci V. Ozone as a bioregulator. Pharmacology and toxicology of ozone therapy today. Journal of Biological Regulators and Homeostatic Agents. 1998;**10**:31-53

[26] Johansen-JS J-HS, Price PA. A new biochemical marker for joint injury. Analysis of YKL-40 in serum and synovial fluid. British Journal of Rheumatology. 1994;**32**:949-955

[27] Simonetti L, Agati R, Leonardi M. Anatomia e fisiopatologia dell'unità funzionale disco-somatica. Rivista di Neuroradiologia. 2001;**14**:7-16

[28] Elliott RJ, Gardner DL. Changes with age in the glycosaminoglycans of human articular cartilage. Annals of the Rheumatic Diseases. 1979;**38**:371-377

[29] Carney SL, Billingham MEJ, Muir H. The structure and metabolism of collagen and proteoglycan in normal and osteoarthritic articular cartilage. Degenerative Joint. In: Verbruggen G, Veys EM, editors. Degenerative Joints: Proceeding of the Second Conference on Degenerative Joint Diseases, 1984 (International Congress Series). Vol. 1. Amsterdam: Excerpta Medica; 1985. pp. 117-128

[30] Leonardi M, Simonetti L, Barbara C. The effects of ozone on the nucleus pulposus: Pathological data on one surgical specimen. Rivista di Neuroradiologia. 2001;**14**:57-61

[31] Nietfeld JJ, Wilbrink B, et al. Interleukin-1 induced interleukin-6 is required for the inhibition of proteoglycan synthesis by interleukin-1 in human articular cartilage. Arthritis and Rheumatism. 1990;**33**:1695-1701

[32] Iliakis E, Valadakis V, Vynios DH, Tsiganos CP, Agapitos E. Rationalization of the activity of medical ozone on intervertebral disc and histological and biochemical study. Rivista di Neuroradiologia. 2001;**14**(suppl.1):25-30

[33] Simonetti L, Raffi L, Cenni P, Agati R, Leonardi M. Pharmacological mechanisms underlying oxygen-ozone therapy for herniated disc. Rivista Italiana di Ossigeno-Ozonoterapia. 2003;**2**:7-11

[34] Iliakis E. Ozone treatment in low back pain. Orthopaedics. 1995;**1**:29-33

[35] Pellicanò F, Martinelli F, Tavanti V, Bonetti M, Leonardi M, Muto M, et al. The Italian oxygen-ozone therapy federation (FIO) study on oxygen-ozone treatment of herniated disc. International Journal of Ozone Therapy. 2007;**6**:7-15

[36] Steppan J, Meaders T, Muto M, Murphy KJ. A metaanalysis of the effectiveness and safety of ozone treatments for herniated lumbar discs. Journal of Vascular and Interventional Radiology. 2010;**21**(4):534-548

[37] Czervionke LF. Fenton DS fat-saturated MR imaging in the detection of inflammatory facet arthropathy (facet synovitis) in the lumbar spine. Pain Medicine. 2008;**9**(4):400-406

[38] Perri M, Grattacaso G, Di Tunno V, Marsecano C, Di Cesare E, Splendiani A, et al. MRI DWI/ADC signal predicts shrinkage of lumbar disc herniation after O_2-O_3 discolysis. The Neuroradiology Journal. 2015;**28**(2):198-204

[39] Splendiani A, Perri M, Conchiglia A, Fasano F, Di Egidio G, Masciocchi C, et al. MR assessment of lumbar disk herniation treated with oxygen-ozone diskolysis: The role of DWI and related ADC versus intervertebral disk volumetric analysis for detecting treatment response. The Neuroradiology Journal. 2013;**26**(3):347-356

[40] D'Aprile P, Tarantino A, Lorusso V. Brindicci D fat saturation technique and gadolinium in MRI of lumbar spinal degenerative disease. The Neuroradiology Journal. 2006;**19**(5):654-671

[41] D'Aprile P, Tarantino A, Jinkins JR, Brindicci D. The value of fat saturation sequences and contrast medium administration in MRI of degenerative disease of the posterior/perispinal elements of the lumbosacral spine. European Radiology. 2007;**17**(2):523-531

[42] Bonetti M, Fontana A, Bragaglio G, Marchina I, Guarino G, Pellicanò G. Oxygen-ozone therapy in the treatment of facet synovitis. An observational study of 36 patients. European Journal of Musculoskeletal Diseases. 2016;**5**(1):2-8

[43] Alonso F, Bryant E, Iwanaga J, Chapman JR, Oskouian RJ, Tubbs RS. Baastrup's disease: A comprehensive review of the extant literature. World Neurosurgery. 2017;**101**:331-334

[44] Filippiadis DK, Mazioti A, Argentos S, Anselmetti G, Papakonstantinou O, Kelekis N, et al. Baastrup's disease (kissing spines syndrome): A pictorial review. Insights Into Imaging. 2015;**6**(1):123-128

[45] Meluzio MC, Smakaj A, Perna A, Velluto C, Grillo G, Proietti L, et al. Epidemiology, diagnosis and management of Baastrup's disease: A systematic review. Journal

of Neurosurgical Sciences. Dec 2022;**66**(6):519-525

[46] Kerroum A, Laudato PA, Suter MR. The steps until surgery in the management of Baastrup's disease (kissing spine syndrome). Journal of Surgical Case Reports. 28 Jun 2019;**2019**(6):1-4

[47] Singla A, Shankar V, Mittal S, Agarwal A, Garg B. Baastrup's disease: The kissing spine. World Journal of Clinical Cases. 2014;**2**(2):45-47

[48] Philipp LR, Baum GR, Grossberg JA, Ahmad FU. Baastrup's disease: An often missed etiology for back pain. Cureus. 22 Jan 2016;**8**(1):e465

[49] Bonetti M, Ottaviani GM, Fontana A, Pellicanò G, Della GL, Muto M. Diagnosis and subsequent treatment with oxygen-ozone therapy of Baastrup's disease. European Journal of Musculoskeletal Diseases. 2020;**9**(2):2-8